FAMILIES, HEALTH, & ILLNESS

Perspectives on Coping and Intervention

Carol B. Danielson, R.N., M.S.N.

Health Educator and School Nurse
Monkton Central School
Monkton, Vermont

Brenda Hamel-Bissell, R.N., Ed.D.

Associate Professor
School of Nursing
University of Vermont
Burlington, Vermont

Patricia Winstead-Fry, R.N., Ph.D.

Professor of Nursing
School of Nursing
University of Vermont
Burlington, Vermont

Illustrated

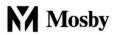 Mosby

St. Louis Baltimore Boston Chicago London Philadelphia Sydney Toronto

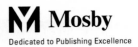

Mosby

Dedicated to Publishing Excellence

Publisher: Allison Miller
Executive Editor: Linda L. Duncan
Editorial Assistant: Becky Sweeney
Project Manager: Patricia Tannian
Production Editor: John P. Casey
Designer: Julie Taugner

Printed in the United States of America

Mosby–Year Book, Inc.
11830 Westline Industrial Drive
St. Louis, Missouri 63146

Library of Congress Cataloging in Publication Data
Danielson, Carol B.
    Families, health, and illness : perspectives on coping and
intervention / Carol B. Danielson, Brenda Hamel-Bissell, Patricia
Winstead-Fry.
        p.   cm.
    Includes bibliographical references and index.
    ISBN 0-8016-0360-9
    1. Family—Health and hygiene. 2. Family nursing. 3. Sick—
Family relationships. 4. Health promotion.   I. Hamel-Bissell,
Brenda.   II. Winstead-Fry, Patricia.   III. Title.
    [DNLM: 1. Adaptation, Psychological. 2. Attitude to Health.
3. Family—psychology.   W 85 D186f]
RT120.F34D35 1993
362.1'0425—dc20
DNLM/DLC
for Library of Congress   92-48736
                                                            CIP

93 94 95 96 97 GW/DC 9 8 7 6 5 4 3 2 1

Contributors

◆

Marilyn A. McCubbin, Ph.D.

School of Nursing
University of Wisconsin
Madison, Wisconsin

Hamilton I. McCubbin, Ph.D.

School of Family Resources and Consumer Sciences
University of Wisconsin
Madison, Wisconsin

To Our Families

Preface

T HE principal purpose of this book is to examine the intricate and complex relationships between health, illness, and families. Despite some progress in integrating a family perspective into the U.S. health-care system, the traditional practice areas continue to focus almost exclusively on the individual. Health-status indicators are reported primarily by individuals, not families. Predictions of health-care utilization patterns are based on individual statistics. This narrow perspective has several critical limitations and fails to recognize the substantial effect families have on the health behaviors of their individual members.

This book explores the importance, viability, benefits, and implementation of family-oriented interventions in the promotion of health and treatment of physical and mental health problems. To understand more fully and more accurately the health behaviors of individuals, health and human service providers need to understand better the critical ways in which family relationships influence such behavior. This book explores and illuminates the need to identify the family, instead of the individual, as the critical unit of health promotion and illness prevention and treatment.

For over 40 years the ABC-X Model of Family Stress, first proposed by Reuben Hill (1949, 1958), has been developed, refined, and expanded for various sociological research pursuits. Today, it provides an impressive accumulation of research on many aspects of the family and family responses to stressors. More factors and interactions have been recognized and further delineated. The theory is currently referred to as the T-Double ABC-X Model of Family Adjustment and Adaptation.

This book presents a variation of the T-Double ABC-X Model called the Resiliency Model of Family Stress, Adjustment, and Adaptation, prepared by Marilyn A. McCubbin and Hamilton I. McCubbin, developers of the T-Double ABC-X Model. The Resiliency Model serves as a framework to determine whether or not a health or illness stressor becomes a family crisis and assists in understanding and predicting the response of different families to similar illness stressors. The Resiliency Model of Family Stress, Adjustment, and Adaptation can be used to document family contributions to health, as well as to plan interventions that decrease family stress during illness. Most of the research on this model is based on studies of healthy families, so insights are particularly germane to the health promotion goals of nursing.

✦ PRIMARY OBJECTIVES

- ✦ To identify the various ways family structure and family relationships influence health maintenance and illness behaviors
- ✦ To delineate the distinctive characteristics of an illness that affect family relationships, functioning, and coping
- ✦ To examine the family as the critical unit in the use and provision of health care
- ✦ To illustrate and discuss specific family-oriented interventions in the treatment of illness and the promotion of wellness
- ✦ To analyze the demands of supporting and caring for an ill family member within the context of a specific illness. This analysis is twofold: (1) to examine the range of coping mechanisms families use when confronted by such situations, and (2) to propose possible family-oriented interventions that might be used in given circumstances.

✦ ORGANIZATION
Part I: Families, Health, and Illness: Background and Rationale

The first part of the book comprises three chapters and provides the background and rationale necessary for the reader to understand the intertwining of the three fundamental concepts around which the book is constructed: health, illness, and families. The advantages of a family orientation in the treatment of illness and the promotion of wellness are discussed. The Resiliency Model of Family Stress, Adjustment, and

Adaptation, which demonstrates family management of illness stressors, is introduced in this portion of the book.

Part II: Family Coping in Health and Illness

Part II builds on the theoretical foundations of Part I, offering specific detail regarding the impact of illness and family coping skills. The purpose of this section is to explore the many facets of illness and highlight more completely the reciprocal relationship between physical and mental health and family functioning. Chapter 4 identifies the specific dimensions of illnesses that influence the degree to which families feel stress. Chapter 5 examines successful and unsuccessful coping characteristics of families and discusses their importance to health and illness.

Part III: Family Interventions for Health-Care Delivery

The principal objectives of the chapters in this section of the book are (1) to describe the foundations for a family perspective in the health-care delivery system and to propose modifications that would further enhance the significant role of families; and (2) to present and create models of family-oriented interventions. Those chapters reviewing specific intervention strategies address the following questions:
1. What is the rationale behind the intervention?
2. What is the intended purpose of adopting this particular strategy?
3. How is the intervention program organized or implemented?
4. What is the role of the health professional vis-a-vis the family when implementing this strategy?
5. What are the inherent obstacles to implementing the strategy?

Part IV: Families and Specific Illnesses

Each chapter in Part IV is constructed around a vignette describing a specific illness, its impact on a fictitious family, and the interventions useful for the specific illness and family situation. It is *not* the goal of these chapters to present comprehensive reviews of the literature on the etiology, course of the disease, or methods of treatment of each illness discussed. Rather, the vignettes are only a mechanism for illustrating, within a particular context, the impact of the illness of a single family member on the entire family system. Then examined are the alternatives for family intervention available to the health-care provider. This part of the book integrates, restates, and reinforces the information and implications offered throughout the book.

Glossary and Appendix

A glossary of key terms and an appendix including family assessment tools have been added to complement information offered in the book. The five family assessment tools can be used separately or together in health and illness situations to evaluate the level of resiliency present in the family that would be available to manage health and illness stressors.

Acknowledgments

✦

T HE creation of this book is the fruitful labor of many years of work and struggle. We would like to thank all those whose support, patience, and encouragement made it possible to continue when difficulties made no apparent end to the project seem possible.

First, we would like to thank Mosby–Year Book's fine editorial staff for fostering quality production of this book. Linda Duncan, Executive Editor, deserves specific mention for her belief in this book and support through difficult times. Becky Sweeney's multiple phone conversations, which offered support, information, and organizational assistance, were pivotal in completing this project. John Casey's editorial talents enhanced the readability of the book and sharpened the visual appeal.

Second, we would like to thank various staff of the University of Vermont for their assistance. David Punia, computer expert, went beyond the call of duty in assisting us in eradicating the "brain virus" that could have destroyed much of the work on our disks. As medical illustrator, Gary Nelson's creativity in assisting us in developing a pictorial representation of the Family Cycle of Health and Illness was inspiring. Our gratitude to Rita Weston for the many hours she spent typing and copying the numerous versions of this manuscript. Also, the assistance offered by the reference librarians and Gail Fisher, graduate student, in locating and updating references was extremely valuable.

Last but *not* least, we acknowledge our families for all they have taught us, firsthand, about family dynamics and its relation to health and for their patience throughout this project. Also, we appreciate the emotional support provided by friends, enabling us to bring this book to fruition.

Carol B. Danielson
Brenda Hamel-Bissell
Patricia Winstead-Fry

Contents

✦

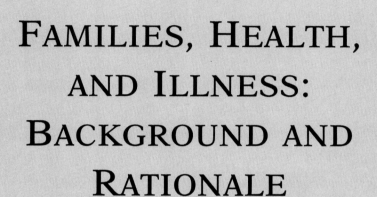

Families, Health, and Illness: Background and Rationale

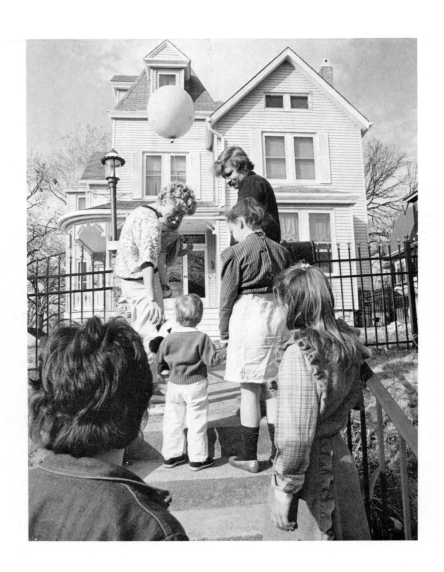

1

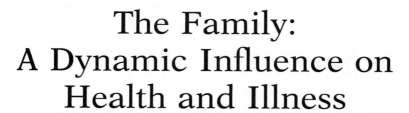

The Family: A Dynamic Influence on Health and Illness

CHAPTER GOALS

✦ To introduce the concept of the family as a critical unit in determining health and illness behaviors

✦ To illustrate the varied influences of the family on health maintenance and illness behaviors

✦ To introduce concepts that are basic to the ideas presented in this book, specifically the family as consumer of health care, the family life cycle, systems theory, and family roles

✦ To discuss the importance of health professionals adopting a family perspective

OVERVIEW

THIS book explores the significant advantages of using the family unit to understand health and illness and to implement health care. The individual is the current focus of health care in the United States (Baird & Doherty, 1990); data about illness and health-care utilization and status are based on individual behaviors. How families influence the health-related behaviors of their members needs to be better understood, since definitions of health and illness form during childhood in a family context.

Definitions

For purposes of this book the family is defined as a unique social group involving "generational ties, permanence, a concern for the total person, heightened emotionality, caregiving, qualitative goals, an altruistic orientation to members, and a primarily nurturing form of governance" (Beutler, Burr, Bahr, & Herrin, 1989).

In discussions on families the terms *nuclear family* and *extended family* are used. *Nuclear family* refers to a family form composed of a husband, wife, and children (Ross & Cobb, 1988). Today that term includes couples without children, single parent households, reconstituted families (second marriages), unmarried couples with or without children, homosexual couples, and people living in communes.

The *extended family* refers to the group of individuals beyond the nuclear family that are usually related by blood, such as aunts, uncles, and grandparents. They usually do not live with the nuclear family.

Historical Perspective

Today's prevailing nostalgia for the family of the past, which is perceived as a happy, intact group, is coupled with the familiar themes of family decline and dissolution. However, historical analysis of family life reveals a less romantic picture. Kain (1990), a historian of family life, makes many interesting points in *The Myth of Family Decline*. He states, "When we have actual data about family life in the past, it often presents a picture of family life that is drastically different from the image that is common in popular mythology" (p. 6). He cites demographic data to show that children are not more likely to live in single parent households today than 100 years ago because of the dramatic increase in life expectancy. This increase in life span has offset the divorce rate of today.

Single parent families were not particularly uncommon in the past. Although the decline of the extended family is a popular idea, little empirical evidence supports this view, primarily because the extended family was never the norm. Laslett's (1972) historical study of family practices demonstrated that the nuclear family was the norm for most of history. The image of several generations living under one roof and always ready to help one another is a fiction. Only the upper class was able to approach this idealized version of extended family life.

Our picture of the "normal" family is clouded by the lack of historical understanding. In spite of the fact that 20% of women worked outside of the home in 1900 (Kain, 1990), the idea of the working father and the domestic mother remains a treasured perception. By 1950 75% of American families consisted of a working husband and a working wife with children. In 1980 that number increased to 84% (U.S. Bureau of Census, 1952, 1982). Therefore to uphold the idea of a husband who works and a wife who stays at home with a couple of children as the norm of American family life is inaccurate and does not withstand scrutiny. Moreover, there is a serious lack of research on the experience of minority group families and single parent families.

When one excludes the myths about families, two trends emerge from recent census data: household size is decreasing and family style is more diverse. In 1950 40% of households consisted of one or two persons. Thirty years later 54% of households had one or two occupants (U.S. Bureau of Census). Over the same 30 years the number of new households that included a husband and a wife dropped from 50% to 12%. Reasons offered for these changes include divorce, persons marrying later, and unmarried persons living together (the diversity of household phenomena). For families and for persons who work with families, the meaning of these changes is developing. It is also important to remember that recent census data have been skewed by the "baby boom" generation, the large number of children born in the late 1940s and early 1950s. The life-style and living patterns of this group may indicate future patterns of family life or may be a temporary aberration. It is essential to note that the census inquires about households, not families: a divorced family occupies two households, whereas two families can share one household.

✦ BASIC CONCEPTS
Family Life Cycle

Reuben Hill and Evelyn Duvall pioneered the idea of a family life cycle in a paper prepared for the National Conference on Family Life in 1948. Duvall continued the work, defining eight stages of family life (Duvall, 1957, 1977). Over the years there have been many commentaries on the number of stages, the tasks of each stage, and the importance of various stages. For the purposes of this book, the stages identified by Carter and McGoldrick (1980) are used. Their book is a classic, summarizing all of the previous work in the field. In addition, it presents the shift in the life cycle that occurs with divorce, and this inclusion makes Carter and McGoldrick's life cycle timely for contemporary American life.

Family life cycle refers to various stages of family development. Each stage involves change and accomplishing tasks for the successful transition from one stage to another. Carter and McGoldrick have defined six stages with associated tasks (see box below).

The most recently added stage of the life cycle is *no. 6, later life.* Today, people are living longer and having fewer children. This is the least understood phase, and for most families it is the stage with the greatest duration.

The family life cycle takes a different course if divorce occurs. The developmental challenges also differ from those of a nondivorced family. The stages and the associated tasks are listed in the box on p. 7.

When children are involved in a divorce, each spouse enters a new life cycle stage, either *single parent family* or *noncustodial single parent.* Both of these roles have tasks, including maintaining parental contact with the former spouse and with children. The custodial parent needs to maintain a

---

Six Stages of the Family Life Cycle

Stage	Major Task
1. Unattached young adult who is between families	Parent and young adult successfully separating from one another
2. New marriage	Committing to a new family system
3. Family with young children	Accepting new members into the system
4. Family with adolescents	Remolding the boundaries of the family to allow the children independence
5. Launching the children and moving on	Accepting many exits and entrances into the family
6. Later life	Accepting shifting generational roles and death

relationship with former in-laws, and both former spouses need to rebuild a personal social network.

If the divorced person remarries, a new life cycle stage is entered, that of the reconstituted family (see second box below).

These life cycle stages are useful for assessing some families. However, the diversity of family life today precludes establishing these stages and accompanying tasks as norms that every family must follow. Nevertheless, the concept of family life cycle is important in understanding family stresses

Stages of the Family Life Cycle During Divorce

Stage	Major Task
1. The decision to divorce	Accepting the inability to resolve marital discord
2. Planning the break up in the system	Creating viable arrangements for all members of the system
3. Separation	Resolve attachment to spouse; develop cooperative co-parenting relationship
4. Divorce	Resolve the emotional divorce

Stages of the Family Life Cycle for the Reconstituted Family

Stage	Major Task
1. Entering a new relationship	Recovery from the loss of the first marriage
2. Planning a new marriage	Accepting fears of all system members; accepting complexities with patience
3. Remarriage and reconstitution of family	Final resolution of attachment to former spouse; acceptance of a different type of family with permeable boundaries

and therefore an integral part of the Resiliency Model of Family Stress, Adjustment, and Adaptation presented in the next chapter.

Systems Theory

Many approaches to family study have developed: structural-functional, interactional, legal, anthropological, developmental, psychoanalytical, and systems. Of these approaches, systems theory is basic to understanding family stress and the impact of illness on the family. Systems theory has been widely used in a number of fields including those as diverse as computer science and family theory (Friedman, 1986). During the past decade, systems theory gained widespread acceptance in the health-care field. According to the principles and concepts of general systems theory, health or illness is always a potential and may be the product of interaction among family members. The systems theory is flexible and may be used to study many aspects of family life including crises. The systems perspective may offer insights into which, if any, family member will become ill during a crisis. On the other hand, illness and health may not be a result of family behavior but may simply be an accident or environmental influence. However, the family can influence the course of recovery or adaptation to illness regardless of its cause. Because of the reciprocal nature of family behavior, one member's intervention in illness may affect the rest of the family (Hathway, Boswell, Stanford, Schneider, & Moncrief, 1987).

The systems approach views the family as a complex social system and as a holistic unit from which individual behaviors flow. The family unit constantly exchanges information, energy, and materials with its environment (von Bertalanffy, 1986). What each member learns from the family partially determines future relationships with self and others, as well as affecting overall health. The family unit socializes its members by establishing roles and by influencing the basic values, beliefs, attitudes, hopes, and aspirations of each individual. How this socialization is achieved directly affects the mental health of the individual and the family.

In addition to socialization the family provides physical maintenance in the form of food, clothing, shelter, and medical care. Even though young family members are educated at school, the family unit contributes to intellectual development. Family members share intense emotional ties that directly influence the emotional development of children and the experience of the whole family. Spiritual needs are also met during family interaction.

In essence, the family can either facilitate or repress growth in the social, physical, emotional, intellectual, and spiritual dimensions of its members.

With the systems approach illness is always a potential hazard that may be the product of family interactions. Illness may be predicted by the level of differentiation (the balance between intellectual and emotional systems; see Chapter 5) of individual family members and by the general level of anxiety within the family. Some researchers even note a direct relationship between physical illness and family emotional processes (Bowen, 1978; Kerr & Bowen, 1988).

Systems-oriented practitioners are interested in the process of verbal and nonverbal interactions within the family, since these influence health and illness (Kerr & Bowen, 1988). Family interactions are complex; they are influenced by the individual family members and by society. To illustrate the systems perspective, consider the Robertson family. The family consists of Bob, the father; Nancy, the mother; Beth, 15 years old; Tom, 10 years old; and Carol, 8 years old. Each of these persons has a relationship with the other (Fig. 1-1).

In addition to the relationships among the family members, each one has relationships with the outside world. For example, Bob plays tennis and

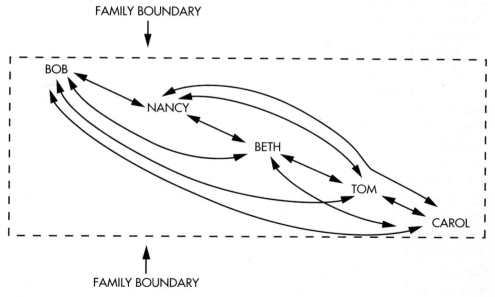

FAMILY BOUNDARY

FAMILY BOUNDARY

FIGURE 1-1
The complexity of family interactions.

belongs to a political organization. Nancy belongs to the same political organization as Bob and to a consciousness-raising group. The children have school friends, sport activities, and piano lessons. If Bob's tennis tournament conflicts with Tom's swimming meet, the whole family will feel tension until some resolution is reached. The outside social world also influences the family through laws, television, religion, and political values. The potential interactions within the family and between the family and society increase exponentially. Tensions that result from stressors during interactions influence family relationships. Unresolved tensions may be increasingly disruptive.

Family Roles

Research about the roles of family members and the role of family in society is value laden and difficult to synthesize. Before the women's movement sociological research discussed the expressive role of the mother/wife and the instrumental role of the husband/father (Parsons & Bales, 1955; Reece, 1964). The mother/wife was expected to perform a nurturing role and care for the children, whereas the father/husband was expected to provide for his family and focus on his job. However, as more women entered the work force these traditional roles were challenged and subsequently seen more as stereotypes than as roles.

Today, the family places less importance on which roles are appropriate for males and females. Of more importance is the interactive nature of various roles and how successful families are in accomplishing their goals. For example, someone must prepare dinner for the family. In the past the family researcher or practitioner assumed this was the mother's role. Today, the father, mother, and children may share this task. As long as the family is fulfilling the responsibility of feeding its members, specifically who does the task is not generally an issue.

Family structure is established by successfully assigning and performing roles. Families may be rigid or flexible in role assignments. Generally, families function better when roles are clearly communicated and when expected role behaviors are established. Most family therapists advocate the creation of generational boundaries within a family (Bowen, 1978; Holman, 1983; Minuchin, 1974); parents should be the architects of the family and should set and enforce rules for themselves and for their children. Rules should change as children mature. This concept also applies to single parent families.

The role of the family in society is changing. In earlier generations family land and other property was passed on. Today, few families have land to pass on. Not all families have children; not all families stay together until death. Families that function well have a sense of purpose, whether that purpose is child-rearing or companionship. They are further characterized by intimacy, relatively equal power, comfort with autonomy, ease in relating, ability to negotiate, and some transcendent beliefs (Beavers, 1982; Haley, 1976).

◆ THE FAMILY AND HEALTH AND ILLNESS BEHAVIORS

Baranowske and Nadar (1985) reviewed research on the relation of families to health and illness behaviors. They described the family as having the potential to play important roles in all levels of prevention. In primary prevention the family can influence life-style choices that may prevent illness. In secondary prevention the meaning the family attaches to symptoms can influence the decision to seek care. In tertiary prevention families influence how members comply with treatment regimens. Family research related to these three levels of prevention are discussed in subsequent sections.

Primary Prevention

Recent research on life-style makes it clear that illness or wellness does not just happen (Justice, 1987). We participate in primary prevention by choosing a specific life-style. Two facets of life-style that influence our health are the development of nutritional behaviors and health-promoting behaviors.

One of the major components of life-style is eating. A family's ethnic background, socioeconomic status, and satisfaction with family life influence nutritional status. In 1985 Baranowski and Nadus reviewed selected literature related to family and eating behaviors. Generally, obesity in children could be related to family eating patterns. In one study 27.5% of the obesity in sons and 24.1% of obesity in daughters could be predicted if all members of the family were obese. In families without obese adult members the predictions of childhood obesity fell to 3.22% for sons and 5.4% for daughters. The study did not consider genetic variables.

Hartz, Giefer, and Rimm (1977) studied 73,532 members of a weight-reducing organization. They found 32% to 39% of obesity in children was related to family environment variables, whereas genetics accounted for 11% of the obesity. Likewise, Khoury, Morrison, Laskarzewski, and Glueck (1983) found a strong relationship between family environment and body mass. These studies support the importance of including the family in primary prevention measures designed to improve nutritional life-style patterns.

Another illustration of the family's influence in primary prevention behaviors is from the child development literature. As early as 1965, Rashkis demonstrated that children have an idea of what constitutes health and illness. Following developmental patterns the child's idea of health and illness develops with age; that is, as the child ages the concepts become more mature. Lasky and Eichelberger (1985) reported that children as young as 4 years old understood health behaviors and practiced them in their lives. Parents who educated and supported their children in actively engaging in self-care behaviors were especially effective in bringing up children who were active agents in behalf of their own health.

McCubbin, Needle, and Wilson (1985) studied stress in families with adolescents and the negative health behaviors of smoking cigarettes, drinking alcohol, and smoking marijuana. The research found that the best predictor that adolescent boys and girls would not engage in these three negative health activities was the family's ability to solve problems. Excessive demands within the family may have created stress for the adolescent and could be ameliorated if the adolescent and the family could communicate and resolve conflicts and differences. Surprisingly, adolescent peer support did not prevent these negative behaviors nor did complaining about family members to friends or other adults.

Secondary Prevention

Secondary prevention refers to the meaning attached to symptoms and decisions to seek care. There is a growing body of literature on family patterns of health-care utilization, some of which is reviewed here.

Family patterns in health-care usage demonstrate that mothers are the gatekeepers concerning their children's access to care (Cunningham, 1990; Mechanic, 1964). Cunningham used the 1977 National Medical Care Expenditure Survey (NMCES) to assess health-care costs at different stages of family life. Generally, employed mothers used less care; more educated mothers used more; single parents had more physicians' visits during the young children phase of the life cycle; poor women used less care during the first years of their children's lives. Although there are some weaknesses in the database Cunningham used, his findings do support the idea that dependent children's access to care is controlled by the family, especially the mother.

Two studies found a positive relationship between the mother's use of physician services for herself and for her children (Newacheck & Halfon, 1986; Schor, Starfield, Stidley, & Hankin, 1987). That is, mothers who used more health care personally also took their children to visit physicians more often than mothers who used less personal health care. In both of the studies the visits were paid for by the husband's insurance. Two interesting questions arise from these studies: (1) What process do mothers use to decide when to seek health care? and (2) Who is educating mothers about when to visit a physician? The answers to these questions would shed further light on family patterns of health-care utilization and may have implications for family education.

In regard to family influences on the decision to seek health care, some preliminary studies suggest that family approaches to consumption of health-care resources vary greatly. Schor, Starfield, Stidley, and Hankin (1987) studied 80,000 ambulatory visits made by 693 families who participated in a prepaid health-care plan over a 6-year period. They found that 5% of the families accounted for 12.3% of the visits. Similarly, Hayes (1989), the medical director of Burlington Industries, reported that 10% of insured employees accounted for 80% of the utilization. Bowen and other family therapists contend that emotional dysfunction can result in physical illness. (See Chapter 5 on family vulnerability for a further discussion of these ideas.) If patterns of health-care usage are related to the emotional health of the family, a stronger argument could be made for the family's influence in health-care consumption. An exploration of these ideas would have to refrain from "blaming" the victim and the family and would have to be undertaken in a respectful, fair manner.

Tertiary Prevention

Tertiary prevention refers to overcoming illness and returning to health. The family influences recovery in numerous ways: by the medical care it can afford, by the caregiving functions it serves, and by the support it gives ill members.

The Working Group of the National Heart, Lung, and Blood Institute on Compliance in Hypertension Treatment (1982) stated that family involvement in compliance with drug and diet regimens is one of the most important predictors of successful patient follow through on health-care plans. Similarly, family units are looked to as the best place to detect cholesterol and triglyceride elevation (Morrison, Namboodiri, Green, Martin, & Blueck, 1983).

In a direct study of psychosocial factors in physical illness, Browne, Arpin, Fitch, and Gafni (1990) studied oncology, rheumatology, and gastroenterology patients. When the patients were divided into how well or how poorly they had adjusted to their illnesses, differences were striking. The poorly adjusted patients, regardless of diagnosis or prognosis, used over 200% more services. Including insurance payments, the 1987 annual cost for a well-adjusted patient was $9791 compared with $31,291 for a poorly adjusted patient. The authors did administer a family assessment scale but did not discuss the relationship between family assessment and adjustment.

Because of a lack of family data, it is difficult to present a conclusive argument about the family as a consumer of health care. However, the preceding material documents family involvement in all phases of an illness. The data strongly suggest that health and illness are family matters. Some carefully controlled demonstration projects are needed to demonstrate the cost effectiveness, humaneness, and outcomes of family-centered care.

Family Patterns and Illness

One of the contributions of the family systems perspective to the understanding of illness is the theory that the multigenerational emotional process (the transfer from generation to generation of family relationship systems) can lead to patterns of family interaction associated with physical, emotional, or social illnesses (Bowen, 1987; Kerr & Bowen, 1988;

Father/son drinking?

Minuchin, Rosman, & Baker, 1978). Schizophrenia, diabetic acidosis, and alcoholism, as well as such diseases as lupus erythematosis, have been related to family patterns.

Minuchin's (1978) classic study of diabetic children illustrates this point. A group of diabetic children were seen in a state of acidosis with predictable frequency in the emergency room. This is a rare event because once the child and the family learn to recognize the symptoms of acidosis they can treat it at home with supplemental insulin injections. This situation was further complicated by the fact that when the child was admitted to the hospital for an exploration of other possible causes of the acidosis or for regulation of their insulin dosage, no confounding problems were found and the child responded well to insulin. The family and the child were given intensive education about diabetes and its treatment. Shortly after the hospitalization the pattern repeated itself. Some of these children were admitted to the hospital for acidosis as often as 15 times a year.

Finally, a psychiatric consultation was sought. The consultation involved three girls who were serendipitously admitted within the same time period. The girls were model patients, gentle and pleasant. Their families were concerned, appeared stable, and were eager to cooperate. At first individual therapy for each child was pursued to enhance their ability to handle stress. However, there was no improvement in the incidence of acidosis.

The pediatric team was then increased to include a family therapist. The family therapist focused on the fact that free fatty acids (FFA) are both a measure of emotional arousal and a substrate from which the liver produces ketone bodies. Too many ketone bodies result in ketoacidosis, generally referred to as acidosis. It was possible, therefore, to set up a study that linked the biological and the emotional factors in these girls' lives.

When the girls were exposed to a fight between their parents, the FFA levels increased dramatically and they became resistant to insulin. The family pattern generated a state of physical illness (acidosis) in the child.

Health-care providers do not want to use the family systems theory of disease to blame families for illnesses. However, family systems theory and the literature on life-style document that the family is a potent influence on health and illness.

◆ CONCLUSION

Readers will note that up to this point few suggestions for intervention have been made. The reason for this is that many families go through even catastrophic crises without seeking professional help. Certainly, most families go through the normal transitions of the life cycle without seeking professional guidance. Olson, McCubbin, Barnes, Larsen, Muxen, and Wilson (1989) studied 1000 "normal" families and reported that few ever consider seeking professional help. All of them rely on spiritual strength and on friends and relatives. The sample was composed mainly of practicing Lutherans. When the families were asked about their interest in 30 workshops, services, or courses, only 15% to 25% of the families expressed some interest in 22 of these programs. With the exception of premarital counseling and childbirth preparation classes, most of the proposed programs did not focus on health. Generally, families participated in no organized programs.

It is the authors' contention that part of the reason families do not readily seek professional help is that the help is not family oriented and does not meet family needs. It is also likely that there are groups of families who do not need professional help to cope with life. Throughout the book interventions will be discussed that are family centered and that call for a collaboration between the family and the health professional.

The material presented in this chapter alerts the health-care worker to the fact that the family is the matrix in which we all live. It is the first agent of socialization for children and the first teacher about matters of health and illness. Within the family the child develops a sense of mastery and meaning about life. Interactions within the family may lead to disease states and affect recovery from illness.

The health-care provider who recognizes the influence of the family will have a powerful ally in healing. If professionals ignore the family, the health-care system and the family may be at cross purposes. For example, educating a male cardiac patient about decreasing his salt intake without instructing his wife, who does the cooking, will not lead to success. Indeed, if the wife feels blamed or slighted, she may respond by cooking more of her husband's "favorite foods," too many of which may be high in salt. Even if the husband and wife agree about reducing salt intake, ethnic factors may blind them to the high sodium content in some favored traditional foods.

The succeeding chapters of this book further explore family dynamics related to health and illness. The value of family involvement will be highlighted from different perspectives. Chapter 2 presents the Resiliency Model of Family Stress, Adjustment, and Adaptation. This model serves as the basis for discussion of family reactions to illness and for family involvement in all phases of health.

REFERENCES

Baird, M. A., & Doherty, W. J. (1990). Risks and benefits of a family systems approach to medical care. *Family Medicine, 22*(5), 396-403.

Beavers, W. R. (1982). Healthy, midrange, and severely dysfunctional families. In F. Walsh (Ed.), *Normal family processes* (pp. 45-66). New York: Guilford Press.

Beutler, I. F., Burr, W. R., Bahr, K. S., & Herrin, D. A. (1989). The family realm: Theoretical contributions for understanding its uniqueness. *Journal of Marriage and the Family, 51*, 805-816.

Bowen, M. (1978). *Family therapy in clinical practice.* New York: Jason Aronson.

Branowski, T., & Nader, P. (1985). *Family health behaviors.* In D. C. Turk & R. D. Kerns (Eds.), *Health, illness, and families* (pp. 93-107). New York: John Wiley & Sons.

Browne, G. B., Arpin, K., Corey, P., Litch, M., & Gafnie, A. (1990). Individual correlates of health service utilization and the cost of poor adjustment to chronic illness. *Medical Care, 28*(1), 43-58.

Carter, G. A., & McGoldrick, M. (1980). *The family life cycle: A framework for family therapy.* New York: Gardner Press.

Cunningham, P. J. (Ed.). (1990). Medical care use and expenditures for children across stages of the family life cycle. *Journal of Marriage and the Family, 52*, 197-207.

Dixon, M. A. (1986). Families of adolescent clients and nonclients: Their environment and health-seeking behaviors. *Advances in Nursing Science, 8*(2), 75-88.

Duvall, E. (1977). *Marriage and family development* (5th ed.). Philadelphia: J. B. Lippincott.

Friedman, M. M. (1986). *Family nursing theory and assessment.* Norwalk, CT: Appleton-Century-Crofts.

Garn, S. M., Bailey, S. M., Solomon, M. A., & Hopkins, P. J. (1981). Effect of remaining family members on fatness prediction. *American Journal of Clinical Nutrition, 34*, 148-153.

Haley, J. (1976). *Problem-solving therapy.* San Francisco: Jossey-Bass.

Hartz, A., Giefer, E., & Rimm, A. A. (1977). Relative importance of the effect of family environment and heredity on obesity. *Annals of Human Genetics, 41*, 185-193.

Hathway, D., Boswell, B., Stanford, D., Schneider, S., & Moncrief, A. (1987). Health promotion and disease prevention for hospitalized patient's family. *Nursing Administration Quarterly, 11*(3), 1-7.

Holman, A. H. (1983). *Family assessment.* Newbury Park, CA: Sage.

Justice, R. (1987). *Who gets sick?* New York: Simon & Schuster.

Kain, J. (1990). *The myth of family decline.* New York: W. W. Norton.

Kerr, M. (1980). Emotional factors in physical illness. *The Family, 7,* 59.

Kerr, M., & Bowen, M. (1988). *Family evaluation.* New York: W. W. Norton.

Khoury, P., Morrison, J. A., Laskarzewski, P. M., & Glueck, C. J. (1983). Parent-offspring and sibling body mass index associations during and after sharing of common household environments: The Princeton school district family study. *Metabolism, 32,* 82-89.

Laslett, P. (1977). Characteristics of the Western family considered over time. *Journal of Family History, 2,* 89-115.

Mechanic, D. (Ed.). (1964). The influence of mothers on their children's health attitudes and behavior. *Pediatrics, 33,* 444-452.

Minuchin, S., & Fishman, H. C. (1981). *Family therapy techniques.* Cambridge, MA: Harvard University Press.

Minuchin, S., Rosman, B. L., & Baker, L. (1978). *Psychosomatic families.* Cambridge: Harvard University Press.

Newocheck, P. W., & Halfin, N. (1986). The association between mother's and children's use of physician services. *Medical Care, 24*(1), 30-38.

Olson, D. H., McCubbin, H. I., Barnes, H., Larson, A., Muxen, M., & Wilson, M. (1989). Families: what makes them work. Beverly Hills, CA: Sage.

Parsons, T., & Bales, R. F. (1955). *Family socialization and interaction process.* Glencoe, IL: Free Press.

Reece, M. M. (1964). Masculinity and femininity: A factor-analytic study. *Psychological Reports, 14,* 123-139.

Ross, B., & Cobb, K. (1988). *Family nursing: A nursing process approach.* Redwood, CA: Addison-Wesley Nursing.

Schor, E., Starfield, B., Stidley, C., & Hankin, J. (1987). Family health: Utilization and efforts of family membership. *Medical Care, 25*(7), 616-626.

von Bertalanffy, L. (1968). *General system theory.* New York: George Braziller.

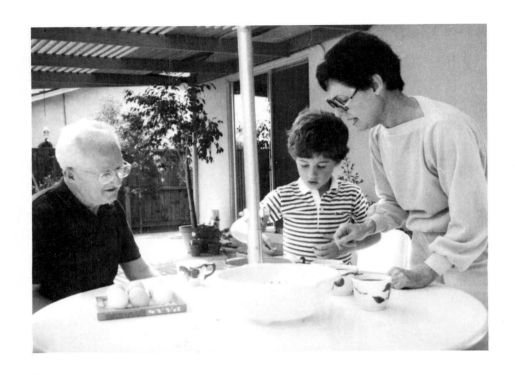

2

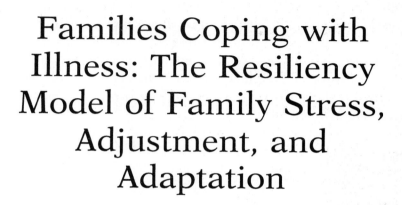

Families Coping with Illness: The Resiliency Model of Family Stress, Adjustment, and Adaptation

MARILYN A. MCCUBBIN AND HAMILTON I. MCCUBBIN

✦

CHAPTER GOALS

✦ To describe the Resiliency Model of Family Stress, Adjustment, and Adaptation and its ability to enhance understanding of family adjustment and adaptation responses to illness situations

✦ To demonstrate the use of the Resiliency Model of Family Stress, Adjustment, and Adaptation as a framework that assists in determining whether or not an illness stressor may cause family crisis

✦ To provide clinical guidelines for application of the Resiliency Model of Family Stress, Adjustment, and Adaptation in assessing critical elements of family functioning during illness

OVERVIEW

E XPERIENCE tells us that two families faced with the same illness stressor can respond in dramatically different ways; one family rallies its members and mobilizes itself to deal constructively with the demands it faces, whereas the other family is immobilized by the situation and begins to unravel as demands are placed on it. How can these differences in coping be understood and predicted by health professionals? The Resiliency Model of Family Stress, Adjustment, and Adaptation provides a framework that assists in determining whether or not an illness stressor may cause family crisis. This chapter describes the Resiliency Model and its application in understanding family responses to illness situations. Also examined is the usefulness of this model as a guide to assessing critical elements of family functioning, the knowledge of which can be useful in planning family interventions during illness.

The Resiliency Model of Family Stress, Adjustment, and Adaptation (Fig. 2-1) is based on the work of Reuben Hill (1949, 1958), the Double ABCX Model (H. I. McCubbin & Patterson, 1981, 1983a, 1983b), and the more recent Typology Model of Family Adjustment and Adaptation (McCubbin & McCubbin, 1987, 1989). These efforts focused on a stressor, the family's efforts to use resistance resources, the family's appraisal of the situation, and the family's coping patterns and problem-solving abilities to maintain function while dealing with a stressor. The Resiliency Model, an expansion of these earlier efforts, emphasizes family *adaptation*.

This presentation of the Resiliency Model focuses on illness as a stressor affecting family life. A fictitious family, the Smiths, is used as an example to address key elements of assessing families struggling to adjust and adapt to illness. Family adaptation rather than adjustment is emphasized, since it is often the most needed response to illness. The discussion demonstrates the importance of the family schema level of appraisal (the family's blueprint for functioning) as a force that can facilitate family coping and adaptation. This appraisal level can produce optimal problem solving for managing illness situations.

In the context of health-care settings the Resiliency Model (McCubbin & McCubbin, 1987, 1989) assists health professionals in assessing family functioning and intervening in the family system to facilitate both family adjustment and, in most illness situations, family adaptation. The Resiliency Model attempts to guide health professionals in determining what family types, capabilities, and strengths are needed, called on, or created to manage illness in the family. The model also is designed to help health-care practitioners develop strategies for intervention based on a systematic diagnosis and evaluation of the family functioning under stress. The

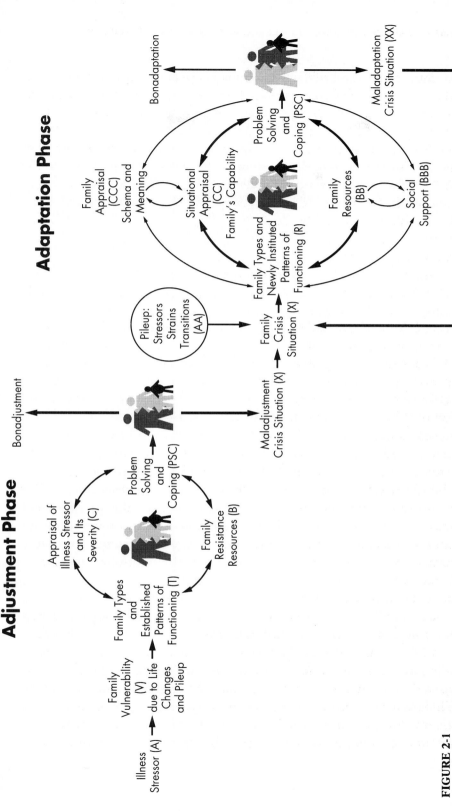

FIGURE 2-1

The Resiliency Model of Family Stress, Adjustment, and Adaptation.

following vignette introduces the Smith family and the illness that confronts them.

✦ ✦ ✦ ✦ ✦

Mr. and Mrs. Smith are sitting quietly, holding hands, shocked by their physician's diagnosis that their younger daughter, Jamie, has cystic fibrosis. After an hour of discussing, questioning, expressing doubts, and seeking explanation, it is evident that the diagnosis has been checked, rechecked, and affirmed. They have received detailed information from Dr. Thomas about cystic fibrosis and its long-term course, but they are too upset to absorb all of the information. They do realize, however, that the treatment will place heavy demands on the family over time and that many of their future plans will be altered. Mr. Smith, age 37, is troubled by the expense involved in the long-term care of his daughter and wonders how they will make ends meet. Mrs. Smith, age 35, struggles with the realization that, in all likelihood, she will need to find full-time work. She wonders whether it is possible for them to handle all the pressures.

At this difficult time, the Smiths' thoughts of the anticipated hardships and pressures are set aside and are not discussed so that they may have the energy to support each other, Jamie, and their two older children, 11-year-old Jonathan and 12-year-old Alice.

How will the Smith family face this diagnosis? How will the family be able to work together to deal with the challenges involved in the long-term care of a child with cystic fibrosis, a chronic condition demanding considerable family investment of time, commitment, and interpersonal and financial resources? How will the two older siblings respond to the situation and what role will they play in the family's efforts to cope? How do families faced with an illness or a chronic health condition manage to respond to the situation and at the same time promote the individual development of all members? What are the coping strategies and changes in the family's organization and patterns of functioning that will be needed to manage the illness over time? Will the family accept all these changes? Will these changes in family patterns be congruent with the family's values, goals, and expectations? If the changes are not congruent, how will the family achieve congruency and thus reestablish stability? Could the family fail as a unit? What would the key factors be in shaping the outcome of either successful adaptation or family maladaptation? What do health professionals focus on in evaluating family functioning during adjustment and adaptation? What are the critical factors that health professionals need to try to influence and shape to facilitate the family's adaptation leading to a successful outcome over time?

Note that these questions stress the role of the family. It would be far too simplistic and too narrow an emphasis for the health professional to focus only on the parents' reactions to the illness without a careful and thorough assessment of the *family system's* reaction to the illness. The family system and its functioning involve a very complex process of interacting individuals, personalities, and family unit characteristics, all of which influence each other to shape the family's course of changing itself. These changes may lead to successful adaptation, *bonadaptation*, meaning that the family is able to stabilize with instituted patterns in place, promote the individual development of its members, and achieve a sense of coherence and congruency even when faced with an illness and major changes in the patterns of family functioning. However, the changes could also result in unsuccessful adaptation, *maladaptation*, where family members sacrifice personal development and growth, the family unit functions in a more chaotic state, and the family's overall sense of well-being, trust, and sense of order and coherence becomes very low.

✦ ✦ ✦ ✦ ✦

The Smith family accepted the diagnosis as a temporary condition. Given the advances in the treatment of cystic fibrosis, the Smiths believed that a cure was just around the corner. From their perspective, whatever adjustments the family might need to make to cope with the illness would be only temporary. Their daughter would soon be back to normal. On the basis of this appraisal of the situation, the family agreed that for the next 6 to 8 months they would devote attention to Jamie and that each family member would chip in to make the tasks easier.

Jamie's home care regimen involved the expenditure of extensive time and energy to clear the mucus from building in her lungs. The family had to vigilantly ensure that Jamie could breathe. Therefore family routines were set aside.

The family's normal functioning could not, of course, come to a complete halt. Many pressures and demands accumulated during the first months: Alice expressed interest in dating (at an early age, from the parent's perspective); Jonathan was having academic difficulty in school; and caring for Jamie was starting to take its toll on the Smiths' limited savings.

The Smiths viewed themselves as a close-knit family, with strong bonds of unity keeping the family together and at the same time promoting flexibility in family functioning. The family's emphasis on bonding and flexibility as integral parts of the family's established patterns of functioning was clear to the nursing staff that worked with them. Mr. and Mrs. Smith were able to talk things through, to be intimate, and to support each other. They showed a willingness to share tasks and responsibilities. The family seemed to agree to make personal sacrifices to allow the family to adjust to the illness. The family communication patterns emphasized affirmation and support for members, and the family took full advantage of the pediatrician's willingness to work with them and the nurse's support and guidance. They viewed such outside help as being in their best interest.

The family chose, however, to avoid making any substantial or lasting changes in the family's established way of doing things. They made only the necessary adjustments to attend to the needs of their youngest member.

The Smiths typify the dynamics of family adjustment. Their making of small adjustments in roles, tasks, routines, and communication sheds light on the complex elements of family functioning that come into play to promote family adjustment.

The family adjustment phase of the Resiliency Model may be described as a series of interacting components that shape the family process and outcomes of adjustment. Outcomes vary along a continuum from the more positive *bonadjustment* — in which established patterns of functioning are maintained — to the other extreme of *maladjustment* — a family crisis that demands changes in the established patterns of functioning.

✦ THE ADJUSTMENT PHASE AND ITS COMPONENTS

In the face of a stressor — in the Smiths' case, an illness — a successful or unsuccessful family adjustment is determined by many interacting components. The *stressor (A) and its severity* **interacts with** the family's *vulnerability (V)*, which is shaped by the pileup of family stresses, transitions, and strains occurring in the same period as the stressor. Family vulnerability **interacts with** the family's typology, which is the *established patterns of functioning (T)*. These components, in turn, **interact with** the family's *resistance resources (B)*. Quality communication between husband and wife and a family's willingness to work together as a family are examples of re-

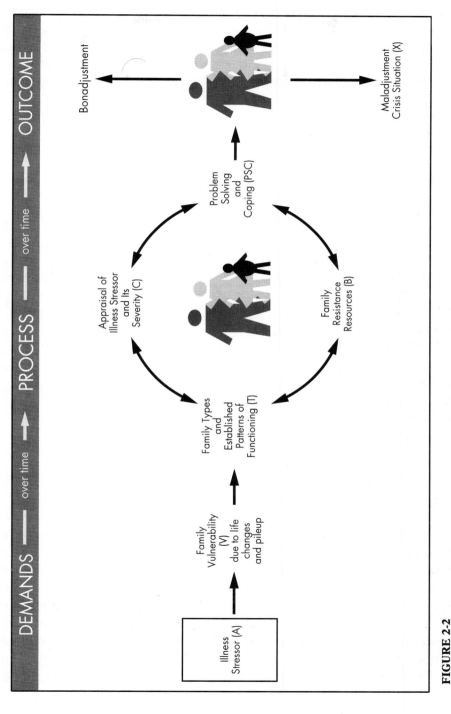

FIGURE 2-2

Adjustment Phase of the Resiliency Model of Family Stress, Adjustment, and Adaptation.

sistance resources. This, in turn, **interacts with** the family's *appraisal (C) of the stressor* (for example, catastrophic, manageable, of short duration). The family appraisal **interacts with** the family's *problem-solving and coping strategies (PSC),* such as adopting an affirming communication style, seeking help from the medical community, and taking advantage of the learning opportunities made available by the pediatrician and the nurse (Fig. 2-2).

Although these components interact with one another to shape the level of adjustment in the family, it nevertheless would be instructive to examine each separately and describe its relative importance in family adjustment.

The Stressor (A) and Its Severity

A *stressor* is a demand placed on the family that produces, or has the potential of producing, changes in the family system. This change, or threat of change, may affect areas of family life besides health—the marital relationship, the parent-child relationship, the sibling relationship, the family-system boundaries (who is in or out of the family unit), the family's goals, the family's established patterns of functioning, and the family's values. The severity of the stressor is determined by the degree to which the stressor threatens the stability of the family unit or places significant demands on the family's resources and capabilities. The stressor could threaten the family's integrity and well-being over time (see M.A. McCubbin, 1986, 1990).

Family Vulnerability (V)—Pileup and Family Life Cycle Changes

Vulnerability is the fragile interpersonal and organizational condition of the family system. This condition, ranging from "high" to "low," is determined by (1) the accumulation, or *pileup*, of demands on or within the family unit, such as financial debts, poor health status of relatives, and changes in a parent's work role or work environment, and (2) the trials and tribulations associated with the family's particular life-cycle stage with all of its demands and changes. For example, the effect of the diagnosis of cystic fibrosis is likely to cause more problems for families at the adolescent or launching stage of the family life cycle because of the accumulation of life changes or strains associated with raising an adolescent and the depletion of family interpersonal, social, and economic resources at this stage (Olson, et al., 1983; H.I. McCubbin, Thompson, Pirner, & M.A. McCubbin, 1988).

Family Types (T) — Profile of Family-Established Patterns of Functioning

A family's *typology* is defined by a set of attributes that explain how the family system operates or behaves. The family type is the predictable and discernible patterns of family functioning. Recent investigations indicate how important it is to understand the wide range of family types and established patterns. In the face of normative transitions, resilient families (those with established patterns of family bonding and flexibility) are better able to manage hardships and promote other family strengths of hardiness, coherence, and predictability, as well as marital and family satisfaction (see Fig. 5-3) (H.I. McCubbin, Thompson, Pirner, & M.A. McCubbin, 1988). In the face of a severe chronic illness situation, balanced families (those with established, but not extreme, patterns of cohesiveness and adaptability) appear to have more positive health outcomes for the chronically ill child (see Fig. 5-2) (M.A. McCubbin, 1986, 1988).

Family Resistance Resources (B) — Capabilities and Strengths

The family's *resistance resources* have been described as a family's abilities and capabilities to address and manage the stressor and its demands by preventing the situation from creating a crisis or disruption in the family's established patterns of functioning (Burr, 1973; Hansen & Johnson, 1979; McCubbin & McCubbin, 1989). The goal of adjustment is to manage the stressor without introducing major or lasting changes in the family's established patterns of functioning. Resources or family strengths then become part of the family's capability for resisting a crisis and promoting family adjustment. The critical family resources are economic stability, cohesiveness, flexibility, hardiness, shared spiritual beliefs, open communication, traditions, celebrations, routines, and organization (Curran, 1983; Olson et al., 1983; H.I. McCubbin et al., 1988).

Family Appraisal of the Stressor (C)

The Smith family's subjective definition of the illness of the younger daughter and the hardships accompanying the illness shaped the family's response and thus became critical to the course of family adjustment. Although there are objective cultural definitions of the seriousness of particular illnesses, such as cancer or heart disease, representing the collective judgment of the community as a whole, the family's *appraisal of the stressor* is the family's definition of the seriousness of a stressor and its related hardships. The family's appraisal of a stressor may range from interpreting it as being uncontrollable and forecasting the family's disintegration to viewing it as a challenge to be met with growth-producing outcomes (H.I. McCubbin & Patterson, 1983b; M.A. McCubbin, 1988).

Family Problem Solving and Coping (PSC)

The problem-solving and coping component in the Resiliency Model indicates the family's management of illness through the use of problem-solving and coping skills. *Problem solving* refers to the family's ability to organize a stressor into manageable components, to identify alternative courses of action to deal with each component, to initiate steps to resolve the discrete issues, as well as the interpersonal issues, and to develop and cultivate patterns of problem-solving communication needed to bring about family problem-solving efforts. *Coping* refers to the family's strategies, patterns, and behaviors designed to maintain or strengthen the family as a whole, maintain the emotional stability and well-being of its members, obtain or use family and community resources to manage the situation, and initiate efforts to resolve family hardships created by a stressor. Coping refers to a wide range of behaviors that family members use to manage a stressor (M.A. McCubbin & H.I. McCubbin, 1989).

Family Response — Stress and Distress

A stressor such as an illness produces tension, a *response,* in the family that calls for management (Antonovsky, 1979). Stress emerges when this tension is not reduced or brought within manageable limits. A state of tension, characterized as family stress rather than as a stressor, arises when there is an actual or a perceived imbalance between the demands placed on the family and the family's resistance resources and capabilities. Family stress is then depicted as a nonspecific demand for adjustment behavior. Therefore the amount of stress in a family varies, depending on the nature of the illness, the resources and the capabilities of the family to deal with the illness, and the psychological and physical well-being of its members at the time of onset of the illness. Family distress describes a negative state in which the family defines the demand-resources imbalance as unpleasant or even destabilizing to the family. In contrast, eustress is a positive state characterized by the family's defining the demands-resources imbalance as desirable and a challenge that family members accept and, in some cases, appreciate (H.I. McCubbin & Patterson, 1983b).

Family Bonadjustment, Maladjustment, and Crises (X)

Some stressors do not create major hardships for the family system, particularly when mediated by the family's typology of established patterns, resources, and coping and problem-solving abilities, appraisals, and strengths. In situations of *bonadjustment*, the family moves through the situation with relative ease, which leads to a positive outcome. In most cases this involves minor adjustments and changes in the family system.

In illness situations, however, especially chronic illness, hardships are often numerous and severe, demanding more substantial changes in the family system — in its roles, goals, values, rules, priorities, boundaries, and patterns of functioning. Families in this situation are not likely to achieve stability with ease. New patterns are called for. In situations involving this disruption in established patterns, the family will, in all likelihood, experience *maladjustment* and a resulting state of *crisis*.

Family crisis has been conceptualized as a continuous condition of disruptiveness, disorganization, or incapacitation in the family social system (Burr, 1973). Whereas family stress is a state of tension brought about by the demand-capability imbalance in the family, crisis is a state of disorganization in the family system. Families in crisis are unable to restore stability, are often trapped in cyclical trial-and-error struggles to reduce tensions (which tend to make matters worse), and make only small changes in the family structure and in patterns of interaction where new patterns of interaction are needed (H.I. McCubbin & Patterson, 1983b). A family in crisis should not carry the stigmatizing value judgment that somehow the family unit has failed, is dysfunctional, or is in need of professional counseling (H.I. McCubbin & Patterson, 1983b). A family crisis may be viewed as an expected, if not a necessary, condition for the family to adapt to a difficult situation.

Family crisis denotes family disorganization and a demand for basic changes in the family patterns of functioning to restore stability, order, and a sense of coherence. This movement to initiate changes in the family system's pattern of functioning marks the beginning of the adaptation phase of the Resiliency Model. The adaptation phase is fully addressed later in the following section.

✦ THE FAMILY ADAPTATION PHASE AND ITS COMPONENTS

✦ ✦ ✦ ✦ ✦

The Smith family made every effort to cope with their younger daughter's illness while maintaining the family's routines and patterns of functioning. But this resistant, adjustment behavior was not sufficient to achieve a satisfactory level of functioning.

Five new patterns or decisions were instituted to cope with the situation:
1. Mrs. Smith reentered the work force, as a secretary, to cope with the economic demands
2. Housekeeping duties were reallocated within the family to minimize pressures on Mrs. Smith
3. Mrs. Smith's plans to complete her college degree were postponed
4. A family vacation that had been planned for 2 years, with all family members very much invested and involved in the planning, was put off
5. The older children, Alice and Jonathan, were called on to help with Jamie's home health care, previously performed by the parents.

These changes created tensions for all family members. There was a growing realization that family roles, expectations, priorities, and goals had been altered and that the changes might be lasting.

Alice and Jonathan resented the changes and complained to their father. Mrs. Smith was made to feel guilty. Support from her friends at work and Mr. Smith's willingness to deal with the children helped to ease the family's tension to a great degree.

The health-care professional's assessment of the family adaptation calls for a more dynamic model than that provided by Hill's (1949) **ABCX** framework, which focused on adjustment. The Resiliency Model, which focuses on family change and adaptation over time, emerged from studies of war-induced family crises (H.I. McCubbin, Boss, Wilson, & Lester, 1980; H.I. McCubbin & Patterson, 1981, 1982, 1983a, 1983b; McCubbin & McCubbin, 1987, 1989). The Resiliency Model adds a host of postcrisis or adaptation-oriented components in an effort to understand and describe the following:

1. The additional life stressors and changes that may influence the family's ability to achieve adaptation in the face of an illness
2. The critical psychological, family, and social factors that families call on, are shaped by, and call into use in their effort to achieve a satisfactory level of family adaptation
3. The unique process of family appraisal that gives "meaning" to changes in the family and facilitates coping and adaptation
4. The processes families engage in to achieve satisfactory adaptation to an illness
5. The outcome of these family efforts to achieve a satisfactory level of adaptation, which brings congruency between the family's values, goals, rules, priorities, and expectations and the family's new patterns of functioning. In fostering congruency the family develops a shared sense of coherence vital to successful adaptation.

The adaptation phase of the Resiliency Model is outlined in Fig. 2-3. When an illness becomes a family crisis, it initiates the beginning of the adaptation phase. The level of family adaptation is determined by a number of interacting components. The pileup (AA) of demands on or in the family system created by the illness, family life-cycle changes, and unresolved strains **interacts with** the family's level of regenerativity or resiliency (R). This resiliency is determined in part by newly instituted patterns of family functioning and retained established patterns of functioning. These components **interact with** the family's resources (BB) such as strengths and capabilities, which are **supported by** family and friends (BBB) in the community and by the family's appraisals. A situational appraisal (CC) is formed from the perceived relationship between the family's resources and the demands of the situation. This family appraisal of the crisis situation (CC) **interacts with** the family's schema appraisal (CCC) (the family's blueprint for functioning—their values, goals, priorities, and rules) to achieve congruency. This interaction creates a family meaning that is attached to the illness and the changes it produces. The resource and appraisal components **interact with** the family's problem-solving and coping repertoire (PSC) to facilitate family adaptation to the crisis situation.

Central Importance of Family Adaptation in Clinical Practice

Illnesses have the unique characteristic of promoting (if not demanding) changes in the family's established patterns of functioning. Illnesses in the

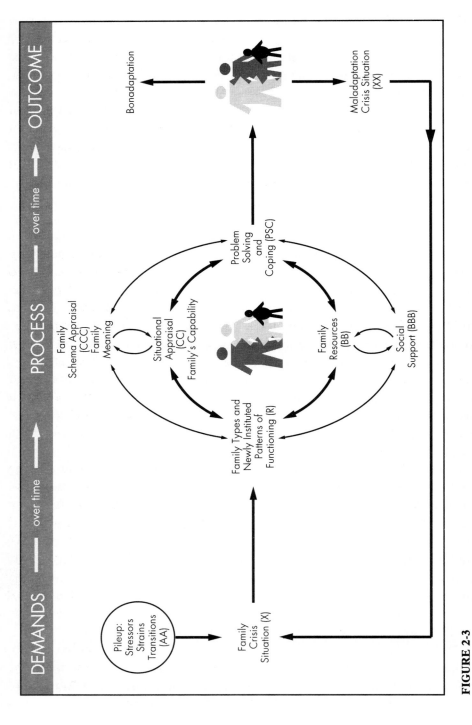

FIGURE 2-3

Adaptation Phase of the Resiliency Model of Family Stress, Adjustment, and Adaptation.

family system often cause family crises and thus set into motion the process of family adaptation. Therefore, with the exception of the common cold or other short-term illnesses, when health professionals examine illness in the family context they need to focus their assessments and interventions on the process of family adaptation. For this reason, at appropriate points in the presentation and discussion of family adaptation, "clinical application guidelines" are introduced to facilitate application of the Resiliency Model to clinical situations. These guidelines summarize theoretical concepts in applied contexts and relate the family knowledge to a clinical plan. Clinical assessment tools that may be useful in this process are suggested.

Family Adaptation

Since family adaptation becomes the central concept in understanding the family's struggle to manage the situation created by the illness, it is used to describe the *outcome* of family efforts to bring a new level of balance, harmony, coherence, and functioning to a family-crisis situation. In that family bonadaptation involves positive change in the family and positive transactions between the family and the community and its agencies—in this case, the health care system—it is reasonable to argue that the family struggles to achieve a balance and a fit at both the *individual-to-family* and the *family-to-community* levels of functioning. Family efforts directed toward adaptation involve consideration of and response to both levels of functioning because the change at one level of family functioning affects the other (Antonovsky, 1987).

A balance between meeting the needs of individual members of the family and the well-being of the family as a whole is sought at the first level of interaction. In the case of the Smith family, a balance is sought between meeting the needs of the individual child with cystic fibrosis, the needs of the family as a whole, and the needs of other family members. As already noted, the medically guided home-care regimen and the family's new patterns of functioning required to cope with the illness (the change in family routines, the demand for continuous and predictable involvement of other family members) reveal the complex interplay needed between the individual and the family unit for successful family adaptation.

Because long-term care of a chronically ill child calls for a collaborative arrangement between the family and the health-care community, the family-to-community level of adaptation, including the health-care community, must also be achieved. The Smith family's success in caring for a child with cystic fibrosis also depends on receiving quality care from the health-care system. The two institutions, the family and the health-care professionals involved, must work as a team. The family benefits from the support and professional care and guidance received on a continuous basis. To be effective, the health-care team and the treatment prescribed depend on the family unit to follow through. A breakdown in the team effort may create difficulties for the child and the family. Family adaptation is enhanced when a mutually supportive relationship develops between the family and the health-care team. This type of relationship is best achieved through shared commitment, mutual respect, and effective communication.

Although all components of the adaptation phase interact with one another to shape the level of family adaptation, it nevertheless would also be instructive to examine each of the components separately. The relative importance of these components is described as they relate to adaptation. Ways are suggested in which a clinical plan for assessment and intervention incorporate this family adaptation–oriented knowledge base.

Pileup (AA) of demands. Because family crises evolve and are resolved over time, families are seldom dealing with a single illness-induced crisis. Our research indicates that the experience of pileup of demands is commonplace and a critical factor that should be taken into account as part of the clinical assessment process. This is particularly important to do in the case of a prolonged illness, such as caring for a child with a physical disability or family member with a chronic illness (M.A. McCubbin, 1988, 1989). Demands or needs of individuals, families, and communities change over time. In the case example of the long-term care of a child with cystic fibrosis, a family will need to stabilize the family environment at the initial phases of the treatment regimen in the home. As technology advances and children with cystic fibrosis move into the young adult or adult stages of the life cycle, the family again is called on to rearrange its functioning, to cope not only with the development of an individual young adult (and all the trials and tribulations that entails), but also with a changing family, created by changes in the parents and in other members. The family may have fewer resources and strengths. There may be changes in roles, with a mother's return to the work force (as in the case of the Smiths); there may be divorces, separations, other illnesses — all occurring at the same time. See the box on p. 37 for a clinical guideline related to pileup.

There are at least six broad categories of stresses and strains contributing to a pileup in a family's adaptation to an illness:

1. The illness and related hardships over time
2. Normative transitions in individual family members and the family as a whole
3. Prior family strains accumulated over time
4. Situational demands and contextual difficulties
5. The consequences of family efforts to cope
6. Intrafamily and social ambiguity that provides inadequate guidelines on how families should act or cope effectively (H.I. McCubbin & Patterson, 1983a; M.A. McCubbin, 1989, 1990) with the illness-related crisis and its hardships.

The illness and related hardships over time. The first category of stresses and strains leading to a pileup is the illness and related hardships over time. When a family experiences an illness-induced family crisis—having a child with a birth defect, having an adolescent member with a spinal cord injury, having an adult member faced with a life-threatening illness—the family also experiences specific hardships associated with that illness that increase or intensify the difficulties families face (McCubbin & McCubbin, 1989).

Clinical Application Guideline: Pileup of Life Changes and Adaptation

Family Knowledge Base

The greater the pileup of life changes overlapping with the course of the illness and the family's effort to change, the greater the family's vulnerability and, thus, difficulty in adapting to the situation.

Clinical Plan

Assess all the life changes, hardships, concurrent hassles, prior strains, situational demands, efforts to cope, ambiguities, and normal life-cycle issues affecting the family.

Clinical Assessment Tool

Clinical interview complemented by the use of the Family Inventory of Life Events and Changes (FILE) (H.I. McCubbin, Patterson, & Wilson, 1981, form B).

The additional illness-related hardships associated with a family crisis may include ambiguity surrounding the diagnosis, the course of the illness, or the outcome of treatment; increased marital or sibling relationship strains; parent-child conflicts; and decreased emotional or financial resources. These hardships may also include frequent disturbing, but necessary, visits with the attending physician or medical staff, follow-up treatment regimens in the home environment (such as the case of children with cystic fibrosis), the revamping of the entire family environment to accommodate home treatment, and the side effects of the treatment itself. These hardships create additional burdens on the family system above and beyond the diagnosis and therapy. See the box below for a clinical guideline related to illness, severity, and adaptation.

Normative transitions. The second broad category of stresses and strains leading to pileup is normative transitions. Families are not static social units. They go through predictable transitions as the result of the normal growth and development of their young members (for example, the need for nurturance and supervision, or increasing independence and autonomy), the development of adult members (career development, return to school for more education, returning to the work environment, commitment to a career and independence), the changes in the extended family system (illness and death of grandparents), and the predictable

Clinical Application Guideline:
Illness, Severity, and Adaptation

Family Knowledge Base

The greater the severity of the illness and hardships created by the illness, particularly the demands placed on the family as a whole, the greater the difficulty in achieving a satisfactory level of family adaptation.

Clinical Plan

Assess the severity of the stressor (illness) in terms of the immediate or anticipated consequences for the family unit.

Clinical Assessment Tool

Clinical interview.

family life-cycle changes (children entering school, adolescence, the empty-nest stage, retirement).

These normal transitions may occur at the same time as the crisis–precipitating illness event. The simultaneous occurrence of normative transitions and an illness stressor event often creates a family crisis, which necessitates an adaptation response. Intervention with families faced with an illness-induced crisis must take into consideration not only the specific hardships of the illness itself, but also the concurrent normative transitions that may spin the family out of a stable situation into a disturbing, disorienting style of functioning.

Prior family strains accumulated over time. The third category of stresses and strains leading to pileup is prior family strains. Most family systems carry residual strains, which may be the result of unresolved hardships from earlier stressors, transitions, crises, or which may be inherent in ongoing roles, such as parenthood and employment (Pearlin & Schooler, 1978; H.I. McCubbin et al., 1988; H.I. McCubbin & Thompson, 1989). Prior strains may be exacerbated in the face of a new illness stressor and, consequently, contribute to the pileup of difficulties families are called upon to face.

These prior strains may surface under the pressure of new demands and therefore require management in a crisis situation (H.I. McCubbin & Patterson, 1983a). Prior strains become an important target for professional intervention for two reasons. First, the illness situation may mask family difficulties (prior strains) that need attention. Second, prior strains may mask the major hardships of the illness crisis, which also demand attention.

Situational demands and contextual difficulties. The fourth category of stresses and strains leading to pileup is situational demands and contextual difficulties. Medical or social agencies may create additional demands that undermine the functioning of the family as it attempts to adapt to a crisis situation.

Family decisions regarding illness are often complex, calling for negotiation with several medical agencies and a variety of health professionals. For example, the decision to sustain a family member's life with the continued use of life-support equipment and open-heart surgery calls for a complex consideration of many factors and major financial responsibilities. In the case of organ transplants the decision often involves other family members, whose well-being may be threatened by the final decision.

Additionally, patterns of health-care delivery may change, prompting the family to alter the way it has traditionally functioned. These changes in patterns of health-care delivery certainly applies in the case of a family with a child with cystic fibrosis. Moreover, medical needs change as the child becomes a young adult. Basic care is transferred from the attentive and well-informed pediatrician, from the parents' point of view, to the "less-informed" internist. Because the family's relationship with the pediatrician has been well-established and has provided a sense of continuity and coherence, the change in care creates an additional burden for the family and disrupts its equilibrium.

Consequences of family efforts to cope. The fifth category of stresses and strains leading to pileup is the consequences of family efforts to cope. These stresses and strains emerge from specific behaviors or strategies that a family may have used in the adjustment phase, such as increased rigidity or suppression of anger, or that the family uses currently in their effort to adapt to the illness situation (H.I. McCubbin & Patterson, 1983a; M.A. McCubbin, 1990).

Some coping strategies, such as taking on a job to handle the financial demands of the family situation (as Mrs. Smith was called on to do) or consuming alcohol to manage psychological tension (which may lead to psychological or physical dependency), may produce additional burdens on the already overtaxed family. These demands, some created initially as a result of seemingly positive effort, must also be considered in the assessment of family demands and pileup in an illness crisis situation. Because successful coping is often the direct result of trial-and-error efforts and the result of individual family members' coping skills and abilities, as well as the family coping as a unit, the health-care professional should not be surprised to discover families struggling with what they perceive to be a good coping effort or strategy, only to discover that the short-run benefits may lead to long-term difficulties. The health care professional assists families in deciphering and determining for themselves the difficulties and hardships they face as a direct result of the illness situation and whether they confront challenges in a manner that fosters positive long-term outcomes.

Intrafamily and social ambiguity. The sixth category of stresses and strains leading to pileup is intrafamily and social ambiguity. Every illness-induced crisis situation has a certain amount of ambiguity and uncertainty. Any change in demand for family adaptation, as in the case of the long-term care of a terminally or chronically ill member, has an element of uncertainty because the family needs to alter its structure, rules, roles, and responsibilities. It is suggested that boundary ambiguity (Boss, 1977, 1980) within the family system is a major stressor because a family system needs to be sure of its components, that is, who is inside of the family boundaries, physically and psychologically, and who is outside. Is a family member who is ill treated as a contributing member to the family or is that member isolated and perceived as being only physically present? This intrafamily ambiguity may create additional pressures.

Given the expectation that society will offer families guidelines for coping with illness, it is probable that families will face the additional strain of social ambiguity in those situations where needed social prescriptions for illness-crisis resolution and family adaptation are unclear or absent (H.I. McCubbin & Patterson, 1983a). For example, how families behave toward a member who has survived a major heart attack and bypass surgery is not well prescribed. While the medical regimen will call for a change in diet, exercise, and a carefully monitored home regimen, society, with its emphasis on high productivity, fast pace, and demand for commitment to the company goals rather than to health promotion, may not encourage the long-term self-care that is in the employee's best interest. Given our economy, in which dual wage earners have become the norm, the availability of a spouse for administering ongoing care may be a luxury. For families with two wage earners, it is more efficient to consume high-caloric and fatty meals. Thus the patterns of functioning may not support the home regimen for the patient recovering from a heart attack. The prescriptions for coping may not be clear.

In the absence of guidelines family adaptation is often a trial-and-error process, with potentially deleterious side effects and additional demands on the family system. If the culture or community can provide the family with adequate solutions, the family's ability to manage the accumulation of demands will also be enhanced; if the community is lacking or insufficient in its guidelines or supports, the family is likely to face additional struggles in its efforts to adapt to an illness-induced crisis.

Family Types and Newly Instituted Patterns of Functioning (R)

The Resiliency Model of Family Stress, Adjustment, and Adaptation has been shaped by David Olson and colleagues at the University of Minnesota (Olson, 1986; Lavee, 1985; M.A. McCubbin, 1990) and by their efforts to introduce and document the importance of family types developed on the basis of family strengths that explain, and predict, family adaptation. By taking two family strength dimensions — cohesion and adaptability — these scholars have emphasized the importance of the Circumplex Model, comprising 16 family types (see Fig. 5-2).

Our efforts have underscored the importance of various family types, in addition to the Circumplex Model, which may help us understand which instituted and established patterns of family functioning emerge to be of greatest importance under different circumstances. In our research on both normative families and families faced with an illness-induced crises (H.I. McCubbin et al., 1988; H.I. McCubbin & Thompson, 1989; M.A. McCubbin, 1989; McCubbin & McCubbin, 1989), several family types or instituted patterns were introduced for consideration, each emphasizing different aspects of family functioning. We introduced the regenerative family type, which involves family coherence (appraisal) and family hardiness (internal strengths and locus of control) as an important set of patterns that instill a sense of integrity and strength in family units faced with an illness (see Fig. 5-3). Additionally, we underscored the importance of a rhythmic pattern of family functioning and introduced the rhythmic family type, which focuses on family time and routines as the family's way of maintaining family life in relatively predictable patterns of family living in an effort to cope with life changes (see Fig. 5-3). Finally, the resilient family typology highlights patterns of family flexibility (the degree to which the family is able to change roles, rules, and boundaries) and family bonding (the degree of emotional bonding to form a meaningful and integral family). Family bonding and flexibility are significant patterns for managing and adapting to illness stressors (see Fig. 5-3). In the context of families under stress, these instituted patterns provide a process by which family unity and durability are maximized.

These three family typologies gain added importance in our approach as health practitioners to assessing and diagnosing family functioning in what might become viable targets for intervention (McCubbin & McCubbin, 1989). These typologies represent an attempt to classify families into unique groups that we assume characterize how families function and suggest processes operative within the family system. The current literature on family strengths (Curran, 1983; H.I. McCubbin, Patterson, & Lavee, 1983; Olson, H.I. McCubbin, Barnes, Larson, Muxum, & Wilson, 1983; Stinnet & DeFrain, 1985) points to the importance of family attributes and patterns

Clinical Application Guideline:
Family Types, Established Patterns, and Adaptation

Family Knowledge Base

The greater the breadth, depth, and efficacy of the family's established patterns of functioning that can also manage the illness and its hardships, the greater the ease with which families are able to adapt to the crisis situation.

Clinical Plan

Assess the family's established patterns of functioning and types.

Clinical Assessment Tools

Clinical interview complemented by the use of the Family Hardiness Index (H.I. McCubbin, M.A. McCubbin, & Thompson, 1986a); Family Adaptability and Cohesion Evaluation Scales (Olson, Portner, & Lavee, 1985); Family Time and Routines Scale (H.I. McCubbin, M.A. McCubbin, & Thompson, 1986b).

---

that emphasize family integrity, unity, flexibility, and predictability. See the box above for a clinical guideline related to family types, established patterns, and adaptation.

The importance of newly instituted patterns in adaptation. Families have a wide range of established patterns of functioning that give meaning and stability to the family's way of life. A family's established patterns may not be adequate to manage illness in the family system, and so newly instituted patterns are called for to keep the family functioning with a sense of unity and stability while managing the illness and related hardships.

Although we have chosen to focus on critical family strengths and the patterns families adopt to develop and maintain these enduring qualities, we are also interested in what newly instituted patterns of functioning families create and maintain to achieve adaptation.

The Smith family, for example, made the following five major changes in the family pattern of functioning:

1. Established an "at home" regimen for Jamie's care that caused a major change in family routines and the home environment

2. Established a pattern of shared work rules and responsibilities to distribute the burden of tasks needed to keep the home in order and functioning smoothly; all family members, particularly Mr. Smith, had more home responsibilities
3. Established a dual–wage earner family routine, with Mrs. Smith reentering the workforce; this change created a major shift in family routines and in the emotional climate in the home (mother's fatigue, shared family responsibilities, reduction in intimacy, reduced tolerance for small problems, and children feeling less cared for)
4. Established a closer relationship with the health-care professionals involved in Jamie's care
5. Established a pattern of being more isolated from the community and friends until the family feels more in control and fully understanding of the situation.

It is important that health-care professionals assess new family patterns and use this knowledge to determine strategies for intervention. In addition to assessing instituted patterns, which promote resiliency in families, it is equally important to focus on those instituted patterns of functioning that are tailored to address the illness situation and related hardships. By assessing these new or modified patterns of family functioning, we can begin to understand what these families identify as important to them, the strengths and resources they value. This type of assessment begins to shed light on what meaning the family attaches to itself, the illness, and its future.

Harmony in the marriage of old, established family patterns and newly instituted patterns is not achieved over night. Families struggle to make these changes fit into the family's well-developed schema for family functioning that has evolved over time. As will be discussed more fully under the concept of family appraisal, the family's schema plays a key role in determining the legitimacy, value, and longevity of the family's newly instituted patterns of functioning. These patterns are matched against the family's values, priorities, expectations, goals, and rules. Family adaptation calls for changes in the family system in an effort to address the illness and its hardships while creating a family environment that promotes the development of its members and creates a climate of predictability and stability. How effective these new patterns of family functioning are is determined by the degree to which they are congruent with the family's values, priorities, expectations, goals, and rules—the family's schema. See the box on p. 45 for a clinical guideline related to family schema, congruency, and adaptation.

Clinical Application Guideline: Family Schema, Congruency, and Adaptation

---

Family Knowledge Base

Changes in the family's patterns of functioning made to address the demands created by an illness do not guarantee a satisfactory level of adaptation. The level of family adaptation is determined, in part, by the degree of congruency between the family's schema (its values, priorities, expectations, goals, and rules that have evolved over time) and the family's newly instituted patterns of functioning.

The greater the degree to which the family's newly instituted patterns of functioning address the hardships created by the illness and are congruent with the family's schema, or blueprint, for functioning, the greater the ease and the more positive the level of family adaptation.

Clinical Plan

To conduct a review and assessment of changes in the family patterns of functioning intended to reduce tensions and better manage the hardships of the illness. Review and assess the effect of these changes and the degree to which these changes are congruent with the family's shared values, priorities, expectations, goals, and rules.

Clinical Assessment Tools

Clinical interview tailored to address the family's values, priorities, expectations, goals, and rules and the changes in patterns of the family functioning.

Family Resources (BB) — Strengths and Capabilities

In the Resiliency Model of Family Stress, Adjustment, and Adaptation, *capability* is defined as a potential the family has for meeting all of the demands it faces. We emphasize two sets of capabilities: (1) resources and strengths, which are what the family has and (2) coping behaviors and strategies, which are what the family does as individual members and as a family unit. Just as there are three sources of demands (individual members, the family unit, and society), there are three potential sources of resources: individual family members, the family working as a unit, and the community, which includes the medical community. An adaptive resource is a characteristic, trait, or competency of one of these systems (individual, family, community) that facilitates adaptation. Resources may be tangible, such as money, or intangible, such as self-esteem. A listing of potential resources is nearly infinite. Those resources that have emerged in the family stress literature as being crucial for meeting demands during illness in the family are discussed below.

Personal resources. Six kinds of personal resources that may be used by the family in adaptation are:

1. The innate intelligence of family members, which can enhance awareness and comprehension of demands and facilitate the family's mastery of these
2. Knowledge and skills acquired from education, training, and experience so that individual family members and the family unit can perform tasks with greater efficiency and ease
3. Personality traits (for example, a sense of humor) that facilitate coping
4. Physical and emotional health so that intact faculties and personal energy may be available for meeting family demands
5. A sense of mastery, which is the belief that one has some control over the circumstances of one's life
6. Self-esteem, that is, a positive judgment about one's self-worth.

These latter two personal resources, a sense of mastery and self-esteem, have been emphasized by many researchers of family stress as important factors in the stress process because their presence is critical for effective efforts at managing demands. Yet these are the resources most threatened when the pileup of demands, which implies a failure at mastery, becomes too large. One of the important pathways that may link stresses and strains to negative family outcomes, such as the psychologic depression of its members or intrafamilial conflict, is the weakening of self-esteem (Pearlin, Menaghan, Lieberman, & Mullen, 1981). Time is an important resource that should not be overlooked. It is unique among family members because all individuals and families have an equal amount of it. However, the allocation and use of time are important in the management of family demands.

Family system resources. Family resources for family adjustment and adaptation have been intensely studied in the past decade. Social and behavioral scientists and lay people yearn to identify the traits of "healthy, normal, invulnerable, resilient, well-functioning" families.

Two of the most prominent family resources identified by several investigators (see review by Olson, Sprenkle, & Russell, 1979) are cohesion (the bonds of unity running through the family life) and adaptability (the family's capacity to meet obstacles and shift course). Other aspects of cohesion that have been emphasized include trust, appreciation, support, integration, and respect for individuality (Stinnet & Sauer, 1977).

Family organization is another resource that has received attention (Hill, 1958; Moos, 1974). Family organization includes agreement, clarity, and consistency (not to preclude fluidity) in the family role and rule structure. Shared parental leadership and clear family generational boundaries are additional resources related to organization (Lewis & Looney, 1984). Communication skill is a critical resource. Different aspects of communication ability such as clear and direct messages (Satir, 1972), instrumental and affective communication capability (Epstein, Bishop, & Baldwin, 1982), and verbal-nonverbal consistency (Fleck, 1980) have been emphasized. Family problem-solving is also significant. Some families adopt a problem-solving style that underscores affirmation of family members' worth and self-esteem, whereas other families adopt an incendiary style that exacerbates family tensions (M.A. McCubbin, H.I. McCubbin, & Thompson, 1987).

Family hardiness also emerges as an adaptation resource. Family hardiness specifically refers to the internal strengths and durability of the family unit. It is characterized by sense of control over the outcome of life events and hardships, a view of change as beneficial and growth producing, and an active orientation in responding to stressful situations (M.A. McCubbin, 1989). A buffer, a mediating factor in mitigating the effects of stresses and demands, family hardiness helps a family adjust and adapt over time.

Family time together and family routines in daily living are relatively reliable indicators of family integration and stability. When faced with a medical crisis, families that make an effort to maintain family routines to create some degree of family continuity and stability have a higher probability of enduring (H.I. McCubbin, Thompson, Pirner, & M.A. McCubbin, 1988). See the box on p. 48 for a clinical guideline related to family resources and adaptation.

Social Support (BBB)

Community resources and supports include all persons and institutions that the family may use to cope with a stressor situation. Resources and supports include friends and a range of services, such as medical or

Clinical Application Guideline: Family Resources and Adaptation

Family Knowledge Base

The greater the breadth, depth, and efficacy of the available personal and family resources, the greater the ease with which the family is able to adapt to the illness situation.

Clinical Plan

To conduct a systematic assessment of the family's strengths and capabilities.

Clinical Assessment Tools

Clinical interview complemented by the use of the Family Inventory of Resources for Management (FIRM) (H.I. McCubbin, Comeau, & Harkins, 1981).

community services. Schools, churches, and employers are also resources for the family. At the broad social level, government policies that support families may also be viewed as community resources.

In the study of family adaptation, social support is the one community resource that has received the most attention in literature on stress. It is most often viewed as one of the primary buffers or mediators between stress and health breakdown (see reviews by Cassel, 1976; Cobb, 1976; Pilisuk & Parks, 1983).

What is social support? There have been many conceptualizations of social support (see Caplan, 1974; Cassel, 1976; Granovetter, 1973; House, 1981; Pinneau, 1975), but we believe Cobb's (1976) definition is the most useful in the context of the Resiliency Model for the family faced with an illness. Cobb (1976) defines social support as information exchanged at the interpersonal level that provides: (1) emotional support, leading the individual family members in the family unit to believe that they are cared for and loved; (2) esteem support, leading family members to believe that they are respected and valued; and (3) network support, leading the family members to believe that they belong to a network of communication involving mutual support and mutual understanding.

Clinical Application Guideline:
Family Social Support and Adaptation

Family Knowledge Base

The greater the breadth, depth, and efficacy of the family's support network and quality of affirming social support, the greater the ease with which the family is able to adapt to the illness situation.

Clinical Plan

To conduct a systematic assessment of the family's support network and quality of social support.

Clinical Assessment Tools

Clinical interview complemented by the use of the Social Support Inventory (H.I. McCubbin, Patterson, Rossman, & Cooke, 1982) and the Social Support Index (H.I. McCubbin, Patterson, & Glynn, 1982).

Drawing from the stress literature, we have added to Cobb's three forms of support to include: (4) appraisal support, which is information in the form of feedback allowing family members to assess how well they are doing with life tasks in the medical crisis; (5) altruistic support, which is information received in the form of goodwill from others for having given something of oneself.

In the health-care literature and publications on clinical intervention with illness-related family crises, a distinction is made between social support and the concept of social network. The latter focuses on all the people who the individual or the family unit has contact with and from whom they potentially may get support but who may, in fact, be more a source of demand than a source of support. Social support implies more than superficial contact with people; it involves a qualitative exchange of communication in an atmosphere of mutual trust. See the box above for a clinical guideline related to family social support and adaptation.

Family Appraisal — Situational (CC)

In the adjustment phase described earlier, the single C component was limited by Hill to the family's definition of the stressor. In introducing and refining the Resiliency Model of Family Stress, Adjustment, and Adaptation, we have come to realize that family appraisal includes two additional levels that come into play in managing a family crisis situation and shaping the course of family adaptation. At the second level, we refer to the family's situational appraisal (the CC component) of the family's capability: the critical relationship between the demands on the family (created by the illness and its hardships) and the family's capabilities and strengths to manage these demands. The family's situational appraisal (CC) would reveal the adequacy or inadequacy of the family unit to manage the situation and serve as the basis for additional coping or changes in the family patterns of functioning.

When demands are experienced, families are constantly in the process of evaluating and interpreting their experience in an effort to break the problem situation into specific manageable tasks and choosing the strategies that they may use to cope with or manage the situation. The assessments families make include many components of the stressor, such as the intensity, the degree of controllability of the situation, the amount of change expected of the family system, and whether or not the family is capable of responding to the situation. In some instances the illness exists only by virtue of their perception, as in the case of families struggling with whether the diagnosed tumor is malignant or benign. In the absence of confirmatory medical information, should the family decide to act on the basis of the information they may have, the crisis situation would be viewed as purely one of their appraisal or judgment. The resources and the coping options are also appraised by the family in relationship to illness and its hardships. When the family appraises its overall capability and skills as being inadequate or insufficient relative to the illness-induced crisis and all the hardships, there emerges an imbalance in the family system that contributes to, or becomes the cause of, family tensions and stress. In some situations the lack of a clear definition on how to manage or cope with the illness creates ambiguity and, thus, greater tensions. Although there is an amount of uncertainty and ambiguity inherent in all illness-induced family crises and the management of stress involves a reduction of this ambiguity, it is understandable why the family's appraisal, at a situational level, becomes so crucial in shaping the family's response. It is through the process of situational appraisal, involving the evaluation of the illness, an assessment of the family capabilities and strengths, and the evaluation of alternative courses of action and coping strategies, that the family

Clinical Application Guideline:
Family Situational Appraisal of Family Capability and Adaptation

Family Knowledge Base

The more constructive and positive the family's appraisal of an illness and the capabilities and strengths families have to manage the demands, the greater the ease with which families are able to develop effective problem solving and coping, make effective use of resources, and ultimately adapt to the situation.

Clinical Plan

To encourage families to share their appraisal of an illness and its hardships. Focus on both agreed upon appraisals and divergent appraisals among family members.

Clinical Assessment Tool

The clinical interview focusing on the family's shared or divergent definition of the illness and the family situation.

ultimately comes together as a unit to cope with the illness. See the box above for a clinical guideline related to the family's situational appraisal.

Family Appraisal—Schema and Meaning (CCC)

The third level of appraisal is family schema and meaning. In the face of an illness-induced family crisis demanding changes in rules and organization and patterns of functioning, the family is called on to appraise its past and its future in an effort to give meaning to the illness and to the resulting changes in the family system. This meaning can facilitate adaptation. Over time, families develop, shape, and attach value to a set of shared or accepted values, rules, goals, priorities, and expectations, which compose the individual family's schema. This worldview level of family appraisal has been influenced by the seminal work of Reiss and colleagues (Reiss, 1981; Reiss & Olivari, 1980), who have emphasized the importance of family paradigms in the stress process. Other theorists concerned primarily about individual responses to stress and who have emphasized the central importance of global orientations as in the concept of coherence (Antonovsky, 1979) have also influenced this concept.

✦ ✦ ✦ ✦ ✦

After a year and a half, the Smith family had settled into new roles and patterns of functioning. Tensions surfaced with intensity when it became a shared viewpoint that this situation, particularly Mrs. Smith's working, was not likely to change. Up to this point, Jamie's older siblings had endured the changes by believing that things would return to what they had been before. For them, the old family routines, which gave them more individual attention and nurturance, were better.

The Smiths struggled to give meaning, and thus legitimacy, to the new family patterns. They hoped that the children would come to accept the situation as it was without conflict or resentment. They emphasized the need to accept Jamie's condition as a fact of life. It was "God's will," they would say to bring a sense of order or congruity to the situation.

This was not sufficient to justify the changes in family roles, goals, priorities, and expectations. Over time Mr. and Mrs. Smith introduced new meaning to the changes the family struggled with. They pointed to the family's need to build a stronger and a more secure financial base to prepare for Alice's and Jonathan's college education. Jamie's diagnosis helped the family to get an earlier start, the parents argued. Mother's working was inevitable and done for the well-being of all members. "We must be grateful for what good fortune we have," the parents emphasized. The parents also pointed to the valuable lessons they had learned as a family: the illness had brought them closer together and had "taught the old dog (dad) new tricks." These new meanings, which did more than explain Jamie's illness, brought legitimacy and value to the family changes and seemed to give the children a sense of purpose and meaning beyond the need to care for Jamie or to accept mother's employment. With this, the overall changes in the family unit gained both meaning and acceptance and seemed to be the basis of the family's emerging sense of calm and commitment. Over time, the family seemed to gain a greater sense of congruity and coherence.

Families who reveal a strong schema emphasize their investment in their family unit, their shared values and goals, and their investment in the family's collective "we" rather than "I." They share a sense of orientation that guides their appraisal of a stressor, their appraisal of a situation, as well as their established patterns of family functioning. These investments are guided by a relativistic view of life circumstances and a willingness to accept less-than-perfect solutions to all their demands (McCubbin & McCubbin, 1989; H.I. McCubbin, M.A. McCubbin & Thompson, 1991). The family schema, unlike other components of the Resiliency Model, is relatively stable because it is used as a major reference against which situational and stressor level appraisals are contrasted and shaped. In turn, the family schema may also be shaped, molded, and remolded over time in response to crisis situations and experiences in which the family's established patterns of behavior are challenged and new patterns are called for. The family schema is more stable and enduring than situational appraisals because it captures the family's values and internal sense of identity and goals.

The importance of family meanings. Because family adaptation is likely to call for possible changes in the family schema—particularly the family's values, goals, rules, priorities, and expectations—as well as changes in the family's patterns of functioning to achieve the optimum fit, the third level of appraisal takes on critical, and some would argue central, importance. In contrast to the stressor level of appraisal (C, level 1) and the situational appraisal (CC, level 2), the family's schema appraisal (CCC, level 3) surfaces in the family context to give *meaning* to the illness and the family's changes. This third level of appraisal serves to foster a congruency between changes in the family's schema and the family's instituted patterns of family functioning. Developing a shared sense of family meaning to changes created by a family crisis is a difficult and a demanding (of the family) process, and the family's shared sense of congruency is achieved only through perseverance, patience, negotiation, understanding, and shared commitment to the family.

The Smith family made a concerted effort to give meaning to the changes in the family unit. The family's schema that included mother's role as the caretaker was challenged by her return to the work force. The resulting incongruency was difficult to resolve. The parents' effort to give meaning to these changes in schema and patterns of functioning proved to be successful. Reframing the changes as "inevitable and helpful" to the family's commitment to the other children's future, and to the benefit of all, put the family's adaptation in a more positive, meaningful, and acceptable light. What meanings families give to the newly reshaped family unit are important to health-care professionals seeking to foster family adaptation. By reinforcing meanings that give the family a positive outlook, health professionals provide the incentive and framework for successful adaptation. See the box below for a clinical guideline related to family changes, schema, meaning, and adaptation.

Clinical Application Guideline: Family Changes, Schema, Meaning, and Adaptation

Family Knowledge Base

The family's appraisal of changes in the family's patterns of functioning and their congruency with the family's schema (values, goals, rules, priorities, and expectations) plays a critical role in shaping the course and outcome of family adaptation.

In the case of great incongruency between the family's schema and newly instituted patterns of functioning, family appraisal may serve to foster additional changes in both the schema and patterns of functioning. In the case of incongruency, complemented by the appraisal that these changes are the most appropriate and additions or changes are not called for, family appraisal at the third level serves a vital role in giving meaning to these changes, thus over time, rendering legitimacy and support to the family's new level of functioning.

When there is great congruency between the family's schema and the family's new patterns of functioning, supported by the family's shared meaning attached to these changes, there will be greater ease and potential for a positive level of family adaptation.

Clinical Plan

To assess the instituted changes in family functioning, the degree of fit or congruency between these changes and the family's schema. Assess the family's satisfaction with these changes.

Clinical Assessment Tools

Clinical interview tailored to shed light on the family's schema and its congruency with the changes in the family's new patterns of functioning. Seek understanding and efficacy of the family's effort to develop a shared meaning and understanding of the family situation with its changes.

Problem Solving and Coping (PSC)

The process of acquiring, allocating, and using resources for meeting illness-induced demands is a critical aspect of family stress, adjustment, and adaptation. Researchers, family practitioners, and health care professionals who use a resource-management framework to view both human and material resources also understand and recognize that resources are limited. Therefore resources must be allocated to manage multiple goals and demands (Deacon & Firebaugh, 1975; Paolucci, Hall, & Axinn, 1977). The Resiliency Model of Family Stress, Adjustment, and Adaptation characterizes the family system as a resource-exchange network in which problem solving and coping occur. In this model problem solving and coping are the actions for this exchange.

In the context of the Resiliency Model, we define a coping behavior as a specific effort (covert or overt) by which an individual family member or the family functioning as a whole attempts to reduce or manage a demand on the family system and bring resources to bear to manage the situation. Specific coping behaviors may be grouped into patterns, such as coping directed at "maintaining family integration and cooperation," which is one of the coping patterns that has emerged as important for families who have a chronically ill child (M.A. McCubbin, 1984). Coping patterns, on the other hand, are more generalized ways of responding that transcend different kinds of stressful situations. When coping is viewed in the context of multiple demands, it seems more useful and relevant to view coping as a generalized, rather than a specific, response.

Although coping most often has been conceptualized at the individual level, we also consider family-level coping, for obvious reasons. Family coping may be viewed as coordinated problem-solving behavior of the whole system (Klein & Hill, 1979), but it could also involve complementary efforts of individual family members, which fit together in a synergistic whole. This creates a balance between demands and resources and at the same time eliminates stressors and hardships. In our view the function of coping is to maintain and restore the balance between demands and resources and at the same time remove or lessen the intensity of the illness and its accompanying hardships. In our work with families faced with an illness-induced crisis, we have identified four broad headings that characterize the ways in which coping facilitates adaptation to an illness.

1. Coping may involve direct action to eliminate or reduce the number and intensity of demands created by the illness. For example, a family could decide to place its terminally ill grandmother in a nursing home rather than keep her at home with them. The pressures of home care may often disrupt the family. The placement of the grandmother in a nursing home may reduce the tensions in the illness situation.

2. Coping may involve direct action to acquire additional resources not already available to the family. Finding medical services for a member with a chronic illness or developing self-reliance skills when a spouse dies suddenly are examples of coping to increase resources.

3. Coping may involve managing the tension associated with ongoing strains. This is necessary because of the inevitable residual of family strains resulting from an illness. Physical exercise is a commonly recognized coping mechanism. Taking time out as a family for talking and enjoying each other's company, using humor appropriately, and openly expressing emotion and affect in a responsible, nonblaming manner are other ways for families to reduce tension and to place the medical crisis into a more constructive and manageable form.

4. Coping may involve family-level appraisal to create, shape, and evaluate meanings related to a situation to make it more constructive, manageable, and acceptable. This strategy for coping interacts directly with what is labeled as family schema appraisal in the Resiliency Model. It may be directed at changing individual family members or the total family schema of the situation, such as reducing role strain by lowering home expectations of a family member who spends a majority of time at the hospital. Reframing the home environment or sections of it as a "hospital setting" helps the family to label the situation in a manner that has more meaning and thus is more acceptable. Maintaining an optimistic outlook and acceptance of the situation and fostering the belief that this is the best the family can do under the circumstances are also important appraisal-oriented coping strategies.

In summary, coping and problem solving may be directed at the reduction or elimination of stresses and hardships, the acquisition of additional resources, the ongoing management of family system tension, and shaping the appraisal at both the situational and the schema level. These coping strategies are vitally important and often operate simultaneously in an illness-induced family crisis. See the box on p. 57 for a clinical guideline related to family coping and problem solving.

Clinical Application Guideline:
Family Problem Solving and Coping Repertoire and Adaptation

Family Knowledge Base

The greater the family's repertoire of coping strategies, complemented by a problem-solving strategy and communication style for managing family tension, the greater the ease with which the family is able to make a satisfactory adaptation.

Clinical Plan

To conduct a systematic assessment of family problem-solving communication and coping.

Clinical Assessment Tools

Clinical interview complemented by the use of the Family Problem-Solving Communication Index (M.A. McCubbin, H.I. McCubbin, & Thompson, 1987); Coping Health Inventory for Parents (CHIP) (H.I. McCubbin, M.A. McCubbin, & Cauble, 1979) and the Family Crisis–Oriented Coping Evaluation Scales (H.I. McCubbin, Larsen, & Olson, 1983).

The Family Adaptation Process—Bonadaptation, Maladaptation, and Crisis (XX)

Family adaptation is a process in which families engage in direct response to the excessive demands of a stressor and depleted resources and realize that systemic changes are needed to restore functional stability and improve family satisfaction. At one level, adaptation involves the process of restructuring and making changes in rules, boundaries, and patterns of functioning. Once changes are instituted as new family patterns, the family efforts at adaptation are complemented by the family's efforts at the appraisal (schema) level. Family efforts at the appraisal level bring family members to value, accept, and affirm changes over time facilitating bonadaptation (H.I. McCubbin & Patterson, 1983b; McCubbin & McCubbin, 1989). On the other hand, families may not achieve a satisfactory level of adaptation (maladaptation). Consequently, they return to a crisis situation (XX) and then must find a new way to adapt.

Coping strategies play a critical role in adaptation. They facilitate synergizing, interfacing, and compromising—vital components of the family's efforts at adaptation (H.I. McCubbin & Patterson, 1983b). *Synergizing* refers to the family's ability to work together as a unit to achieve a life-style and orientation not normally attained by the efforts of only one member but which is achieved by the family's interdependence and mutuality. The synergism is important after the family has instituted a few structural or pattern changes in order that the family may again work as a unit, with mutual support and shared values, goals, rules, priorities, and expectations. As families work to synchronize their appraisals, needs, and resources, they become attuned to one another. The unit becomes more harmonious in its functioning.

The concept of family adaptation is not strictly confined to internal changes. Because the family has transactions daily with other social institutions (the workplace, school, and so on) and the community as a whole, the *interfacing* with the community to achieve a "better fit" is also part of the family's adaptive process.

In our view it is not sufficient for families to restructure and synergize internally; they must also maintain a level of rapport and interaction with the community at large. The family's internal restructuring may also necessitate a new set of rules and transactions for maintaining the complementary relationship between the family and the community. For example, in coping with the long-term care of a child with cystic fibrosis, expenses may prompt the family to seek income through the entry or reentry of a member into the work force. The work environment and all its demands will create additional burdens on the newly employed or dual-employed member, forcing the family to adapt to the added responsibilities. Some employers may be flexible to allow a parent/employee to respond to the illness and the demands of follow-up care. The family may need to chip in and share the home duties and home-care medical regimen to allow the mother or father to cope with work demands and not be stretched too thin.

Even with synergism and interfacing, however, successful adaptation also requires *compromising* because a family cannot always attain perfect functioning either among themselves or with the community at large. The difficult and evercompeting demands require realistic appraisals and a willingness to accept less than perfect resolutions of the various demands. Health professionals must be aware of the competing demands and guide the family toward compromise so that successful adaptation can continue. See the box on p. 59 for a clinical guideline related to family bonadaptation.

Clinical Application Guideline:
Family Adaptation to Illness

Family Knowledge Base

Successful family adaptation is achieved when the family's schema and patterns of functioning are congruent, family members' personal growth and development are supported, the family's integrity maintained, the family's relationship with the community is mutually supportive, and the family develops a shared sense of coherence. The family must use the coping strategies of synergism, interfacing, and compromise.

Clinical Plan

To assess the degree to which the family unit has adapted to the crisis situation.

Clinical Assessment Tools

A clinical interview focusing on the family's instituted patterns of functioning and their congruency with the family's schema, the level of satisfaction with these changes, and the well-being of family members. An assessment of the family's shared sense of coherence is essential. The interview may be complemented by the use of the Family's Sense of Coherence Index (FSOC) (Antonovsky & Sourani, 1988) and the Family Index of Resiliency and Adaptation (FIRA-G) (H.I. McCubbin & Thompson, 1991).

✦ CONCLUSION

Families negotiate change and stressful life events with an innate reaction to fight, to remain stable, and to resist changes in the family's established patterns of behavior. Family adjustment, characterized by relatively minor changes in the family system, is a predictable phase in the family's response to a stressor such as an illness. Many illness stressors may also require family adaptation, even drastic change in the family system. In these situations families are called on to expand and to contract, to incorporate and to release, and to achieve stability by disrupting existing patterns of functioning. In these struggles and particularly in the face of an illness-induced family crisis, families adapt by instituting changes in the family's patterns of functioning, changing its scheme, or blueprint, for functioning, and by changes in the family's relationship to the outside world.

Family stress theory, in particular the Resiliency Model of Family Stress, Adjustment, and Adaptation, attempts to explain this dynamic process by isolating those individual, family, and community properties and processes that interact and shape the course of family behavior over time and in response to a wide range of stressful situations. The Resiliency Model encourages health-care professionals to recognize family resiliency and the natural healing qualities of family life, which, if understood, could become targets for intervention.

Such interventions would be different from the penetrating roles of the family therapist, at least at the beginning. In illness situations the emphasis is placed on family problem-solving strategies, to release the blocks to the family's own natural healing abilities, and enhancement strategies, to promote the natural process of family regenerativity and resiliency. By focusing on the current issues affecting family life—the stresses and hardships, the pileup of demands, and the normative transitions, as well as the side effects of family efforts of coping, the family's own resources and capabilities, and social support—the health-care practitioner is in a better position to manage the family as a whole to facilitate adaptation.

REFERENCES

Antonovsky, A. (1979). *Health, stress, and coping.* San Francisco: Jossey-Bass.

Antonovsky, A. (1987). *Unraveling the mystery of health.* San Francisco: Jossey-Bass.

Antonovsky, A., & Sourani, T. (1988). Family sense of coherence and family adaptation. *Journal of Marriage and the Family, 50,* 79-92.

Boss, P. (1977). A clarification of the concept of psychological father presence in families experiencing ambiguity of boundary. *Journal of Marriage and the Family, 39,* 141-151.

Boss, P. (1980). Normative family stress: Family boundary changes across the lifespan. *Family Relations, 29,* 445-450.

Burr, W.F. (1973). *Theory construction and the sociology of the family.* New York: John Wiley & Sons.

Caplan, G. (1974). *Support systems and community mental health.* New York: Behavioral Publications.

Cassel, J. (1976). The contribution of the social environment to host resistance. *American Journal of Epidemiology, 104,* 107-123.

Cobb, S. (1976). Social support as a moderator of life stress. *Psychosomatic Medicine, 38,* 300-314.

Curran, D. (1983). *Traits of a healthy family.* Minneapolis: Winston.

Deacon, R., & Firebaugh, F. (1975). *Home management: context and concepts*. Boston: Houghton Mifflin.

Epstein, N., Bishop, D., & Baldwin, L. (1982). McMaster model of family functioning: A view of the normal family. In F. Walsh (Ed.), *Normal family processes* (pp. 115-141). New York: Guilford.

Fleck, S. (1980). Family functioning and family pathology. *Psychiatric Annals, 10*, 46-57.

Granovetter, M. (1973). The strength of weak ties. *American Journal of Sociology, 78*, 1360-1380.

Hansen, D., & Johnson, V. (1979). Rethinking family stress theory: Definitional aspects. In W. Burr, R. Hill, F.I. Nye, & I. Reiss (Eds.), *Contemporary theories about the family*, (Vol. 1, pp 582-603). New York: The Free Press.

Hill, R. (1949). *Families under stress*. New York: Harper & Row.

Hill, R. (1958). Generic features of families under stress. *Social Casework, 49*, 139-150.

House, J. (1981). *Work stress and social support*. Reading, MA: Addison-Wesley.

Klein, D., & Hill, R. (1979). Determinants of family problem-solving effectiveness. In W. Burr, R. Hill, I. Reiss, & I. Nye (Eds.), *Contemporary theories about the family* (Vol. 1, pp. 493-548). New York: The Free Press.

Lavee, Y. (1985). *Family types and family adaptation to stress: Integrating the circumplex model of family systems and the family adjustment and adaptation response model*. Unpublished doctoral dissertation, University of Minnesota–St. Paul.

Lewis, J., & Looney, J. (1984). *The long struggle: Well-functioning working-class black families*. New York: Brunner/Mazel.

McCubbin, H.I., Boss, P., Wilson, L., & Lester, G. (1980). Developing family vulnerability to stress: coping patterns and strategies wives employ. In J. Trost (Ed.), *The family and change* (pp. 89-103). Sweden: International Library Publishing.

McCubbin, H.I., Comeau, J., & Harkins, J. (1981). Family Inventory of Resources for Management (FIRM). In H. McCubbin & A. Thompson (Eds.) (1987), *Family assessment inventories for research and practice* (pp. 143-160). Madison, WI: University of Wisconsin–Madison.

McCubbin, H.I., Larson, A., & Olson, D. (1983). F-COPES: Family Crisis–Oriented Personal Scales. In H. McCubbin & A. Thompson (Eds.) (1987), *Family assessment inventories for research and practice* (pp. 193-207). Madison, WI: University of Wisconsin–Madison.

McCubbin, H., McCubbin, M., & Cauble, A.E. (1979). Coping Health Inventory for Parents (CHIP). In H. McCubbin & A. Thompson (Eds.) (1987), *Family assessment inventories for research and practice* (pp. 173-192). Madison, WI: University of Wisconsin–Madison.

McCubbin, H.I., McCubbin, M.A., & Thompson, A. (1986a). Family hardiness index. In H. McCubbin & A. Thompson (Eds.) (1987), *Family assessment inventories for research and practice* (pp. 123-130). Madison, WI: University of Wisconsin–Madison.

McCubbin, H.I., McCubbin, M.A., & Thompson, A. (1986b). Family Time and Routines Scale. In H. McCubbin & A. Thompson (Eds.) (1987), *Family assessment inventories for research and practice* (pp. 131-141). Madison, WI:

University of Wisconsin–Madison.

McCubbin, H.I., McCubbin, M.A., & Thompson, A. (1991). Resiliency in families: The role of family schema and appraisal in family adaptation crisis. In T. Brubaker (Ed.) (in press), *Family relationships: Current and future directions*. Beverly Hills, CA: Sage.

McCubbin, H.I., & Patterson, J.M. (1981). *Systematic assessment of family stress, resources, and coping: Tools for research, education, and clinical intervention*. St. Paul, MN: Department of Family Social Science.

McCubbin, H.I., & Patterson, J.M. (1982). Family adaptation to crisis. In H. McCubbin, A. Cauble, & J. Patterson (Eds.), *Family stress, coping, and social support* (pp. 26-47). Springfield, IL: Charles C. Thomas.

McCubbin, H.I., & Patterson, J.M. (1983a). The family stress process: The Double ABCX Model of adjustment and adaptation. In H. McCubbin, M. Sussman, & J. Patterson (Eds.), *Advances and developments in family stress theory and research* (pp. 7-37). New York: Haworth.

McCubbin, H.I., & Patterson, J.M. (1983b). Family transitions: Adaptation to stress. In H.I. McCubbin & C.R. Figley (Eds.), *Stress and the family: Coping with normative transitions* (pp. 5-25). New York: Brunner/Mazel.

McCubbin, H.I., Patterson, J.M., & Glynn, T. (1982). Social Support Index (SSI). In H. McCubbin & A. Thompson (Eds.) (1987), *Family assessment inventories for research and practice* (283-302). Madison, WI: University of Wisconsin–Madison.

McCubbin, H.I., Patterson, J.M., & Lavee, Y. (1983). *One thousand army families: Strengths, coping, and supports*. St. Paul, MN: University of Minnesota–St. Paul, Family Social Science.

McCubbin, H.I., Patterson, J.M., Rossman, M., & Cook, B. (1982). *Social Support Inventory (SSI)*. Madison, WI: University of Wisconsin–Madison.

McCubbin, H.I., Patterson, J.M., & Wilson, L. (1981). Family inventory of life events and changes (FILE). In H.I. McCubbin & A. Thompson (Eds.) (1987), *Family assessment inventories for research and practice* (pp. 79-98). Madison, WI: University of Wisconsin–Madison.

McCubbin, H.I., & Thompson, A. (1991). Family index of resiliency and adaptation (FIRA-G). In H.I. McCubbin & A. Thompson (Eds.), *Family assessment inventories for research and practice* (2nd ed., pp. 294-312). Madison, WI: University of Wisconsin–Madison.

McCubbin, H.I., & Thompson, A. (1989). *Balancing work and family life on Wall Street: Stockbrokers and families coping with economic instability*. Edina, MN: Burgess International Group.

McCubbin, H.I., Thompson, A., Pirner, P., & McCubbin, M.A. (1988). *Family types and strengths: A life cycle and ecological perspective*. Edina, MN: Burgess International Group.

McCubbin, M.A. (1984). Nursing assessment of parental coping with cystic fibrosis. *Western Journal of Nursing Research, 6*, 407-422.

McCubbin, M.A. (1986). *Family stress and family types: Chronic illness in children*. Doctoral dissertation, University of Minnesota–St. Paul.

McCubbin, M.A. (1988). Family stress, resources, and family types: Chronic illness in children. *Family Relations, 37*, 203-210.

McCubbin, M.A. (1989). Family stress

and family strengths: A comparison of single- and two-parent families with handicapped children. *Research in Nursing and Health, 12,* 101-110.

McCubbin, M.A. (1990). The typology model of adjustment and adaptation: A family stress model. *Guidance and Counseling, 5,* 6-22.

McCubbin, M.A., & McCubbin, H.I. (1987). Family stress theory and assessment: The T-Double ABCX Model of family adjustment and adaptation. In H.I. McCubbin & A. Thompson (Eds.), *Family assessment inventories for research and practice* (pp. 3-32). Madison, WI: University of Wisconsin–Madison.

McCubbin, M.A., & McCubbin, H.I. (1989). Theoretical orientations to family stress and coping. In C.R. Figley (Ed.), *Treating stress in families* (pp. 3-43). New York: Brunner/Mazel.

McCubbin, M.A., McCubbin, H.I., & Thompson, A. (1987). Family problem-solving communication index. In H.I. McCubbin & A. Thompson (1989), *Balancing work and family life on Wall Street: Stockbrokers and families coping with economic instability.* Edina, MN: Burgess International Group.

Moos, R. (1974). *Family environment scales.* Palo Alto, CA: Consulting Psychologists.

Olson, D. (1986). Circumplex Model VII: Validation studies and FACES III. *Family Process, 25,* 337-351.

Olson, D., McCubbin, H.I., Barnes, H., Larsen, A., Muxem, A., & Wilson, M. (1983). *Families—what makes them work.* Beverly Hills, CA: Sage.

Olson, D., Portner, J., & Lavee, Y. (1985). *FACES III. Family social science.* University of Minnesota–St. Paul.

Olson, D., Sprenkle, D., & Russell, C. (1979). Circumplex model of marital and family systems: 1. Cohesion and adaptability dimensions, family types, and clinical applications. *Family Process, 18,* 3-28.

Paolucci, B., Hall, O., & Axinn, N. (1977). *Family decision making: An ecosystem approach.* New York: John Wiley & Sons.

Pearlin, L., Menaghan, E., Lieberman, M., & Mullan, J. (1981). The stress process. *Journal of Health and Social Behavior, 22,* 337-356.

Pearlin, L., & Schooler, C. (1978). The structure of coping.*Journal of Health and Social Behavior, 19,* 2-21.

Pilisuk, M., & Parks, S. (1983). Social support and family stress. In H. McCubbin, M. Sussman, J. Patterson (Eds.), *Social stress and the family: Advances and developments in family stress theory and research* (pp. 137-156). New York: Haworth Press.

Pinneau, S. (1975). Effects of social support on psychological and physiological stress. Unpublished doctoral dissertation. Ann Arbor: University of Michigan.

Reiss, D. (1981). *The family's construction of reality.* Cambridge, MA: Harvard University.

Reiss, D., & Oliveri, M.E. (1980). Family paradigm and family coping: A proposal for linking the family's intrinsic adaptive capacities to its responses to stress. *Family Relations, 29,* 431-444.

Satir, V. (1972). *People making.* Palo Alto, CA: Science & Behavior.

Stinnet, N., & DeFrain, J. (1985). *Secrets of strong families.* Boston: Little, Brown.

Stinnet, N., & Sauer, K. (1977). Relationship characteristics of strong families. *Family Perspective, 11*(4), 3-11.

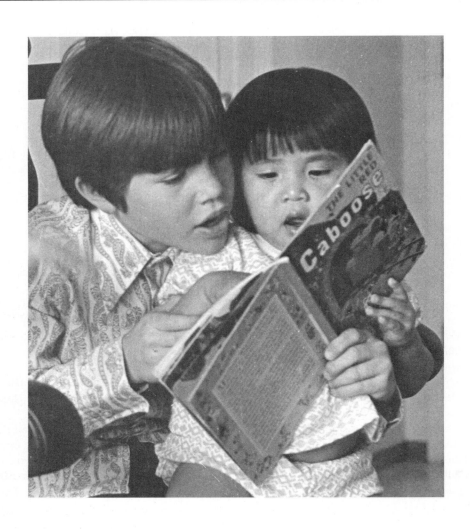

3

Illness and Health Maintenance as Potential Family Stressors

✦

CHAPTER GOALS

✦ To define and illustrate illness and health maintenance as potential family stressors

✦ To describe and illustrate the different phases within the family cycle of health and illness and common family behavior and functioning in each phase

✦ To identify the potential for family crisis within the different stages of illness

OVERVIEW

T HE purpose of this chapter is to discuss the effect of illness and health maintenance routines on the family and the potential each has for becoming a family stressor. The first part of the chapter reviews the terms *stressor*, *family strain*, and *family stress*. Within those definitions, illness and health maintenance are identified as family stressors. The second part of the chapter examines the various phases of the health and illness cycle and offers a graphic representation of that cycle from a family perspective. Each phase of the cycle is described and illustrated with common individual and family system reactions and behaviors particular to that phase. Also identified is the potential for family crisis that can be found in each phase. Within the framework of The Resiliency Model of Family Stress, Adjustment, and Adaptation, this chapter focuses on illness stressor (A) (Fig. 3-1).

✦ ELEMENTS OF THE FAMILY STRESS RESPONSE
The Stressor

The family stress response has three main elements: the event (the stressor/demand), the family's reaction (strain/stress) to the event, and the family's response (outcome, level of adjustment/adaptation) (McCubbin & McCubbin, Chapter 2). The first element, the stressor, is a life event that affects the family unit and either produces, or has the potential to produce, change in the family's social system. Stressors are neither inherently positive or negative but rather are events with inherent demands that challenge the established patterns of the family unit, prompting the need for family adjustment and adaptation. Stressors may have either minor or major consequences depending on the amount of change demanded. Stressors can escalate family stress to crisis proportions, causing family disruption and disorganization, or, on the other hand, the family may be able to resist the stressor and make adjustments with little or no disruption.

Family Strain and Stress

The second element in the family stress response is the family's reaction of strain or stress initiated by the stressor (McCubbin & McCubbin, Chapter 2). Family *strain* exists when a family successfully manages the tension caused by a stressor. The family overcomes or buffers tension by adjusting to the stressor. On the other hand, family *stress* exists when the family cannot manage the tension caused by a stressor. Stress in families arises from an actual or perceived imbalance between a demand (that is, a challenge or threat) and resources capabilities (that is, tangible resources and coping abilities). As a result, the amount of stress at a given time depends on the family's appraisal of the stressor and its demands, the family's present situation, and their capabilities. Both family strain and stress are everyday occurrences with positive and negative effects. Family stress, however, involves a nonspecific demand for change in family function.

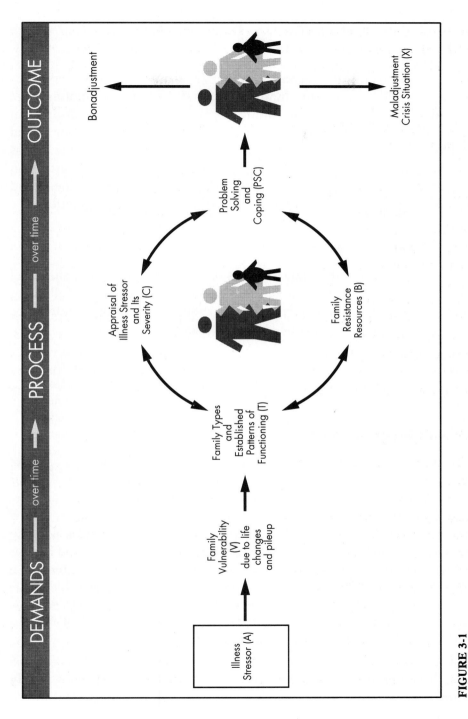

FIGURE 3-1

Adjustment Phase of the Resiliency Model of Family Stress, Adjustment, and Adaptation. This chapter focuses on the illness stressor (A).

✦ HEALTH MAINTENANCE AND ILLNESS AS FAMILY STRESSORS

Illness and health maintenance qualify as family stressors when they produce demands that require family change. If the family cannot manage the strain of the illness stressor, family stress results. Stress resulting from illness and health maintenance events is caused by a perceived or actual imbalance between the family's capabilities and the demands of the illness or health maintenance activity. The imbalance requires family attention and, consequently, family adjustment, adaptation, or both. Illness and health maintenance events can have both positive and negative effects.

Health Maintenance

How can health maintenance events be a stressor? Being healthy and maintaining health are positively linked with a state of well-being (Lancaster, McCance, & Vanderschmidt, 1986). Yet, health maintenance events can be a stressors, as the following anecdote illustrates.

✦ ✦ ✦ ✦ ✦

Joe and Sally are a young married couple with two small children, 5 and 7 years old. Joe exercises very little and has been contemplating the need to exercise more frequently. His family has a history of heart problems, which increases Joe's chance of having similar problems. His doctor advised him to participate in an adequate exercise program to prevent heart problems. One of his friends has been running daily after work and has been encouraging Joe to join him. Joe decides to do so.

Joe enjoys running and feels better because of it. However, his wife resents it. She is accustomed to Joe coming home after work to take care of the children while she prepares dinner; now, she must perform both duties. The children are used to eating earlier and therefore demand her attention because they are hungry and tired. Also, they miss "their time" with their father. Sally really feels it's important for the family to eat dinner together, since it is the only time they spend together during the day. As a result, she is reluctant to feed the children earlier. The idea of cooking and cleaning up after two separate meals does not please her either.

In this situation a health maintenance activity has upset a family routine, thus creating family tension and demanding change within the family system. Joe's health maintenance activity has become a family stressor with demands the family will need to manage. Joe, Sally, and the children need to adjust or adapt to the situation. The ramifications of this situation are further discussed later in this chapter. The important point here is that even "healthy activities" — ones our society values — can be stressors depending on the family system in which they occur.

Illness

Illness is an event usually considered as a stressor. The biophysical and psychosocial components of illness imply a limited capacity to engage in appropriate or usual task and role performances (Lubkin, 1990). Therefore when a family member becomes ill and is unable to fulfill usual tasks or roles, the family must change its established patterns and roles. Bahnson (1987) describe illness of a family member as constituting "an attack on the unconscious expectations of the existing family structure" (p. 36). Illness creates a demand for change in the family system and requires family members to adjust and adapt. The tasks or roles relinquished by the ill individual can be eliminated, ignored during the illness, or redistributed within the system. Since this need for change within the family can be an inherent part of a family member's illness, it establishes illness as a family stressor (McCubbin & McCubbin, Chapter 2).

Sometimes the changes called for by illness stressors can be relatively insignificant and transitory, and the family adjusts patterns and tasks easily or temporarily. For example, conjunctivitis (pink eye), commonly seen in children, can be a relatively minor illness resolved by a visit to the doctor and treatment with medication. This illness stressor requires family resources of money for the medical appointment and medication and the personal resources of the parents' time and energy. If using these resources is not *perceived* as a problem, their use is valued and adjustment to the situation will be eased (McCubbin & McCubbin, Chapter 2). Therefore the temporary change in family tasks is considered positive.

On the other hand, an illness stressor can require larger demands and more long-term adjustment and adaptation of family patterns. Families may or may not feel capable of fulfilling the demands of the illness (McCubbin & McCubbin, Chapter 2). This feeling often occurs with chronic, long-term illnesses. For example, Parkinson's disease, a chronic neurological illness, is progressively disabling and long-term in nature. Managing the initial symptoms of Parkinson's disease may require few resources (routine doctor visits and daily medication) and therefore only minimally disrupts the family routine. However, as the illness progresses and neurological deficits increase, these ill family members become less able to care for themselves; eventually, they need physical care at the most basic levels (feeding, toileting, dressing). Now the family needs not only to redistribute or eliminate the tasks relinquished by the ill family member but also to learn and master the skills and tasks involved in the care of their ill family member or find alternative sources of care (for example, nursing home or in-home nursing care). The need for an alternative source of care in turn increases the need for financial resources (Quinn, 1986). The necessary shifts in family pattern and the need for resources will be ongoing, long-term, and permanent, increasing in demand as the disease progresses. Parkinsonism can lead to death anywhere from 5 to 30 years after diagnosis (Hoehn, 1990; Mckeique & Marmot, 1990). The length and magnitude of demands this stressor puts on the family can exhaust many family resources especially time, energy, and finances. As resources are continually taxed over time and pileup of strains and stressors occurs, family stress and crises may be produced (M.A. McCubbin, 1988, 1989). Initially, this illness stressor may involve pattern changes for only one or two family members. However, as disabilities increase, more family members are likely to become involved in supportive and physical care and financial assistance. The effects of long-term illness on the family will be discussed in greater depth later in this chapter and in Chapters 4 and 11.

Illness stressors have variable effects on the family, and these effects, regardless of the stressor's magnitude, are seldom confined to the ill family member. Inevitably, changes in one member of the family affect the entire family system. This "rippling effect" (Glick, Clarkin, & Kessler, 1987) is not confined to any particular stage of an illness; the entire family can be affected by such changes throughout all phases of illness. In fact, the effects of the illness can last a lifetime (Bahnson, 1987).

✦ THE FAMILY CYCLE OF HEALTH AND ILLNESS

Since the family unit is not a static system, the impact of an illness stressor on the family is multifaceted and complex (Turk & Kerns, 1985).

When illness strikes an individual family member, its effect on the individual and family depends on the following factors:

1. The developmental stage of both the individual and the family
2. The emotional and physical state of the ill individual, the individual family members, and the family as a whole
3. The socioeconomic status of the family
4. The cultural, ethnic, religious, and health beliefs of the individual and the family
5. Individual, family, and community resources
6. Other simultaneous significant events happening to the individual and the family
7. The characteristics of the disease itself

An illness stressor produces both the positive effects of drawing the family closer together and the negative effects of family disorganization (Martinson, Gilliss, Colaizzo, Freeman, & Bossert, 1990; M. A. McCubbin 1988; Musial, 1989). The course taken by the family will depend on the nature of the illness and the family's ability to manage the situation (McCubbin & McCubbin, Chapter 2).

Various models or phases of illness have been established to facilitate discussion of illness and its effect on the individual and family (Good, DelVecchio Good, & Burr, 1983; Kemp, Pillitteri, & Brown, 1989; Miller, 1988; Reiss & De-Noir, 1989). For the purpose of our discussion we chose to draw from Doherty and McCubbin's Family Health and Illness Cycle (1985), and Coe's Stages of the Illness Experience (cited in Dery, 1983) to establish a model of health and illness relevant to the family. Eight phases of the Family Cycle of Health and Illness are listed below and are also presented in Fig. 3-2.

1. Family and Family Member Health
2. Family Vulnerability and the Symptom Experience
3. The Sick Role and Family Appraisal
4. Medical Contact—Diagnosis
5. Illness Career and Family Adjustment/Adaptation
6. Recovery and Rehabilitation
7. Chronic Adjustment/Adaptation
8. Death and Family Reorganization

Typical patterns of behavior, as well as illness-specific crises, occur during each phase of illness (Aguilera, 1990; Burns, 1988; Cleveland, 1980/1989). The following sections define each phase of the Family Cycle

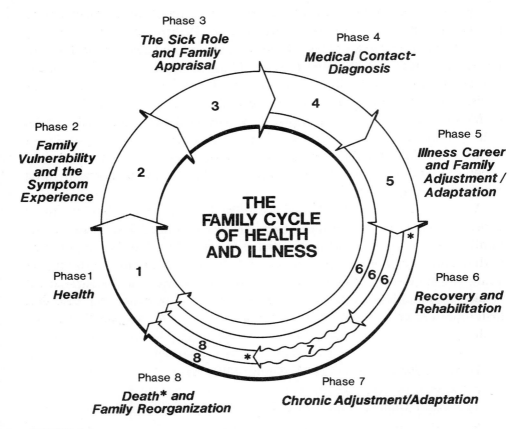

FIGURE 3-2
Eight phases of the Family Cycle of Health and Illness.

of Health and Illness and describe common family reactions and potential for family crisis within each phase of illness. Kaplan, Smith, Grobstein, and Fischman (1973/1977), Goldberg (1973/1977), and Reiss and De-Noir (1989) have assigned specific family coping tasks to certain illness phases. With this in mind, we have compiled a list of coping tasks for each phase of the Family Cycle of Health and Illness. It is best, but not always possible, for the family and its ill family member to accomplish the coping tasks specific to each phase *during* that phase of the cycle (Reiss & De-Noir, 1989). The following presentation of the Family Cycle of Health and Illness Model will become a vehicle for illustrating the impact health and illness stressors can have on family systems.

Although the phases of the health and illness model will be discussed in sequential order and are depicted in a sequential, cyclical order, (see Fig. 3-2) the actual process for the ill family member and the family does not necessarily follow an exact order. More often, the nature of the illness or the family's reaction to the illness determines the order. For example, a car accident can cause the family to go directly from Phase 1 (Health) to Phase 4 (Medical Contact). An illness such as the common cold that can be managed by the family starts with Phase 1 (Health), passes through Phase 3 (the Sick Role and Family Appraisal), and then continues to Phase 6 (Recovery and Rehabilitation). Medical contact is unnecessary, thereby eliminating Phases 4 and 5.

We have chosen a circle to represent the family health and illness experience to demonstrate the presence of a continuum that exists for the family despite the death of an ill family member. The family's experience with illness does not end with death of the ill family member; rather, the death can be the beginning of family reorganization with the subsequent return to Phase 1 (Health), or it can initiate a family stress response that fosters illness and thereby returns the family to the illness portion of the cycle.

Phase 1: Family and Family Member Health

COPING TASKS
1. *Participation in health-promoting behaviors*
2. *Participation in risk-reduction behaviors*

In Phase 1 the family and its members are in a state of well-being. Roles and patterns that meet the family's needs are established (Doherty & McCubbin, 1985). Health-promotion and risk-reduction behaviors necessary for family functioning have been incorporated into family life. Family members feel vital and vigorous and directive in their pursuits. Since family coping involves the integration of the various skills and abilities of family members (McCubbin & McCubbin, Chapter 2), these behaviors of each member contribute to family health and in turn decreases family vulnerability to stress. Family resources and capabilities also include the psychological and physical well-being of individual family members (McCubbin & McCubbin, Chapter 2), which assists in accounting for the impact a family member's illness can have on the family system.

In Phase 1 activities that promote health and reduce risk are potential family stressors, as demonstrated by the story of Joe and Sally at the beginning of this chapter. In this situation Joe tries to incorporate a new health-promotion activity—daily running—into family patterns. His new routine requires other family members to tolerate changes around established family mealtime patterns. Consequently, his health activity can become a source of family tension, a family stressor.

Families find it difficult to change established patterns for many reasons. Montgomery (1982) described four reasons for these family difficulties; his ideas have been verified by McCubbin and McCubbin (Chapter 2) and Olson et al. (1989). First, current patterns are the family's first choice. The family is comfortable with them and deems other patterns as less desirable. Sally demonstrates this in her dislike of the changes taking place around the dinner hour. She believes eating dinner together is a vital part of family functioning and a way of enhancing family relationships. A family dinner together is her first-choice pattern concerning this aspect of family life. Therefore she resists changing this pattern especially when she considers the extra work involved in preparing two meals.

Families are invested in their established patterns, and this investment is the second reason why families have difficulties changing (Montgomery, 1982; Olson et al. 1989). In our anecdote, even the children, who are used to eating earlier, are affected and disgruntled by the change. They had enjoyed "their time" with their father and find waiting for dinner difficult.

Third, changing patterns involves rethinking present patterns and taking risks in forming new behaviors, a process of family reorganization that is unsettling (Montgomery, 1982; McCubbin & McCubbin, Chapter 2). Sally and Joe will have to rethink the situation and may need to establish different values, priorities, and behaviors to meet new demands. For example, is there a better way the family can meet both Joe's health needs and Sally's desire to eat together? Can Joe run at a different time? How does the value of Joe's exercising compare with that of eating meals together?

Finally, new family patterns appear inefficient when compared with old patterns (Montgomery, 1982). The present loss is certain and clear, whereas the long-term gain is questionable. Will running prevent heart problems for Joe? Will the sacrifice in family time and energy, as well as family disruption, be worth the investment? This scenario demonstrates how a "health" stressor can cause family disruption and can demand change in family patterns.

Phase 2: Family Vulnerability and the Symptom Experience

COPING TASKS

1. *Awareness of symptoms indicating possible illness*
2. *Application of folk medicine — self-medicine*

Phase 2 begins when the family and its ill family member become aware of symptoms of possible illness (Dery, 1983; Hirsch, 1988). Unpleasant or painful sensations, fever, chills, shortness of breath, loss of vigor and stamina, or changes in behavior are frequent symptoms indicating illness. These symptoms alert the family to the possibility of illness. The importance given to the symptoms depends on the ill family member's ability to carry on normal activities, the family's medical knowledge, family members' experiences with similar symptoms, and the family's present situation.

Upon hearing an ill family member's description of symptoms, family and friends frequently offer home remedies and advice — folk medicine (Lubkin, 1990). Family members and friends, not health professionals, are the major source of health information during the early phases of illness (Becker, 1989). Kosa and Haggerty's research (1967) concluded that six out of every seven symptoms were handled without seeing a doctor (cited in Becker, 1989). Lay remedies are put into action in an attempt to ward off the illness. Offering folk remedies and advice is the family's way of showing support and concern. Family resources of time and support are directed toward the ill individual. The amount of attention and support offered by individual family members depends on the roles, tasks, and other insistent demands in each one's life (McCubbin & McCubbin, Chapter 2; Turk & Kerns, 1985). Through the bonds of love and empathy, the illness of a family member affects the family unit.

Berkanovic and Telsky (1982) discovered that the family and the individual's social network established whether it was advisable to seek medical advice (cited in Becker, 1989). The decision to visit a physician was based on the perceived seriousness of the signs and symptoms and on the belief that seeing a doctor would help.

Family vulnerabilities play a large role in Phase 2 (Doherty & McCubbin, 1985). Since families often function as buffers against stress, breakdown of this function may increase vulnerability to stress and illness. Normative transitions of the family life cycle, pileup of demands, and other problems of family life (for example, divorce) may decrease family buffering capacity and increase family vulnerability. Families with few strengths are particularly vulnerable (McCubbin & McCubbin, Chapter 2), thus setting into motion a vicious circle of increased vulnerability to stress leading to more stress. Such vulnerabilities can predispose family members to further illness or actually precipitate the onset of illness (Doherty & McCubbin, 1985).

Crisis in Phase 2 — maladjustment — occurs when coping tasks are not completed by either the family or the individual. For example, if the first task — awareness of symptoms indicating possible illness — is completed by the family but not by the individual, or vice versa, a potential conflict arises over the appraisal of the situation. Families with an aging parent may face this conflict as the aging process causes disabilities that prevent the parent's performance of adequate self-care. The parent may deny these disabilities, fearing loss of independence or placement in a nursing home. However, the family clearly recognizes something wrong and cannot ignore the situation. Yet, the parent's behavior may prevent the family from taking any action. The family may feel ambivalent and antagonistic toward the parent because of the parent's failure to understand, or admit, observed changes (Robinson & Thurnher, 1979/1986). Family fear and exhaustion may occur as the family conceals or compensates for the aging parent's behavior (Laurence & Gass, 1987). These disruptions can lead to family crisis. Clearly in this situation the denial of the aging parent hampers movement through Phase 2 of the health and illness cycle.

Although the signs and symptoms of illness are physically felt and experienced by the ill individual, the family nevertheless feels the impact of illness. Both the meaning and impact of an illness in this phase are determined by the give-and-take relationship between the ill member and the family.

Phase 3: The Sick Role and Family Appraisal

COPING TASKS
1. *Acceptance of the sick role by the family and ill family member*
2. *Formation of a family appraisal of and response to the situation*
3. *Adjustment or adaptation of the family to the sick role*

The sick role. In Phase 3 the family appraises the possible illness situation and provides the ill family member with the "right" to assume the sick role (Birchfield, 1985; Turk & Kerns, 1985). This validation is provisional, since American society requires a health professional to legitimize entrance into the sick role (Lubkin, 1990; Hirsch, 1988). Movement toward this role implies that the ill family member is (1) exempt from established responsibilities, (2) obliged to seek help, (3) obliged to comply with the advice of a competent person, and (4) expected to surrender the sick role as soon as possible (Hirsch, 1988; Kemp et al., 1989; Lubkin, 1990). The sick role supersedes other roles, even those as important as mother and breadwinner (Leventhal, Leventhal, & Van Nguyen, 1985). Because of this prominence, illness can have a devastating effect on family systems.

The family accommodates to the sick role by adjusting or adapting to the roles and tasks relinquished by the ill member. At the same time the family must deal with the moods and feelings (helplessness, dependence, discomfort, insecurity) of the sick family member, whose focus has become illness-oriented and self-centered (Rowat & Knafe, 1985). Support becomes a one-way street as the ill family member usually has only limited concern for the family and its affairs. At this point the family begins to experience the illness. The extent to which the family becomes a "victim" of the illness depends on its ability to manage the situation (Turk & Kerns, 1985). Therefore the components of the Resiliency Model of Family Stress, Adjustment, and Adaptation—resources, family vulnerability, resiliency, typology, appraisal, and problem-solving capacities, all of which determine the family's ability to manage stressors—become important.

The family appraisal. In the United States illness is most often viewed as a weakness (Olson et al., 1989). Illness can also be perceived as a threat, a loss, a gain, or as insignificant (Good et al., 1983; Olson et al., 1989). The family appraisal of the illness stressor is determined through the interchange of ideas, feelings, and circumstances between the ill family member, the family, and their social support systems. The formation of the family's appraisal of the illness begins in this phase and continues to evolve and adapt, changing as the family progresses through the health and illness cycle.

If the family appraisal of the illness indicates a potential for threat or loss that may be uncontrollable, the family may begin mobilizing to meet the demand (Leventhal et al., 1985; McCubbin & McCubbin, Chapter 2; Reiss & De-Noir, 1989). This type of appraisal indicates an awareness of impending change and of potentially inadequate resources. The appraisal acknowledges a demand-resource imbalance that causes family stress.

Feelings of fear, which are common in the presence of illness, can escalate (Bahnson, 1987; Leventhal et al., 1985). Fear, then, can become a source of maladjustment. For example, if the signs and symptoms indicate possible cancer, a disease associated with pain and potential loss through death, feelings akin to panic in both the ill family member and the family may lead to family crisis.

As the illness progresses, the family coping process of reframing (changing the meaning or point of reference to viewing the illness as a challenge) can alter the above appraisal and make it more manageable (McCubbin & McCubbin, Chapter 2; Olson et al., 1989). In this process the family schema (the family's goals, priorities, expectations, values, and rules) is central in establishing a meaning and a positive appraisal, and the illness can then be seen as beneficial. The perceived demand for change in response to the illness can be viewed as an opportunity to gain a renewed closeness through a shared experience that fosters growth of interrelationships (M. A. McCubbin, 1988). Illness may become a positive experience, bringing value to family efforts of adjusting or adapting to the illness (McCubbin & McCubbin, Chapter 2). The changes incurred are then less likely to be perceived as a burden.

On the other hand, the family can benefit from a member's illness by using the sick role as a scapegoat or as another way of coping with (ignoring) other family stressors (Lubkin, 1990). Illness makes it acceptable to relinquish other responsibilities and can become a vehicle for avoiding other problems or conflicts within the family.

Families also cope by using the passive appraisal process (Olson et al., 1989). The family appraises the situation as one that will take care of itself over time. The family considers the illness insignificant, indicating little or no need for adjustment. This minimizing process makes resources appear adequate for the situation, fostering a perceived demand-resource balance. Minimization or denial involves misinterpretation of selected facts to reduce the threat of the illness. Family denial can occur when the present life situation hinders the ability or willingness to notice signs and symptoms (Leventhal et al., 1985; Pearlin & Turner, 1987). This is especially true when current stressors pileup. In this case the family may choose to ignore or minimize the illness until there is a better time to deal with it—an attempt to conserve their resources for the present situation. This coping strategy may cause guilt feelings later, especially if the illness is eventually diagnosed as serious (Good et al., 1983).

When not carried to extremes, denial is a successful coping mechanism with positive effects. Denial can increase the amount of time available for the family to adjust and accept the illness. However, extreme denial produces negative effects. For example, denial can stifle family communication regarding the illness, thus decreasing the availability of support (Colen, 1988). More important, denial can prevent the family from accomplishing the coping tasks of this phase and therefore impede movement toward medical advice and treatment.

Phase 4: Medical Contact — Diagnosis

COPING TASKS

1. *Establishment of a relationship with health professionals*
2. *Gathering of information about the diagnosis*
3. *Acceptance of the diagnosis*

Diagnosis, a medical act of classification, socially legitimizes the sick role (Lubkin, 1990; Hirsch, 1988). Family hopes and fears surface during prediagnostic testing. There may even be a period of negotiation around the patient-family's perception as opposed to the doctor's perception of the problem (Gerhardt, 1985; Wright & Leahey, 1987). This negotiation usually concerns acceptance of the diagnosis and the proposed treatment plan. Second opinions concerning the diagnosis are sought, and alternative treatment plans are weighed and chosen.

Because of multiple and conflicting messages generated in the diagnostic process, a relationship of mutual trust is essential between health professionals and patients and their families (Lubkin, 1990). Health professionals need to encourage family coping by involving patients and their families in the diagnostic process. Families gain control through investigation, understanding, and attaching meaning to situations (Leventhal et al., 1985; Olson et al., 1989). Lack of information may create a sense of disorder and helplessness that reinforces similar feelings the patient and family may already have. Furthermore, family consensus regarding the appraisal of the situation is crucial to making necessary adjustments and adaptations (Leventhal et al., 1985; McCubbin & McCubbin, Chapter 2). A family consensus that is realistic about the situation is difficult to reach if the patient or the family has inadequate information. Families seek information from many sources to redefine the appraisal of the illness formed in Phase 3. Problems may arise if communication between patients, families, and health professionals is blocked (Bozetti, 1987; McWhinney, 1989); it certainly makes it difficult to accept the diagnosis, one of the tasks of this phase. To foster family adaptation, health care professionals need to impart information that encourages the family to form a positive appraisal of the illness (McCubbin & McCubbin, Chapter 2).

The moment of diagnosis is often remembered by patients and their families as the single most difficult incident of the illness (Cleveland, 1980/1989). The diagnosis can produce shock, alarm, self-pity, shame, guilt, anger, depression (Clements, Copeland, & Loftus, 1990; Bozett, 1987), or relief in finally knowing what is wrong (Wright & Leahey, 1987). Family crisis commonly occurs at the time of diagnosis, especially when the diagnosis is perceived as a threat or loss and the family fears its resources will be inadequate in meeting demands. Some families may find feelings around the diagnosis so overwhelming that they choose to deny the diagnosis (Leventhal et al., 1985; Reiss & De-Noir, 1989). Even when the prognosis is excellent, the diagnosis can produce serious uncertainty about the future (Leventhal et al., 1985). Health professionals who diagnose illness should consider these factors and explore what the illness means to the family when offering their diagnosis and its explanation (Reiss & De-Noir, 1989).

Open communication during the diagnostic process can lead to shared mourning over anticipated losses and renew family closeness (Cleveland, 1980/1989; Leventhal et al., 1985). This closeness offers support to sick family members and access to a collective coping experience that makes the illness less difficult to confront. Integral to the collective coping process is the expectation that all family members help meet the demands of the situation. Failure to share responsibility and information during this phase limits openness, and support, thereby defeating the collective coping process. Cooperative relationships lessen the family's struggle through this phase. If family members fail to assist each other in meeting the needs of the illness situation, resentment often results.

Phase 5: Illness Career and Family Adjustment/Adaptation

COPING TASKS

1. *Acceptance of the treatment plan*
2. *Family reorganization and role changes*
3. *Maintenance of a positive relationship with health-care professionals*

Phase 5 involves further family adjustment or adaptation to acute or chronic illness. Once the sick role has been legitimized by the health-care professional's diagnosis, the patient and family move into the *illness career* (Gerhardt, 1985). Patients may feel helpless and a loss of control over their lives. These feelings may trigger excessive complaints, demands, and aggressive behavior, all of which create turmoil for the family (Leventhal et al., 1985). In turn, the family mirrors the reactions of its ill family member; the family may try to gain more control over the situation or may feel helpless itself (Figley, 1983; Rowat & Knafe, 1985). Previous family relationships change; new patterns emerge, and some old, established patterns may disappear. Finding new patterns that work involves a trial-and-error process (McCubbin & McCubbin, Chapter 2) that absorbs family energy and time. Lengthy involvement in this process dissipates family energy as each new pattern is attempted. Therefore, the speed with which the family is able to appraise, adjust, or adapt to the illness stressor influences the expenditure of energy (Montgomery, 1982). Quickness enables the family to conserve energy and resources for other demands.

When ill family members enter the illness career, it implies expected cooperation with the treatment plan established by the health professional (Gerhardt, 1985; Hirsch, 1988; Kemp et al., 1989). They expect the treatment plan to assist them in "getting better" and leaving the sick role. Acceptance of the treatment plan by both the patient and family is desirable because families exert a great deal of influence in fostering compliance or noncompliance (Becker, 1989). If illness already prevents a sick family member from participating in certain essential family activities and roles, the treatment plan may further remove them from family functioning. Moreover, the family may need to learn new skills to carry out the treatment plan. Family acceptance of the treatment plan makes it easier for the ill individual to accept these changes (Anderson & Holder, 1989). For example, the patient may not comply with medication regimens if the family is not supportive (Storer, Frate, Johnson, & Greenberg, 1987). If the family believes the medication is unimportant or a waste of money, the individual may then not attach importance to the medication (Becker, 1989). Consequently the ill member either "forgets" or neglects to take it. This neglect can be fatal with certain illnesses such as diabetes or cardiac dysfunctions. When families are not consulted or involved in the formation of treatment plans, plans may be formed that are impractical or impossible for the health-care professional to implement.

Crisis situations may occur in this phase when the family finds existing patterns and roles inappropriate for the illness situation. The family may respond in one of two ways (McCubbin & McCubbin, Chapter 2). They may continue to resist change by adjusting patterns further so that the existing family patterns can be retained or returned to. This approach can be successful if the illness is mild or temporary and demands few role changes. Conversely, the family may choose to, or need to, adopt new patterns and roles, thereby producing a functionally different family system. For example, if illness prevents the father from working, the mother may need to find a job. This change requires adaptations throughout the family system, since the mother's roles (for example, child care and housekeeping) must be performed by other family members or hired out. The result is a new functioning family system.

Phase 6: Recovery and Rehabilitation

COPING TASKS

1. *Relinquisment of the sick role*
2. *Establishment of and adjustment/adaptation to a new definition of "normal" or reestablishment of the original family system.*
3. *Reentering of Phase 1: Individual and Family Health*

The recovery phase of the Family Cycle of Health and Illness can occur at two separate points in the cycle. First, it can occur after Phase 3, The Sick Role and Family Appraisal (Fig. 3-3). About 80% of all health problems are solved by families without seeing a physician (Hennen, 1987). Although the ill family member assumes the sick role in this situation the family does not consider the signs and symptoms of the illness serious enough to warrant medical intervention. The family applies folk medicine successfully, and the ill family member returns to health. An illness such as the flu or common cold fits into this category. The recovery phase also can occur after Phase 5 – Illness Career and Family Adjustment (see Fig. 3-3).

The family experiences further demands for change once the recovery phase begins. The family may reestablish the patterns and roles that existed before the illness. However, some family members may resist this change, since they wish to keep their now familiar responsibilities or patterns of functioning developed during the illness (Leventhal et al., 1985). For example, a mother may be reluctant to let her child resume normal activity following surgical intervention and recovery from congenital cardiac

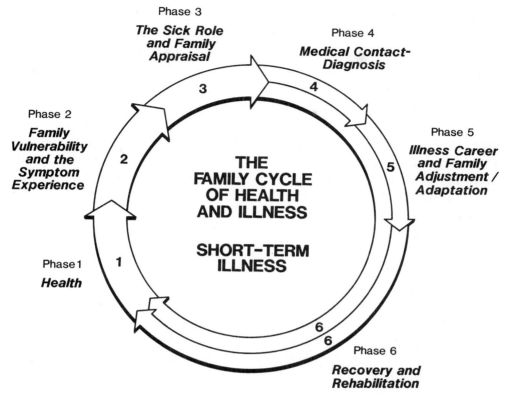

FIGURE 3-3
The Family Cycle of Health and Illness: short-term illness.

problems (Good et al., 1983). The mother has difficulty giving responsibility back to the child. In such situations the patient may need a clearly assigned "recovered" label by the health care professional to encourage family movement out of the sick role and to minimize psychosocial problems (Leventhal et al., 1985; Hirsch, 1988). This labeling process gives the family the social confirmation to relinquish its own sick role behaviors. Moreover, the family needs to be willing to relinquish any secondary gains the sick role has brought. For example, a family can use the illness to avoid other responsibilities or other family problems. It may be necessary for the health professional to help the family understand the meaning the illness has for them to persuade them to return to "normal" (Kerr & Bowen, 1988).

Recovery takes three forms, which are well described by Good et al. (1983). First, there is *complete* recovery. This includes abandonment of the sick role and return to health by both the ill family member and the family. The family acquires confidence from this kind of recovery; it has learned new coping skills during the illness experience, and these skills are now available for use against future stressors (Figley, 1983). A period of rehabilitation may be necessary for complete recovery, but a return to "normal" can be realized.

Partial recovery, the term used by Good et al. (1983) for the second form of recovery, is also described by Leventhal et al., 1985. The recovery is partial because the ill family member awaits the return of the disease and may ask: Did they get all the cancer? Is the cure permanent? The result is an inability to return to a total sense of well-being, which reduces personal resources and family coping skills. A sense of vulnerability pervades.

Finally, the third form of recovery occurs with a disability (Good et al., 1983; Leventhal et al., 1985). In this case some form of rehabilitation may be needed before recovery can be complete. Family support and encouragement during the rehabilitation program are vital (Steinbauer, 1989) because these contribute greatly to the motivation and compliance of the disabled family member to the rehabilitation program. The rehabilitation process has many successes and failures with accompanying emotional swings. Family support can be key to stabilizing the process and producing a successful outcome.

With a disability, recovery occurs but the return to "normal" is not always possible. The disabled family member may not be able to reassume all previously held family responsibilities, and the struggle between dependence and independence may persist (Cleveland, 1980/1989; Leventhal et al., 1985). Because of this the family may not be able to return to its former state. Instead, the family may need to reorganize its system, redefine its identity, and develop a new "normal."

Grief will be experienced by the family as the losses associated with permanent disability become more evident (Damrosch & Perry, 1989). This upheaval in the family system and the accompanying grief may precipitate family crisis (Leventhal et al., 1985). If the disability is static (unchanging) or minor, it is possible for the family to adjust or adapt successfully and progress through the illness cycle to health. However, if the disability can randomly change, produce other randomly occurring medical complications, or becomes more severe, the family may enter into the chronic adjustment / adaptation phase of the Family Cycle of Health and Illness.

Phase 7: Chronic Adjustment/Adaptation

COPING TASKS

1. *Reestablishment of new definitions of normal as the illness requires:*
   a. Modify and learn new patterns, regimens, skills, and roles
   b. Maintain a sense of control
2. *Adjustment and adaptation to altered social relationships and stigma of the disability*
3. *Maintenance of a positive relationship with health and allied health care professionals*
4. *Completion of the tasks of the grieving process in relation to losses incurred and anticipated from the disability*

In Phase 7 the ill family member is described as having a chronic illness or disability. This includes: (1) a long-term *disease* such as diabetes that requires constant monitoring or a disease such as multiple sclerosis with disabilities that become more severe with time and eventually lead to death, or (2) a severe *disability* such as a paraplegia from an accident or the cognitive and neuromuscular deficits from a stroke. Family members with these kinds of chronic illnesses or disabilities require specialized daily care, the challenge of which is absorbed mainly by the family (Johnson, 1985; Steinbauer, 1989). Constant adjustment or adaptation is necessary in chronic illness situations as either the illness or the family situation changes. This constant need for adjustment and adaptation is depicted in Fig. 3-4, the Family Cycle of Health and Illness, by the wavering arrow used to represent the Chronic Adjustment/Adaptation Phase. Numerous studies demonstrate the direct relationship between families with chronically ill members and increased family emotional and physical illness (Bloom, 1985; Johnson, 1985; McWhinney, 1989; Ramsey, 1989; Rowat & Knafe, 1985). The chronic illness has become an assault on family stability and health. On the other hand, many studies find chronic illness in families can cause renewed family growth, closeness, and return to stability (Johnson, 1985; M. A. McCubbin, 1988; Mishel, 1990). Within the framework of this book, a possible predictor of the family's outcome is the family's ability to manage stressors, prevent crisis, or move through crisis to increased adapation. The Resiliency Model of Family Stress, Adjustment, and Adaptation offers insight into this variation in family outcomes (McCubbin & McCubbin, Chapter 2).

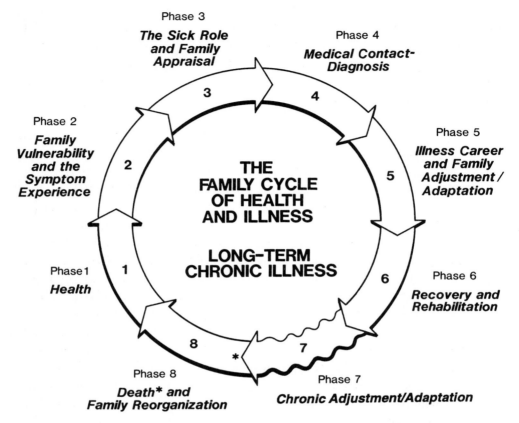

FIGURE 3-4
The Family Cycle of Health and Illness: long-term chronic illness.

In Phase 7 disabled family members may be labeled as *different* either within the sick role or after they relinquish the sick role. This label, *different*, causes feelings of isolation (Cleveland 1980/1989; Gerhardt, 1985). Both friends and, initially, families see the disabled individual as different — a person with different roles, abilities, and habits. Because of this, relationships are strained, awkward, or clouded with the pretense that nothing is wrong (Aadalen & Stroebel-Khan, 1981/1989; Leventhal et al., 1985). Both the disabled member and the family need to learn new skills in managing uncomfortable social transactions such as hostile stares, pity, or judgmental comments (Leventhal et al., 1985; Steinbauer, 1989). For family members, especially those involved in the physical care of the disabled member, feelings of isolation are reinforced by a loss of freedom to come and go as they please. It is difficult to find caretakers qualified to care for a chronically ill individual; this difficulty and the tremendous expense contribute to the family's loss of freedom (Hennen, Seitz, & Seitz, 1989; Johnson, 1985). These conditions intensify the family's feelings of isolation and add to the physical, emotional, and financial challenges of providing care.

The nature of the chronic disease itself may require frequent repetition of the coping tasks of this phase. For example, multiple sclerosis, a neurological disease, causes unpredictable exacerbations and remissions of the signs and symptoms of the disease. These symptoms can include impaired motor and sensory function, dementia, and visual loss. The family adjustments necessary to manage these constantly fluctuating disabilities may increase family tension and feelings of being out of control (Ferrari, Matthews, & Barabas, 1983/1985; LaRocca, Kalb, & Kaplan, 1987). Family resources may be threatened by constant change. Since a steady state in relation to these needs can be short-lived, frustration, anger, and depression can develop. Consequently, family relationships may become strained.

The family with a mentally retarded child is another example of the need to repeat coping tasks, especially as they relate to the grieving process (Wikler, 1981/1983). At the time of diagnosis the family feels grief over the loss of the fantasized normal child. The grief initially felt may be exacerbated with passage of each developmental milestone and loss of expected parenting experiences (for example, the first step, the first word, the twenty-first birthday). These shattered expectations make rearing a mentally retarded child a lifetime of hardships. The term *chronic sorrow*, first used by Olshansky (1962) and more recently by Damrosch and Perry (1989), has been used to describe this normal chronic grieving process that occurs in families with chronic or long-term illnesses. The health care professional needs to refrain from labeling families as *pathological* when they periodically express this grief.

The family with a chronically ill or disabled family member may be constantly adjusting and adapting to manage and balance the needs of the ill family member and the family. To cope with these situations the family needs clear information and assistance from health-care professionals and other resources. These adjustments and adaptations will continue until the death of the chronically ill person. At that time the family will continue to move through the health and illness cycle to Phase 8 — Death and Family Reorganization — and eventually back to Phase 1 — Health (Fig. 3-4).

Phase 8: Death and Family Reorganization

COPING TASKS

1. *Working through both individual family members' and the family unit's grieving process*
2. *Reorganization of the family to fill vacant roles left by the deceased*
3. *Realignment of extrafamilial roles*

Phase 8 requires the ill family member to work through the grieving process toward acceptance of death, as established by Kubler-Ross (1969) (Fig. 3·5). Denial, anger, bargaining, depression, and, finally, acceptance are the stages of the grieving process. Each of these feelings reverberate throughout the family system as the family responds to the ill family member's and each individual family member's emotional response. Each family member will go through his own grieving process at his own rate. However, specific family mourning tasks distinct from what we recognize as individual mourning tasks also need to be accomplished. These tasks were identified by Goldberg (1973/1977) and further described by Kosten, Jacob, and Kasl (1985) and Rosen (1990). These family mourning tasks include:

1. Sharing the experience of grief; allowing mourning to occur by encouraging expression of feelings
2. Establishing a shared acknowledgment of the reality of the death; relinquishing the memory of the deceased (for example, decision making based on the present not on what the departed might have done)
3. Reorganizing the family system; realignment of *intrafamilial* roles by redistributing the roles left vacant by the death
4. Redirecting family relationships and goals, which includes realignment of *extrafamilial* roles such as roles with the community and its organizations.

Health professionals need to monitor and encourage successful completion of these tasks by the family.

Phase 8 of the health and illness cycle is fraught with situations requiring family adjustment and adaptation. Death converts a stressful event to a family crisis in many ways. First, the finality of the loss requires

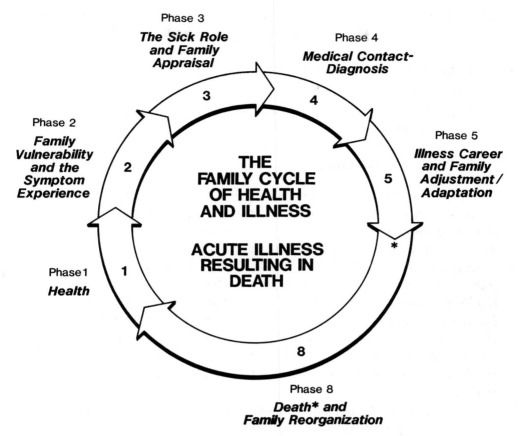

FIGURE 3-5
The Family Cycle of Health and Illness: acute illness resulting in death.

adjustment and adaptation of family roles and tasks (Carter, 1989; Kosten et al., 1985). The amount of change required will depend on the number and significance of roles and tasks held by the dead family member. For example, the death of a father and breadwinner can require extensive family adjustment and adaptation both within the family and in relation to the community (Leventhal et al., 1985). Second, because of longer life spans and improved medical care, death is not experienced as frequently today (Carter, 1989; Perkins & Harris, 1990). Therefore the family may not have established patterns to confront this situation. Third, at the time of death many decisions must be made quickly, causing pileup of stressors. Multiple new contacts need to be made: funeral home, insurance company, cemetery, lawyer, banker, government, and so on. While coping with the mourning process, many families find increased decision making either overwhelming or an escape from the reality of the death (Mandell, McAnulty, & Reece, 1980/1989).

Many studies have been done to measure the impact of death within the family. Holmes and Rahe (1967) determined that death of a spouse was the most stressful of all life events (cited in Olson et al., 1989). Other studies using different assessment scales have supported this (Osterweis, Solomon, & Green, 1984; Stroebe & Stroebe, 1987). However, when comparing the death of a spouse, parent, or child, Sanders (1979) found the death of a child produced the widest range of reactions and the highest grief intensity (cited in Perkins & Harris, 1990). Perkins and Harris attributed this to a lack of normative patterns of grief caused by its infrequent occurrence in American society. Moss and Moss (1983) described the significant impact of the death of a parent on an adult child (cited in Perkins & Harris, 1990). This kind of family death may cause remorse over unresolved conflicts and reminders of mortality as the death places them next in the generational line for eventual decreasing health and subsequent death. On the other hand, relief from the burden of caregiving for an aging parent may be experienced. Perkins & Harris found few studies on the death of a sibling during adulthood. However, studies on adult sibling relationships indicated that death of a sibling would involve loss of a companion and a source of emotional support and practical aid. This relationship is lifelong in its ties and therefore can be the longest of personal ties. Termination of the relationship would then be significant. Osterweis, Solomon, and Green (1984) studied the impact of death on children and adolescents. Generally it is agreed that the coping strategies of children under 4 are too immature to achieve successful mourning. Adolescents can successfully mourn, but the multiple changes going on in their lives makes this difficult. These factors make children and adolescents vulnerable to death of a family member. This is supported by studies demonstrating that death of a parent during childhood causes emotional vulnerability that may lead to both psychiatric and physical illness. The stressfulness to all family members of losses such as aunts, grandparents, and friends depends on the meaning attached to the relationship.

The stress produced by death of a family member in any case has the potential to produce all the physical, psychological, and social repercussions (for example, illness, exhaustion, depression, loneliness, change in social status, crisis) stress has to offer the family unit and its members (Kosten et al., 1985). Yet despite the family stress generated by death, when both individual family members and the family unit complete the coping tasks of this phase, the family passes through Phase 8 to Phase 1, thereby returning to the start of the Family Cycle of Health and Illness (see Fig. 3-5).

✦ CONCLUSION

At whatever phase of illness the health professional encounters the patient, it is clear that dealing with individuals as if they functioned in a social vacuum (devoid of any influence from the family), is akin to treating only the proverbial tip of the iceberg. Family studies referred to throughout this chapter provide evidence that illness is associated with measurable social, psychological, and sometimes physical challenges for families. Moreover, the ability of individuals to cope with the demands of their illness is, in part, a function of the capacity of the collective family system to manage the circumstances either positively or negatively. In this way the family serves either to enable or hinder family members as they attempt to cope with the demands of the illness.

REFERENCES

Aadalen, S. P., & Stroebel-Kahn, F. (1989). Coping with quadriplegia. In R. H. Moos (Ed.), *Coping with physical illness: Vol. 2. New perspectives* (pp. 73-188). New York: Plenum. (Reprinted from *American Journal of Nursing*, 1981, *81*(8), 1471-1478)

Aguilera, D. C. (1990). *Crisis intervention: Theory and methodology* (6th ed.). St. Louis: Mosby–Year Book.

Anderson, C. M., & Holder, D. P. (1989). Family systems and behavioral disorders: Schizophrenia, depression, and alcoholism. In C. N. Ramsey (Ed.), *Family systems in medicine* (pp. 487-502). New York: Guilford.

Bahnson, C. B. (1987). The impact of life-threatening illness on the family and the impact of the family on illness: An overview. In M. Leahey & L. M. Wright (Eds.), *Families and life-threatening illness* (pp. 26-44). Springhouse, PA: Springhouse.

Becker, L. A. (1989). Family systems and compliance with medical regime. In C. N. Ramsey (Ed.), *Family systems in medicine* (pp. 416-431). New York: Guilford.

Birchfield, M. (1985). *Stages of illness: Guidelines for nursing care*. Bowie, MD: Prentice-Hall.

Bloom, B. (1985). *Stressful life event theory and research: Implications for primary prevention*. Rockville, MA: United States Department of Health and Human Services.

Bozett, F. W. (1987). Family nursing and life-threatening illness. In M. Leahey & L. M. Wright (Eds.), *Families and life-threatening illness* (pp. 2-25). Springhouse, PA: Springhouse.

Burns, E. (1988). Crisis intervention. In R. Taylor (Ed.), *Fundamentals of family medicine* (3rd ed., pp. 72-88). New York: Springer-Verlag.

Carter, S. L. (1989). Themes of grief. *Nursing Research*, *38*(6), 354-358.

Clements, D. B., Copeland, L. G., & Loftus, M. (1990). Critical times for families with a chronically ill child. *Pediatric Nursing*, *16*(2), 157-161.

Cleveland, M. (1989). Family adaptation to traumatic spinal cord injury — response to crisis. In R. H. Moos (Ed.), *Coping with physical illness: Vol. 2. New perspectives* (2nd ed., pp. 159-171). New York: Plenum. (Reprinted from *Family Relations*, 1980, *29*(4), 558-565)

Colen, B. D. (1988). The ostrich syndrome: denying the facts about a particular disease or condition. *Health*, *20*(2), 6-9.

Damrosch, S. P., & Perry, L. A. (1989). Self-reported adjustment, chronic sorrow, and coping of parents of children with Down syndrome. *Nursing Research*, *38*(1), 25-30.

Dery, G. K. (1983). Concepts of health and illness. In W. J. Phipps, B. C. Long, & N. F. Woods (Eds.), *Medical-surgical nursing: Concepts and clinical practice* (2nd ed., pp. 5-17). St. Louis: Mosby–Year Book.

Doherty, W., & McCubbin, H. I. (1985). Families and health care: An emerging arena of theory, research, and clinical intervention. In W. Doherty & H. I. McCubbin (Eds.), *Family relations* (pp. 5-10). Minneapolis: National Council of Family Relations.

Figley, C. (1983). Catastrophes: An overview of family reactions. In C. Figley & H. I. McCubbin (Eds.), *Stress and the family: Coping with catastrophe* (vol. 2, pp. 3-20). New York: Brunner/Mazel.

Ferrari, M., Matthews, W. S., & Barabas, G. (1985). The family and the child with epilepsy. In D. H. Olson (Ed.). *Family studies: Review yearbook* (Vol. 3, pp. 63-69). Beverly Hills, CA: Sage. (Reprinted from *Family Process*, 1983, *22*, 53-59)

Gerhardt, U. E. (1985). Stress and stigma: Explanation of illness. In U. E. Gerhardt & M. E. J. Wadsworth (Eds.), *Stress and stigma: Explanation and evidence in sociology of crime and illness* (pp. 161-204). New York: St. Martin's.

Goldberg, S. B. (1977). Family tasks and reactions in the crisis of death. In R. H. Moos (Ed.), *Coping with physical illness* (pp. 421-434). New York: Plenum. (Reprinted from *Social Case Work*, 1973, *54*, 398-405)

Good, B. J., DelVecchio Good, M., & Burr, B., D. (1983). Impact of illness on the family: disease, illness, and the family trajectory. In R. Taylor (Ed.), *Fundamentals of family medicine* (2nd ed., pp. 34-44). New York: Springer-Verlag.

Glick, I. A., Clarkin, J. F., & Kessler, D. R. (1987). *Marital and family therapy.* (3rd ed.) Orlando, FL: Grune & Stratton.

Hennen, B. K. (1987). The family and stress. In D. B. Shires, B. K. Hennen, & D. I. Rice (Eds.), *Family medicine: A guidebook for practitioners of the art* (2nd ed., pp. 37-41). New York: McGraw-Hill.

Hennen, B. K., Seitz, M., & Seitz, B.

(1987). The chronically disabled child and the family. In D. B. Shires, B. K. Hennen, & D. I. Rice (Eds.), *Family medicine: A guidebook for practitioners of the art* (2nd ed., pp. 42-50). New York: McGraw-Hill.

Hirsch, L. L. (1988). Problem differentiation. In R. B. Taylor (Ed.), *Family medicine* (3rd ed., pp. 58-65). New York: Springer-Verlag.

Hoehn, M. (1990). Natural history of the untreated prelevodopa disease. In G. Stern (Ed.), *Parkinson's disease* (pp. 307-314). Baltimore: Johns Hopkins.

Johnson, S. B. (1985). The family and the child with chronic illness. In D. C. Turk & R. D. Kerns (Eds.), *Health illness and families: A life-span perspective* (pp. 220-254). New York: John Wiley & Sons.

Kaplan, D. M., Smith, A., Grobstein, R., Fischman, S. E. (1977). Family mediation of stress. In R. H. Moos (Ed.), *Coping with physical illness* (pp. 81-96). New York: Plenum. (Reprinted from *Social Work*, 1973, *18*, 60-69).

Kemp, B., Pillitteri, A., & Brown, P. (1989). *Fundamentals of nursing: a framework for practice*. New York: Springer-Verlag.

Kerr, M. E., & Bowen, M. (1988). *Family evaluation*. New York: W. W. Norton.

Kosten, T. R., Jacob, S. C., & Kasl, S. V. (1985). Terminal illness, bereavement, and the family. In D. C. Turk & R. D. Kerns (Eds.), *Health, illness, and families* (pp. 311-337). New York: John Wiley & Sons.

Kubler-Ross, E. (1969). *On death and dying*. New York: MacMillan.

Lancaster, J., McCance, K., & Vanderschmidt, H. (1986). A curriculum project for clinical prevention: The role of the nurse. *Family, Community and Health*, *8*(4), 48-53.

LaRocca, N. G., Kalb, R. C., & Kaplan, S. R. (1987). Psychological issues. In L. C. Scheinberg (Ed.), *Multiple sclerosis: A guide for patients and their families* (2nd ed., pp. 197-213). New York: Raven.

Laurence, M. K., & Gass, D. A. (1987). Confusion in the elderly. In D. B. Shires, B. K. Hennen, & D. I. Rice (Eds.), *Family medicine: A guidebook for practitioners of the art* (2nd ed., pp. 275-287). New York: McGraw-Hill.

Leventhal, H., Leventhal, E. A., & Van Nguyen, T. (1985). Reactions of families to illness: Theoretical models and perspectives. In D. C. Turk & R. D. Kerns (Eds.), *Health, illness, and families* (pp. 108-145). New York: John Wiley & Sons.

Lubkin, I. M. (1990). Illness roles. In I. M. Lubkin (Ed.), Chronic illness: Impact and interventions (pp. 43-64, 2nd ed.). Boston: Jones & Bartlett.

Mandell, F., McAnulty, E., & Reece, R. (1989). Observations of parental response to sudden unanticipated infant death. In R. H. Moos (Ed.), *Coping with physical illness: Vol. 2. New perspectives* (2nd ed., pp. 51-60). New York: Plenum. (Reprinted from *Pediatrics*, 1980, *56*(2), 221-225.)

Martinson, I. M., Gilliss, C., Colaizzo, D. C., Freeman, M., & Bossert, E. (1990). Impact of childhood cancer on healthy school-age siblings. *Cancer Nursing*, *13*(3), 183-190.

McCubbin, M. A. (1988). Family stress, resources, and family types: Chronic illness in children. *Family Relations*, *37*, 203-210.

McCubbin, M. A. (1989). Family stress and family strengths: A comparison of single- and two-parent families with handicapped children. *Research in Nursing and Health, 12,* 101-110.

McKeique, P., & Marmot, M. (1990). Epidemiology of parkinson's disease. In G. Stern (Ed.), *Parkinson's disease* (pp. 295-306). Baltimore: Johns Hopkins.

McWhinney, I. R. (1989). The family in health and disease. In I. R. McWhinney (Ed.), *Textbook of family medicine* (pp. 202-227). New York: Oxford University.

Miller, W. (1988). Models of health, illness and health care. In R. B. Taylor (Ed.), *Family medicine* (3rd ed., pp. 58-65). New York: Springer-Verlag.

Mishel, M. H. (1990). Reconceptualization of the uncertainty in illness theory. *Image: Journal of Nursing Scholarship, 22,*(4), 256-262.

Montgomery, J. (1982). *Family crisis as process: Persistence and change.* Washington: University Press of America.

Musial, E. M. (1989). An unsung hero: The living related kidney donor. In R. H. Moos (Ed.), *Coping with physical illness: Vol. 2. New perspectives* (2nd ed., pp. 295-304). New York: Plenum. (Reprinted from *Nephrology Nursing,* 1980, *2,* 21-22, 60-62)

Olshansky, S. (1962). Chronic sorrow: a response to having a mentally defective child. *Social Case Work, 43,* 190-193.

Olson, D., McCubbin, H. I., Barnes, H., Larsen, A., Muxen, M., & Wilson, M. (1989). *Families: What makes them work* (2nd ed.). Newbury Park, CA: Saga.

Osterweis, M., Solomon, F., & Green, M. (Eds.). (1984). *Bereavement: Reactions, consequences, care.* Washington: National Academy.

Pearlin, L. I., & Turner, H. A. (1987). Measurement and methodological issues in social support. In S. V. Kasl & C. L. Cooper (Eds.), *Stress in health: Issues in research methodology* (pp. 167-205). New York: John Wiley & Sons.

Perkins, H. W., & Harris, L. S. (1990). Familial bereavement and health in adult life course perspective. *Journal of Marriage and the Family, 52,* 233-241.

Quinn, J. (1986). Seeking quality alternatives in the community. *Business and Health, 3*(8), 21-24.

Ramsey, C. R. (1989). The science of family medicine. In C. N. Ramsey (Ed.), *Family systems in medicine* (pp. 3-15). New York: Guilford.

Reiss, D., & De-Noir, A. K. (1989). The family and medical team: a transactional and developmental perspective. In C. N. Ramsey (Ed.), *Family systems in medicine* (pp. 435-444). New York: Guilford.

Robinson, B., & Thurnher, M. (1986). Taking care of aged parents: A family cycle transition. In R. Moos (Ed.), *Coping with crisis* (pp. 195-209). New York: Plenum. (reprinted from *Journal of Gerontology,* 1979, *19*(6), 586-593).

Rosen, E. J. (1990). *Families facing death: Family dynamics of terminal illness.* Lexington, MA: Lexington Books.

Rowat, K. M., & Knafe, K. A. (1985). Living with chronic pain: The spouse's perspective. *Pain, 23*(3), 259-271.

Steinbauer, J. R. (1989). Spinal injury: Impact and implications for family medicine research. In C. N. Ramsey (Ed.), *Family systems in medicine* (pp. 458-468). New York: Guilford.

Storer, J. H., Frate, D. A., Johnson, A., &

Greenberg, A. (1987). When the cure seems worse than the disease: Helping families adapt to hypertension treatment. *Family Relations, 36,* 311-315.

Stroebe, W., & Stroebe, M. S. (1987). *Bereavement and health: The psychological and physical consequences of partner loss.* New York: Cambridge University.

Turk, D. C., & Kerns, R. D. (1985). The family in health and illness. In D. C. Turk & R. D. Kerns (Eds.), *Health, illness, and families* (pp. 108-145). New York: John Wiley & Sons.

Wikler, L. (1983). Chronic stress of families of mentally retarded children. In D. H. Olson (Ed.), *Family studies: Review yearbook* (Vol. 1, pp. 143-150). Beverly Hills, CA: Sage. (Reprinted from *Family Relations,* 1981, *30,* 281-288)

Wright, L. M., & Leahey, M. (1987). Families and life-threatening illness: Assumptions, assessment, and intervention. In M. Leahey & L. M. Wright (Eds.), *Families and life-threatening illness* (pp. 45-58). Springhouse, PA: Springhouse.

FAMILY COPING IN
HEALTH AND
ILLNESS

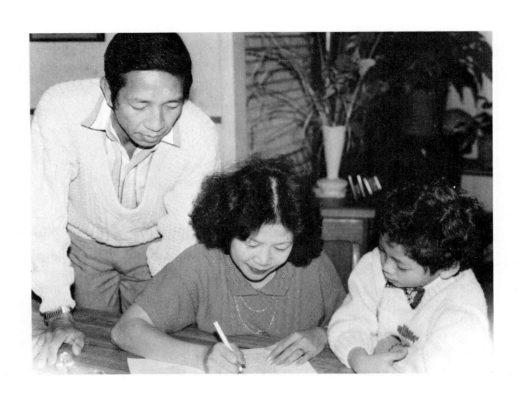

4

Dimensions of Illness That Affect the Family

✦

CHAPTER GOALS

✦ To describe the ten dimensions of crisis classified by Lipman-Blumen (1975) that characterize the nature of a crisis and the influence it has on a social system

✦ To use the ten dimensions of crisis to characterize the nature of an illness stressor and the influence it has on the family system

✦ To discuss the significance and implications this classification of illness stressors offers the health-care professional in creating family interventions for various types of illnesses

OVERVIEW

Not all illnesses have the same impact on families; moreover, the family's reaction is not always a direct function of the medical severity of the illness. This chapter identifies and discusses the dimensions of illness that contribute to or help to predict the effect illness has on the family. Lipman-Blumen's (1975) characterization of crises and their impact on social systems is used as the basis for classifying those dimensions of an illness stressor that affect the family. These dimensions of illness can help health providers identify and understand diverse illnesses and their differential effects on the family. This chapter also focuses on two components of the Resiliency Model of Family Stress, Adjustment, and

Adaptation: the illness stressor (A) and the level of family adjustment to the stressor—bonadjustment/adaptation or maladjustment/adaptation (crisis situation—X) (Fig. 4-1).

✦ TEN DIMENSIONS OF ILLNESS

Studies on the family unit and illness bring together two multifaceted and complex elements. In studying this relationship, researchers in the social sciences have developed a definitive and quantitative analysis of family dynamics especially in the area of stress (M. A. McCubbin & H. I. McCubbin, 1987; H. I. McCubbin & M. A. McCubbin, 1987; McCubbin & Thompson, 1987; Olson et al., 1989). Other studies have explored the impact of a specific disease or type of disease (for example, chronic, catastrophic) on the family or on a specific family situation (for example, developmental stage, siblings, spouse) (Anderson & Holder, 1989; Mercer, May, Ferketich, & DeJoseph, 1986; Rowat & Knafe, 1985; Steinbauer, 1989). Outside of the numerous studies on long-term illness, few studies have documented the effects of specific dimensions of illness and associated problems of family adjustment. One study by Ferrari, Matthews, and Barabas (1983/1985) analyzed families with epileptic children to explore how the *predictability* of an illness stressor affects the family. They focused on the *unpredictable nature* of the child's seizures and related this illness dimension to specific family functioning problems in communication, cohesion, and integration. This study, which will be discussed further in this chapter, provides evidence that some family adjustment problems are specific to certain dimensions of illness. Awareness of the relationship between dimensions of illness and family functioning can alert health-care professionals to potential family difficulties during certain illnesses.

Both Lipman-Blumen (1975) and Berren, Beigel, and Ghertner (1980/1986) developed a classification of crisis that characterizes the nature of a crisis and the influence it has on a social system. The ten dimensions developed by Lipman-Blumen (see box on p. 102) provide a framework to classify the dimensions of an illness stressor that govern the illness's capability to cause family strain, stress, and crisis. Although each illness and family is unique, family crises from illness stressors fall into common groupings (Aguilera, 1990; Kaplan, Smith, Grobstein, & Fischman, 1973/1977).

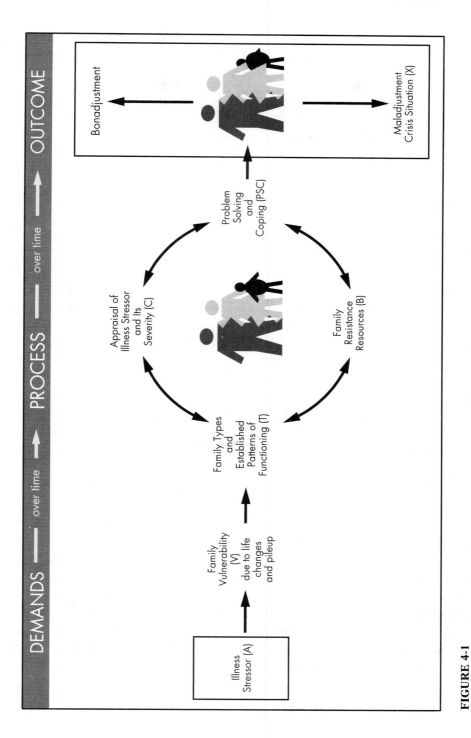

FIGURE 4-1

Adjustment Phase of the Resiliency Model of Family Stress, Adjustment, and Adaptation. This chapter focuses on illness stressor (A) and the level of family adjustment — bonadjustment / maladjustment — crisis situation (X).

Ten Dimensions of Illness

1. *Origin* of the stressor — inside or outside of the family
2. *Extent* of the stressor's impact — on all the family members or only a few
3. *Severity* of the stressor — mild or severe
4. *Duration* of the stressor — short term or long term
5. *Onset* of the stressor — sudden or gradual
6. *Control* of the stressor — manageable or unmanageable
7. *Cause* of the stressor — natural, man-made, or unknown
8. *Predictability* of the stressor — predictable or uncertain
9. *Resource demands* of the stressor — great or small
10. *Stigma* of the stressor — great or small

Modified from Lipman-Blumen, J. (1975). A crisis framework applied to macrosociological family changes: Marriage, divorce, and occupational trends associated with World War II. *Journal of Marriage and the Family, 3,* 889-902.

Each dimension has a varied ability to impact the family. In fact, Lipman-Blumen originally classified the dimensions in terms of polar opposites. For example, *origin* was originally termed *internality vs. externality.* The crisis was characterized as having its origin either "internal or external to the social system affected" (Lipman-Blumen, 1975 p. 89). For the purposes of this book, the dimensions have been renamed to simplify references to the illness stressor's dimension.

1   *Origin* of the Stressor: Inside vs. Outside the Family

Illness stressors originate inside or outside of the family (Leventhal, Leventhal, & Van Nguyen, 1985). Illness stressors originating inside the family consist of (1) an actual illness of a family member or (2) an illness with a cause linked to the family (that is, hereditary disease).

An ill family member indicates that the family may have responsibility in causing, dealing with, and resolving the illness (Leventhal et al., 1985). The family may feel guilt related to the illness (Bozett, 1987). Feelings of obligation may compel the family to meet the demands of the illness, since family ties can instill a strong sense of responsibility. Fulfilling these demands may require changes in family patterns and roles (see Chapter 3). Therefore these demands can generate family strain, stress, and crisis. Role changes have the greatest potential to disrupt the family (Aguilera, 1990; Leventhal et al., 1985).

The second aspect of illness stressors originating within the family concerns cause of the illness. Illnesses with causes that apparently originate within the family create special family problems (Leventhal et al., 1985). For example, hereditary diseases, such as sickle cell anemia and hemophilia, that affect children can initiate family guilt and fear (Black & Weiss, 1988; Hennen, Seitz, & Seitz, 1987). Since children are often seen as physical and psychological extensions of their parents, the ill child may be perceived as a reflection of the parents' inadequacies and imperfections. Also, the family may be stigmatized by the illness (Gerhardt, 1985; Leavitt, 1989; Turnbull & Turnbull, 1985). These factors are detrimental to family self-esteem, as well as to individual self-esteem, both of which are vital resources for successful family functioning (McCubbin and McCubbin, Chapter 2).

On the other hand, illness stressors originating outside the family, such as an ill friend tend to have less affect on the family. Here, the responsibilities are not dictated by family ties, and the requirement to respond in full measure is optional. The magnitude of impact depends on the meaning and intensity of the friend's relationships with family members. In most cases the family may offer assistance and support, but demands for adjustment within the family are usually minimal or transient. Demands for role changes are likely to be nonexistent, as is the potential for family guilt. These factors decrease the capabilities of this kind of illness stressor to cause family strain or stress.

2   *Extent* of the Stressor's Impact: All Family Members vs. Only a Few

Illnesses that directly affect all family members have greater family significance than those affecting only a few members. For example, a toothache may involve only the ill individual and perhaps a family member who provides transportation to and from the dentist. Here, the demands for family change and the use of family resources are minimal. Therefore both family tension and disruption generated are relatively mild. On the other hand, a fatal illness such as cancer may affect few family members initially, but in the end all family members are affected by the death, each according to the significance of the relationship with the deceased (Bozett, 1987). The need for change will be felt by the whole family, and many family resources may be tapped (see Chapter 3). The demand for change and the need for resources, especially support from and for family members, increase the level of family tension and the potential for family disruption and crisis (Kosten, Jacobs, & Kasl, 1985). The greater the extent of involvement and the number of family members entangled in the illness experience, the greater the potential for family disruption, stress, and crisis.

Illness and its demands can affect family members unevenly (Fradkin & Liberti, 1987); that is, the burden of care can fall more heavily on one family member because of that person's nurturing or leadership role in the family, their relationship with the ill family member, or their physical proximity to the ill individual. This situation is common in the provision of care for the elderly. Seventy-two percent of family caregivers are women, twenty-three percent being wives and twenty-nine percent being daughters (Stone, Cafferata, & Sangl, 1987). The responsibilities associated with the illness often are not distributed equally (Cleveland, 1980/1989), thereby causing resentment (Fradkin & Liberti, 1987) that may increase family tension and possibly lead to family crisis.

3 *Severity* of the Stressor: Mild vs. Severe

Severity of an illness can be used as a barometer to predict the impact of an illness stressor on the family (McCubbin & McCubbin, Chapter 2; Turk & Kerns, 1985). Since severely ill family members are generally unable to fulfill their family roles and tasks, the need for change within the family is inevitable. The more severe or disabling the illness, the greater the potential demands on family time, energy, and finances (Leventhal et al., 1985; McCubbin & McCubbin, Chapter 2). M. A. McCubbin (1986, 1990) states that the severity of the illness stressor is established by how seriously the family's stability is threatened or by how many significant demands are placed on family resources and capabilities (cited in McCubbin & McCubbin, Chapter 2). Over time, illness demands can threaten family integrity and well-being, and family crisis may erupt.

On the other hand, an illness of low or little severity may have little or no impact on the family. Strep throat, with proper medical care is a mild illness that causes little family disruption. The demands it may bring will be only temporary and will not threaten family integrity or well-being. Money for a visit to the physician's office and medication will be significantly less than that for more severe illnesses.

Within the context of the Resiliency Model of Family Stress, Adjustment, and Adaptation the family appraisal of the severity of the illness is initially determined by the family appraisal of the illness stressor in the adjustment phase. In the adaptation phase the situational appraisal (CC) and the family's schema (the family's blueprint for functioning) appraisal (CCC) adjust the original appraisal to meet the demand of adapting (McCubbin & McCubbin, Chapter 2). Through the family's schema, the family's community and society influence family appraisals. The number of hardships incurred and the amount of present and anticipated loss will be weighed and evaluated from a family, cultural, and societal viewpoint. The more losses and hardships incurred and anticipated, the more likely the illness will be defined as severe. Objective cultural designations about illness help determine the seriousness of illness events and thereby influence the family schema appraisal. Illness itself is considered a hardship, but certain illnesses are considered more severe than others (M.A. McCubbin & H.I. McCubbin, 1989). For example, illnesses producing disfigurement, limb dysfunction, cognitive dysfunction (for example, stroke), or death (for example, cancer, AIDS) are considered severe hardships. Cultural definitions shape the magnitude of stress experienced by the family (Larkin, 1987).

When the family defines the illness as a severe threat or loss, the appraisal strikes the core of family stability and self-esteem. The family sense of order and safety and its ability to adjust to the situation are imperiled. Anticipatory grief occurs in relation to anticipated losses (Bozett, 1987). The severe stress generated may overwhelm the family and cause disorganization. Family functioning and communication may be impaired. For these reasons, severe illness can be expected to produce severe stress and situational depression in family members (Johnson, 1985; Leventhal et al., 1985; Rowat & Knafe, 1985). In children, acting out behavior, such as physical aggression, is often seen (Hennen, 1987; Walker, 1988). When illness is defined as severe families are receptive to outside support, and coping strategies can be facilitated by the nature of the support received, and not necessarily determined by preexisting family patterns (Aguilera, 1990). This receptivity provides an opportunity for health professionals to intervene and offer support to the family.

The availability of resources can buffer the severity of an illness situation (McCubbin & McCubbin, Chapter 2). A balance between demands and resources minimizes the severity of the situation and decreases the opportunity for family stress and crisis. For example, sufficient financial resources may lessen the threat of the illness and its demands. If emotional support, a resource originating both within the family and outside the family, is plentiful, it significantly diminishes the severity of illness stressors (Dunst, Trivette, & Deal, 1988). When family crisis occurs, as it usually does at the onset or diagnosis of a severe illness, emotional support from within the family and from health-care professionals can help determine how the family will confront a severe illness.

4   *Duration* of the Stressor: Short Term vs. Long Term

The duration of a stressor's impact also predictively contributes to individual and family difficulties. Seyle's classic studies of stress (1956) and its physiological responses in the individual reports that the persistence of stress causes exhaustion, a state of physical and psychological illness. Family studies demonstrate a link between prolonged family stress and a high risk for physical and psychological problems in the family (Gaynor, 1990; Rowat & Knafe, 1985). Johnson (1985), Cleveland (1980/1989), and Ferrari et al. (1983/1985) demonstrated that families struggling with a chronically ill child found one of their biggest problems was dealing with persistent strains, especially intrafamilial strains such as financial burdens, marital discord, and sibling–ill child conflict. Clearly, the longer an illness stressor persists, the greater its impact on the family and its members.

When families are confronted with an illness stressor, they need to adjust or adapt to the situation (McCubbin & McCubbin, Chapter 2). With a short-term illness, adjustment behaviors rather than the more challenging adaptive behaviors may be sufficient to meet the demands of the situation. As demonstrated in Chapter 3, patterns are difficult for families to change. The initial family response is to resist change and keep established roles and patterns of functioning. In other words, the family employs its resistance resources which can include adjustment behaviors such as avoidance, elimination, and assimilation, and uses family strengths to manage the situation (McCubbin & McCubbin, 1989). In the presence of a short-term illness stressor it may be possible to resist pattern change successfully. Since the duration of a short-term illness can be anywhere from a day (for example, 24-hour flu) to several months (for example, fractured femur), the temporary nature of the illness does not demand permanent changes. For example, an ill family member with a fractured femur may only temporarily relinquish family tasks. Because the illness is short-lived, the family may use any of the three adjustment behaviors just listed to manage the situation. Established patterns can remain unchanged or only temporarily adjusted. As a result, family stress and crisis are less likely to be generated by the demand for permanent task or role changes.

In the short-term illness, adjustment behaviors can also be used in relation to family responsibilities. Responsibilities can be ignored, reassigned, or postponed until the eventual return to normalcy. Postponement of responsibilities decreases the chance of stressor pileup during the illness experience; the illness becomes only a temporary annoyance. Less opportunity for pileup means less chance of increased family vulnerability to stress (McCubbin & McCubbin, Chapter 2). This ability to postpone responsibilities can foster a benign family appraisal of the situation and thus more benign family stress levels.

Family resources are usually adequate for meeting the demands of a short-lived illness stressor. With a serious short-term illness or disability stressor, the family may require great energy to buffer and adjust to the situation. However, since the illness is not persistent, the family often manages the demands without exhausting its resources. Also, the burden of caring for acutely ill family members is often provided by health-care professionals in the hospital setting, not by the family at home. If depletion or overextension of family resources exists, it is usually minimal. If the family believes it has adequate resources, then the threat of illness is reduced and a more manageable family appraisal may be produced (McCubbin & McCubbin, Chapter 2).

On the other hand, long-term illness or disability often requires permanent family changes (Johnson, 1985; Steinbauer, 1989). The permanent changes in the ill or disabled family member demand permanent changes in the family. Grief is felt over the losses of the family's previous life-style, their anticipated life-style, and the health of the family member (Kahn, 1990). Ill family members may be unable to return to previous roles, necessitating the emergence of permanent role changes. Old roles may be shifted or discarded, and new roles may develop especially around the physical and emotional care of the ill family member. Minimal opportunity exists for old family patterns of functioning to remain intact. A new definition of normalcy needs to be established.

In the initial efforts to resist changes demanded by the long-term illness, the family's adjustment behaviors may be effective but prove ineffective with time (McCubbin & McCubbin, Chapter 2). Maladjustment and crisis may ensue as a result, indicating the need for adaptive behaviors. Application of the more complex adaptive family behaviors of compromise, synergy (working together for a common good), and interfacing (finding a new "fit" with the community) are needed for family restructuring and consolidation. Family negotiations that use the adaptive behaviors of compromise and synergy may be needed to accomplish role changes. Compromising and interfacing are necessary for realignment of family-community ties and roles. Application of these adaptive behaviors is ongoing as the illness and family life cycle progress.

The duration of a long-term illness stressor can be excessive, lasting through the lifetime of the ill individual and through the reorganization phase for the family after the ill member's death. With some long-term illnesses and disabilities such as Parkinson's disease, multiple sclerosis, cerebral palsy, mental retardation, and spinal cord injury, the illness stressor can endure for 20 years or more. In these situations families cannot postpone responsibilities. A later time to resume responsibilities without the presence of the illness stressor does not exist. The family must deal with the challenges of the illness along with the other daily stressors of life. The family is now more vulnerable to stressor pileup. This pileup often strains family resources leading to maladjustment, family crisis, and unresolved conflicts (McCubbin & McCubbin, Chapter 2). There even may be insufficient time between illness-related stressors and other family crises for the family to reach an equilibrium (Rainsford & Schuman, 1981), thus causing exhaustion and a sense of being overwhelmed.

The duration of an illness stressor also affects family resources. When the length of an illness stressor increases, the possibility that family resources will be depleted and overextended becomes greater (Johnson, 1985; Turk & Kerns, 1985). As resources are exhausted, the threat to the family becomes clear. For example, the high cost of long-term medical care can easily deplete a family's financial reserve. When Bloom, Knorr, and Evans (1985) studied long-term childhood cancer, they found more than one third of the family's gross annual income was spent on the illness. For poorer families the percentage approached 50% (47.97%). Often, additional employment was sought to alleviate the financial burden (Johnson, 1985), which adds further stress to an already stressful situation.

Finances are not the only family resource threatened by a long-term illness stressor. The family's coping skills and energy for buffering against stressors can also be depleted. With long-term illness and disability, family energy for buffering and adjusting / adapting may be expended persistently over time as changes occur in the family and illness situation. The family's ability to buffer and adjust / adapt may be exhausted, leaving its members emotionally and physically drained (Cleveland, 1980/1989; Johnson, 1985; Leventhal et al., 1985). Also, it is likely that the burden of physically and emotionally caring for the ill family member falls almost solely on the family. Caring for the ill member's physical needs is often time consuming (for example, bathing, toileting, dressing, range of motion) and demands skills (for example, urethral catheterizations, injections, postural drainage) that may not be a part of the family's resources. Often, one family member takes on this burden, which can quickly become overwhelming (Cleveland, 1980/1989; Fradkin & Liberti, 1987). This is especially true when the burden of care increases as the disease takes its course.

5   *Onset* of the Stressor: Sudden vs. Gradual

The type of onset of an illness stressor can affect families and their functioning. It influences the meaning families attach to the illness or disability and the family's response. For example, the sudden onset of an illness stressor caused by an accident produces strong emotional and attention-getting reactions from both the patient and family members. The more life-threatening the event, the greater the chance for family crisis (Bahnson, 1989). Even in less severe illness situations, sudden onset of symptoms makes the presence of illness clearly evident; it is obvious that something about the family member has changed. This evident change forces the family to take notice and indicates a possible threat.

With the sudden, threatening onset of illness, the family has little time to investigate or gather information, especially in an accident situation. However, this allows the family to appraise the event at face value. The advantage here is that less family energy is lost in gaining consensus on the definition of the stressor (Montgomery, 1982). The perceived threat defines the event as one requiring family support and action (McCubbin & McCubbin, Chapter 2; Reiss & De-Noir, 1989). As a result, family support and assistance may be readily forthcoming. Mobilization of resources begins in an attempt to buffer and adjust to the threat. The disadvantage caused by this clear definition is the great disruption it produces within the family as, suddenly, resources are mobilized in response to the threat.

The sudden onset of an illness stressor limits the time to develop coping strategies (Bloom, 1985). For example, when cardiac arrest occurs in a family member perceived as healthy, little time is available to gather information vital to family coping and problem-solving. Furthermore, families with little previous illness experience may have poorly developed patterns and coping strategies to meet this kind of situation. They are unprepared to react to the illness and have no time to develop any skills through trial and error. Feelings of disruption and disorganization result, culminating in a sense of lost control and family crisis (Bloom, 1985; Cleveland, 1980/1989). Also, if the family member dies from the cardiac arrest, no anticipatory grief has taken place. Anticipatory grief assists families in dealing with and preparing for a death and may decrease the sense of disorganization (Bozett, 1987).

A gradual onset of illness may produce none of the family behaviors just discussed because the definition of this type of illness is unclear (Hirsch, 1988). This uncertain definition results in a low emotional response making it difficult to establish the need for family support *or* action. The onset can be so gradual that the ill person can make minor adjustments as the symptoms develop. This enables the person to hide the differences, which can then be barely perceivable (Montgomery, 1982).

Examples of the gradual onset of illness are hearing loss in the elderly, mental illness, and alcoholism. Gradual onset of illness with vague, fluctuating symptoms can produce denial (Leventhal et al., 1985). For example, a hearing-impaired family member may deny the very existence of symptoms. Now, mobilizing support and action becomes difficult. Denial creates other family problems, as the family sees the need for action, but the individual refuses to see the problem (see Chapter 3).

The uncertainty of those illnesses with a gradual onset may produce vague anxiety, apprehension, and fearful fantasies (Hirsch, 1988). Families may expend a great deal of energy trying to determine a cause for the symptoms by seeking many opinions and reading widely. When patients with a gradual onset of illness seek medical help, it may be necessary to learn about the fears they have developed around the illness. Understanding these fears can assist in understanding the patient's and family's reaction at the time of diagnosis and also, help in clarifying any misconceptions.

Gradual onset of an illness does not produce the same overwhelming feelings of disorganization as sudden onset. Instead, the family has time to gather information, formulate coping strategies through trial and error, and adjust to new roles and tasks. For example, the gradual onset of an illness such as rheumatoid arthritis gives families time to learn about the illness, gather resources, and adjust to changes, particularly in the ill family member's body image, mobility, and discomfort from the illness. Although family disruption is present, adjustment or adaptation can be gradual, lowering the possibility of overwhelming family stress and crisis.

6 *Control* of the Stressor: Manageable vs. Unmanageable

M. A. McCubbin (1988) states that illness stressors are perceived by families as manageable or unmanageable (cited in McCubbin & McCubbin, Chapter 2). Stressors that appear manageable can contribute positively to the family's sense of control, whereas stressors that appear unmanageable can impact families negatively.

Those families that sense they are in control are less vulnerable to the impact of stressors (McCubbin & McCubbin, 1989). A sense of control assists the family in feeling cohesive and organized. When the family feels in control, more energy is available to buffer against stressors because less family energy is spent trying to establish control. A sense of control also fosters family self-esteem and integrity (McCubbin & McCubbin, Chapter 2). Self-esteem is a coping resource that supports the family's ability to manage stressors and perform other family functions. Family efforts are often aimed at maintaining control to facilitate optimal family functioning.

Studies indicate that a direct inverse relationship exists between a sense of mastery or control and anxiety and depression (Mercer et al., 1986). A decreased sense of control resulting in increased anxiety and depression produce negative effects on family subsystem relationships (Mercer et al., 1986). A lack of communication and understanding hinders the development of cohesive relationships and weakens the family's sense of being held together and organized. The family is now more vulnerable to the effect of stressors.

Illness stressors such as AIDS that appear beyond the family's control often cause disruption and disorganization as attempts are made to bring the situation under control. The family is powerless to postpone or exert control over the course of the illness. The illness has no cure and cannot be resolved except through death, a fear-producing event. This fear can terrorize the family and be a source of disruption and crisis (Leventhal et al., 1985; Walker, 1987). The family often needs tremendous energy to gain control in this situation. Family members may make lavish attempts to find a cure through both medical and nonmedical channels (for example, faith healers, diet). Through this exploration the family attempts to gain control by obtaining information and finding solutions that offer hope. This hope replaces feelings of helplessness, thus fostering some sense of being in control and confident (Kahn, 1990). In these situations the family's ability to have a degree of fatalism (a coping resource) that identifies the situation as being truly beyond their control can be desirable (Olson et al., 1989). Acceptance of this kind of appraisal brings some comfort to the situation.

Some characteristics of diseases contribute to the feeling of being or not being in control. Disease characteristics such as lack of a cure, unknown cause, uncontrollable and progressive deterioration of health, multiple exacerbations and remissions, uncontrollable pain, seizures, and death can contribute to out-of-control feelings and family strain and stress (Ferrari et al., 1983/1985; Leventhal et al., 1985; Rowat & Knafe, 1985). The family may then appraise the situation as unmanageable. Studies of the disease characteristics just listed have shown a high probability of causing depression and anxiety within the family (Ferrari et al., 1983/1985; Rowat & Knafe, 1985; Walker, 1987). These studies verify the relationship between a sense of control and anxiety and depression.

Just as there are many disease characteristics that cause feelings of helplessness and unmanageability, there are also many aspects of the illness situation itself that cause similar feelings. For example, the very essence and definition of illness and the sick role indicate the presence of dependency and helplessness, a sense of lost control (Bloom, 1985). Hospitalization during illness is another good example of losing control (Bozett, 1987; Lovejoy, 1986). On entering the hospital the ill family member is separated from his or her normal routine and normal clothing and from familiar support systems—family and community. Waiting for test results, lacking understanding about the functioning of health services, and noting the apparently poor coordination between health services often cause feelings of lost control. During hospitalization the family has lost control over the care of its family member. Now, the health professional has greater control and often excludes family participation in that care (for example, in intensive care units) or perceives the family as being in the way (Pearlmutter, Locke, Bourdon, Gaffey, & Tyrrell, 1984). In addition, family life and routines are disturbed by visits to the hospital or perhaps by one member remaining at the hospital with the patient. The family has no control over these changes, which are experienced as a necessity and not as a choice.

On the positive side, an illness or disability stressor controlled or resolved successfully can produce family satisfaction and an increased sense of mastery (Mishel, 1990). The family may learn new coping skills, nursing care skills, and health-promotion skills. Because of the success of both old and new coping strategies that were applied to the illness stressor situation, the family may have expanded its repertoire of coping alternatives. Individual family members involved in adjusting, changing, expanding, or developing new roles may have succeeded and grown from the experience. New relationships with increased communication lines may have been developed. As a result, a new sense of closeness and purpose arises. The family is now better equipped and prepared to manage other stressors; its buffering capacity has been expanded. The family has grown from its success and thus increased its sense of mastery.

Characteristics of an illness situation may increase or decrease ability to control or resolve the situation. However, family appraisals of the situation ultimately determine the effect of these characteristics on the family's sense of control (Mishel, 1990). The appraisal depends greatly on the availability of both tangible and intangible (coping) resources. For example, a strep throat is usually a manageable illness in terms of the adequacy of financial resources to meet illness demands. However, a demand-resource imbalance may occur if money is unavailable for doctor visits and medication. The family's appraisal may then consider the situation unmanageable, which can lead to family stress and crisis. Therefore, when assessing families in illness situations, health professionals need to examine the family's appraisal. What may be manageable for one family may be unmanageable for another.

7   *Cause* of the Stressor: Natural, Man-made, or Unknown

In Lipman-Blumen's (1975) original work on crisis and its effect on social systems, the *cause* of a crisis was studied in terms of its emergence from either natural or man-made sources. However, the potential causal factors of illness can be threefold: (1) natural (for example, bacterial or viral infections), (2) man-made (for example, a car accident or man-made chemical source), and (3) unknown (for example, cancer). Illness stressors of unknown cause are particularly important in light of their strong influence on both the family's and society's reaction to the illness situation.

In stressful situations families cope more effectively when they can arrive at explanations (Figley, 1983; Olson et al., 1989). They want to know: (1) what happened, (2) how the event happened, (3) why the event happened, and (4) how they can overcome the undesirable situation. When the cause of an illness is known, as with natural or artificial causes, these questions can be answered. A sense of control is present that enables the family to manage the situation. Information about the cause can be gathered for understanding the situation and the illness's treatment and for planning to prevent reoccurrence. The family then can mobilize its resources in specific directions with predictable outcomes.

Artificial causes of illness elicit some specific family responses. Illnesses or disabilities caused by an artificial agent, such as a car accident, job-related accidents, or exposure to industrial chemicals, often create a great deal of anger and guilt, especially when the situation could have been prevented if others had exercised greater precautions (Flannery, 1990). Lawsuits are common in such situations (Easterbrook, 1987) and provide a channel for the anger and guilt. However, they also absorb a great deal of the family's coping and financial resources. Sometimes this anger is focused toward useful channels such as community movements designed to prevent or control the probability of the reoccurrence of a specific illness or situations that produce illness (Berren et al., 1980/1986). Clearly, family energy focuses intensely on the cause of illness.

When the cause of an illness is unknown, helplessness and loss of control are felt by both the individual and the family. Illnesses of unknown cause, especially those that are fatal, are often socially stigmatized (Leventhal et al., 1985). The unknown component of an illness suggests caution, fear, and avoidance (Walker, 1987). Fear is an emotion that potentially causes family disruption and disorganization (Bahnson, 1987; Leventhal et al., 1985). At the same time the family may feel isolated as society withdraws from these ill individuals and their families because of its fear of the disease (Walker, 1987). This hinders access to support at a time when it is needed most. When the cause of disease is unknown, health-care professionals and families cannot devise plans for successful treatment or prevention of the disease. As a result the health-care professionals, along with the family, may also feel helpless, frustrated, and angry (Murray & Zenter, 1985).

Tuberculosis (TB) is a disease that demonstrates how an unknown cause affects the appraisal of an illness and how this changes when the cause becomes known and a cure found. Years ago the cause of TB was unknown and much fear surrounded the disease because it was fatal. The illness was strongly associated with the lower social class, as it spread rapidly in poorly ventilated, close living quarters. Individuals with the disease were isolated from their families and society in sanitariums for "treatment" and often were there for life.

The cause of TB is now known and its contagiousness understood. Effective methods of treatment and detection have been developed. Families do not panic when a family member is diagnosed with TB. Ill individuals do not have to be separated from their families and society but can receive treatment in the hospital and then at home. Overwhelming fear and isolation are no longer part of the disease. The disease can be managed and controlled through the patient's and family's cooperation with medical treatment.

8   *Predictability* of the Stressor: Predictable vs. Uncertain

An illness stressor that occurs unexpectedly and progresses randomly can have a more serious impact on the family than one that is predictable. Predictable stressors seldom cause family crisis, since families can predict the occurrence and progression of the stressor and plan for the responsibilities and changes (Montgomery, 1982). However, random events allow little time for adjustment and acceptance of change (Mishel, 1990). Illnesses often have uncertain components. To be prepared for all possible uncertainties in an illness situation, the family would need to develop a wide range of coping mechanisms that would meet all possible situations. This is an impossible, unrealistic task for any family.

Several studies of illness events demonstrated the significant role uncertainty plays in causing psychological distress and disruption in important life areas (Ferrari et al., 1983/1985; Mishel, 1988; Rowat & Knafe, 1985). Rowat and Knafe (1985) studied ill individuals with uncontrollable, random pain and the effect this situation had on spouses. The randomness of the pain caused an uncertain family life. When would the pain occur? Where would the family be when it occurred? Would the situation be embarrassing? Would they have to leave the place where they were? Would they be able to control the pain this time? This uncertainty caused anxiety derived from the sense of helplessness and loss of control (see Control of the Stressor).

Rowat and Knafe's study also found the uncertainty of the situation rendered the spouse impotent in managing the pain. Eighty-five percent of the spouses were aware of what increased the pain, yet fewer than 50% attempted to alter the situation with direct physical action. They were uncertain about how to go about helping because none of their developed strategies had worked *all* the time. They also feared doing more harm than good in their attempts to relieve the pain.

In another study designed to document illness-specific family adjustment problems, Ferrari, Matthews, and Barabas (1983/1985) examined the role predictability plays in the impact of illness on the family. Fifteen families with a 9-year-old epileptic child were compared with a similar number of families with a 9-year-old diabetic child and a control group with a healthy 9 year old. They hypothesized that the uncertainty of epileptic seizures caused feelings of helplessness that would generalize to other parts of family life. To show that the psychosocial variables were related specifically to the uncertainty of the seizures and were not just a function of chronic disease, they compared families with an epileptic child with families with a diabetic child. They believed that diabetes had more predictable characteristics that the family could control.

The findings of the study demonstrated that the families of epileptic children had a diminished self-concept when compared with the other groups. The epileptic children perceived themselves as being a problem to the family, having fewer parental expectations demanded of them, and having poor sibling relationships. The family was less close than the others, with poorer intrafamilial communication. A chronic illness with unpredictable characteristics like epilepsy appeared to put a family at risk for poor communication, poor cohesiveness, and poor integration.

A critical examination of this study points out that health professionals should look for the interplay of dimensions within an illness stressor. For example, the stigma of an illness can produce poor family communication (Leventhal et al., 1985). The stigma of epilepsy, rather than the uncertainty of the seizures, may be primarily responsible for poor family communication. Further research is needed to confirm this. When assessing potential family adjustment problems, the health professional needs to examine all the dimensions of the illness stressor and determine which of those seem problematic for the family.

Ferrari et al.'s study also demonstrates several other important points for the health professional. An illness dimension such as predictability can affect family behavior in specific and predictable ways. The illness dimension can give health professionals cues to look for specific family behaviors in specific types of illness. Vigilance in assessing family behaviors linked with interventions to prevent and manage maladaptive behaviors can then be instituted proactively in illness situations that have the potential for causing family difficulty. However, this is not meant to imply the existence of unquestioningly predictable family responses to specific types of illness. Each family's response is unique. In fact, families that do not view a particular illness dimension as a problem and appraise the situation in a positive light may respond in different and more positive ways.

Evidence of this more positive response to uncertainty is recently being uncovered by investigators (King & Mishel, 1986; Mishel & Murdaugh, 1987; Mishel, 1988). In chronic illness situations the longer the ill individual lives with continual uncertainty the more positive the appraisal of the situation can become (King & Mishel, 1986). Uncertainty produces personal growth and more complex orientations and appraisals concerning life (Mishel, 1990). A new ability develops to concentrate on multiple alternatives and choices. Fragility and lack of permanence in situations are appreciated as challenges. The appraisal surrounding uncertainty is altered from *danger* to *opportunity*.

Mishel (1990) states that support from health-care professionals can be a factor influencing the growth of this positive orientation. These studies reiterate the importance family appraisal plays in influencing family response and the need for practitioners to seek out the family appraisal as a clue to patient and family behaviors. These studies also support Palazzoli's (1985) proposal that a patient's response to illness is more strongly linked to the family's response than to the condition itself (cited Wright & Leahey, 1987).

9   *Resource Demands* of the Stressor: Great vs. Small

The importance of family resources when confronting an illness stressor should not be underestimated. In fact, the prominent role resources play in a family's ability to deal with stressors is clearly depicted in the Resiliency Model of Family Stress, Adjustment, and Adaptation. Here, resources—B,

BB, and BBB — stand as components underscored three times in the model (Fig. 4-2).

The Resiliency Model demonstrates that tangible, coping, and social support resources can make a difference to families managing stressors. The perceived balance between stressor demands and resources determines the family's appraisal and response (McCubbin & McCubbin, Chapter 2). With illness stressors it is evident that families with many resources are often more capable of handling the strain caused by illness than those with few resources (Dunst et al., 1988; Johnson, 1985; McCubbin & McCubbin, Chapter 2).

Resources within the context of this book include tangible resources, strengths and coping capabilities within the family, as well as social support (McCubbin & McCubbin, Chapter 2). Since money, a tangible resource, is often ignored in discussions about families dealing with illness, this portion of this chapter focuses on financial resources. This is not meant to downplay the importance of coping capacities and social support; even in the presence of small financial resources the coping capacity of the family and social support can be forces that maintain family stability and prevent crisis (Voydanoff & Majka, 1988). However, family coping strategies useful during illness are discussed in detail in Chapter 5, and the prominent role of social support is highlighted in Chapter 8.

Of the tangible resources a family may possess, money is considered one of the most critical for family adjustment and adaptation (McCubbin & McCubbin, Chapter 2). In studies that recognize the financial burden of illness, money to pay medical bills is cited as a source of stress in the family (Hennen et al., 1987; Johnson, 1985; M.A. McCubbin & H.I. McCubbin, 1989; Olson et al., 1989; Rowat & Knafe, 1985). Even wealthy families with good insurance benefits can become financially depleted, if not exhausted, by the high cost of catastrophic or long-term health care (Hennen et al., 1987). In addition, hospitalization of a family member can impart family expenses beyond medical costs. Families can accumulate extra expenses for transportation of family members to and from the hospital (for example, gas, bus, taxi), for parking fees, for the care of children left at home, and for meals away from home. Often, families with low financial resources lack phone service; without a phone these families may lack a communication lifeline that is vital to handling chronic and life-threatening illness.

Money is a tangible resource necessary for providing the family with basic needs — food, shelter, and clothing. A financial threat is therefore a

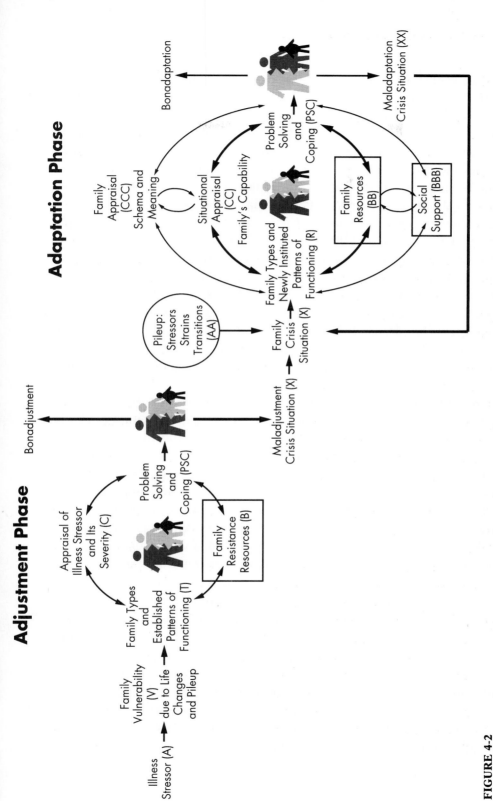

FIGURE 4-2

Adjustment Phase and Adaptation Phase of the Resiliency Model of Family Stress, Adjustment, and Adaptation. The three levels of resources B/BB/BBB play a prominent role in the family's management of stressors.

threat that strikes the very core of family stability and potentially affects every family member. Illness that threatens family income capacity may increase the level of stress and family disruption (Leventhal et al., 1985; Voydanoff & Donnelly, 1988). Since families often pool their resources to meet catastrophic health costs (Wyszewianski, 1986), this burden can extend beyond the nuclear family and also affect the extended family.

The amount of stress generated by the financial burden of illness depends on the family's view of its financial resources and the perceived degree of threat to that resource (McCubbin & McCubbin, Chapter 2). If the capacity is seen as great and the threat small, the stress generated is usually minimal. The ability to meet financial demands can contribute to the family's capacity to have control over the illness situation (Johnson, 1985). Adequate finances therefore may contribute to the family's sense of mastery and control. Stress occurs if financial resources are considered inadequate or are drained (Voydanoff & Donnelly, 1988). The sense of control vital to family functioning is lost.

Strong financial resources also help prevent pileup of demands, especially with long-term health problems requiring home care and expensive equipment. Adequate financial resources not only decrease family stress but also allow the family to purchase equipment and to obtain outside sources of support for the physical care of the ill member and emotional support for the whole family. Money can provide respite for a family caregiver or even relieve the entire family from the responsibility of direct care with around-the-clock nursing care. Moreover, finances available for relaxing and entertaining activities decrease the sense of isolation that may be felt by families during chronic illness (Hennen et al., 1987). Financial flexibility may create less need for change within the family and prevent family members from becoming overwhelmed by the burdens of illness. Family energies then can be applied to the usual tasks instead of being consumed by illness demands. The opportunities for demand pileup may decrease. However, when families try to increase their financial resources to meet illness demands, problems can arise. For example, McCollum (1971) found that families attempting to improve their financial base through supplemental employment may experience pileup because of limited time left to spend with family members (cited in Johnson, 1985).

Even when the community offers financial assistance and provides free or inexpensive resources, families with weak financial resources do not tend to take advantage of the situation because of pride or a lack of knowledge

(Hennen et al., 1987). Ironically, upper-class families are the ones that know of and use these resources. Therefore health-care professionals should explore the family's financial situation and assess its ability to carry the illness burden. Furthermore, health professionals need to increase awareness of free, inexpensive community resources and sources of financial support for lower- and middle-income families. This not only assists the family in dealing with the illness stressor but also it provides the health practitioner with an opportunity to understand another source of family stress in illness situations.

10   *Stigma* of the Stressor: Great vs. Small

An ill family member is medically classified at diagnosis (Wright & Leahey, 1987). This act "spurs off a process of social classification which may often have a limiting or forbidding effect on the patient's previous social participation" (Gerhardt, 1985, p. 192). The ill family member is now considered to deviate from the normal. This stigmatized social role dominates the ill family member's life and pervades the life of the family (Turk & Kerns, 1985).

Within society and a family's schema, illness labels display a wide range of stigmatization. The stigmatized definitions and meanings of different illnesses help to formulate and contribute to individual and family appraisals of illness situations (McCubbin & McCubbin, Chapter 2; Turk & Kerns, 1985). The greater the stigma attached to an illness label the greater its opportunity to negatively influence the family's appraisal and subsequent responses. For example, cancer, AIDS, mental illness, epilepsy, and mental retardation are illness labels with strong negative connotations. These labels produce strong emotional reactions that can lead to family disruption and potential crisis (Gerhardt, 1985; Priestman, 1986; Walker, 1987). In the late 1970s West wrote that physicians treating someone with epilepsy sometimes withheld the diagnosis because of the stigma and its expected family response (cited in Gerhardt, 1985).

Many negative illness labels imply family shame. This shame can be deleterious to self-esteem, an important resource for optimal family functioning. Mental illness is an example of an illness stressor that may produce family shame. The mentally ill are often shunned and regarded with little sympathy (Anderson & Holder, 1989; Chesla, 1989). As a result, families with a mentally ill member develop a sense of shame, guilt, and fear.

Some theories of mental illness place blame or source for the illness on the family. For example, Singer and Wynne (1965) and Wynne (1981) demonstrated that family communication patterns were significantly related to the psychiatric disorder of schizophrenia and its degree of severity (cited in Chesla, 1989). This research validates the family systems therapy approach that theorizes the presence of a multigenerational emotional process that transfers from generation to generation family relationship systems. Theories such as this reinforce the shame that families feel and may bring families to decline therapy that could benefit the patient and help the family deal with the illness label (Anderson & Holder, 1989). Families tend to go to great lengths to hide the illness or explain away the abnormal behavior. The strain of nondisclosure sets a dramatic tone that raises the family stress level and sets up barriers to communication (Leventhal et al., 1985; Chesla, 1989). Communication barriers then prevent development of strong and open intrafamilial relationships and hinder family problem-solving.

AIDS is another highly stigmatized illness that causes feelings of family shame and fear (Musto, 1987; Walker, 1987). The fear of AIDS is derived from many of the characteristics of the disease: it is contagious, incurable, and fatal. This fear coupled with the stigmatization of homosexuality or drug abuse associated with this illness, causes devastating disruptive effects on the family (Walker, 1987). Some families, because of their own family schema, may believe the disease is an act of punishment from God. Others feel responsible because they did not somehow prevent the family member from getting AIDS. This family disruption is then magnified by the isolation promoted by both the family's shame and societal avoidance of the feared disease. In the extreme situation the ill family member may be banished from the family. This ostracism is potent. The stigma of AIDS clearly sets the stage for family stress and crisis.

Families with highly stigmatized illnesses are confronted with a sense of isolation derived from many sources. Families, their friends, and their community can have difficulty relating to family members with illnesses such as cancer, AIDS, or severe disabilities (Aadalen & Strobel-Khan, 1981/1989; Leventhal et al., 1985; see Chapter 11). As people approach families with such illnesses or disabilities, they are afraid of upsetting them or are unable to handle their own feelings about the illness or disability. Because of this, defenses on both sides act as a barrier to meaningful communication. This behavior is not limited to nonmedical individuals. In a breast cancer clinic, Macguire (cited in Gerhardt, 1985) studied nursing staff interactions with patients. He found that nurses made light of or ignored verbal and nonverbal clues offered by patients to discuss feelings. The patients then felt it was inappropriate to express feelings. Gerhardt (1985) attributed this to the inability of hospital staff to face the patient's distress because they themselves were often anxious about the diagnosis. These behaviors promote a sense of isolation in patients and their families that serves to intensify the stress generated by the illness. At the same time it blocks pathways to social support.

✦ CONCLUSION

This discussion has artificially classified the dimensions of illness stressors to identify each dimension and its accompanying family responses. Awareness of these dimensions and related family responses may enable health professionals to predict the possibility of family stress and crisis in illness situations. It also may assist in understanding family behaviors during certain types of illnesses. With knowledge of the relation between the dimensions of illness and family responses, interventions can be developed and implemented for the different types of illness situations. It is possible to create interventions for these illness situations that empower families to prevent and manage stress and crisis.

Illness situations usually encompass at least three or more of the dimensions discussed, plus family situational factors. The combination of dimensions in an illness stressor contributes to the variety and complexity of family responses to illness situations. Usually, those dimensions that demand the most change and adaptation cause the greatest amount of family strain, stress, and potential for crisis. However, the dimensions of the illness stressors are not the sole determinant of family responses. The ultimate key to determining the direction of a family's responses is the family's situational appraisal that governs which, if any, of the illness dimensions are problematic to the family (McCubbin & McCubbin, Chapter 2). Family situational appraisal has this influence because it encompasses input from multiple sources: appraisal of the illness stressor, family vulnerability (pileup and family life cycle stage) at the time, presence of resources, previous experiences with illness, and the family schema and meaning given to the illness. Therefore, when health-care professionals assess the impact of an illness on the family, they must look carefully at both the potential for problems derived from the illness's dimensions and for the appraisal the family attaches to the illness situation.

Although this chapter tends to focus on the negative effects of illness on the family, the opportunity for both individual and family growth during an illness event is present. Family members have the opportunity to expand roles, accept new responsibilities, and learn new organizational and nursing care skills. The family as a whole may become more cohesive, establishing new relationships and strengthening communication lines. The health-care professional is in a powerful position to enhance and reinforce that growth. To enhance family growth in illness situations, practitioners also need to be aware of family strengths and coping strategies used by families who grow from illness experiences. This knowledge of successful family coping enables the health-care professional to identify and foster those positive coping behaviors. The following chapter identifies positive coping strategies used by families that successfully cope with illness.

REFERENCES

Aadalen, S. P., & Stroebel-Kahn, F. (1989). Coping with quadriplegia. In R. H. Moos (Ed.), *Coping with physical illness: Vol. 2. New perspectives* (pp. 73-188). New York: Plenum. (Reprinted from *American Journal of Nursing*, 1981, *81*(8), 1471-1478)

Aguilera, D. C. (1990). *Crisis intervention: Theory and methodology* (6th ed.). St. Louis: Mosby–Year Book.

Anderson, C. M., & Holder, D. P. (1989). Family systems and behavioral disorders: Schizophrenia, depression, and alcoholism. In C. N. Ramsey (Ed.), *Family systems in medicine* (pp. 487-502). New York: Guilford.

Bahnson, C. B. (1987). The impact of life-threatening illness on the family and the impact of the family on illness: An overview. In M. Leahey & L. M. Wright (Eds.), *Families and life-threatening illness* (pp. 26-44). Springhouse, PA: Springhouse.

Berren, M., Beigel, A., & Ghertner, S. (1986). A typology for the classification of disasters. In R. H. Moos (Ed.), *Coping with life crisis: An integrated approach* (pp. 295-305). New York: Plenum. (Reprinted from *Community Mental Health Journal*, 1980, *16*, 103-111)

Black, R. B., & Weiss, J. O. (1988). A professional partnership with genetic support groups. *American Journal of Medical Genetics*, *29*, 21-33.

Bloom, B. (1985). *Stressful life event theory and research: Implications for primary prevention*. Rockville, MD: United States Department of Health and Human Services.

Bloom, B. S., Knorr, R. S., & Evans, A. E. (1985). The epidemiology of disease expenses: The cost of caring for children with cancer. *Journal of the American Medical Association*, *253*(16), 2393-2397.

Bozett, F. (1987). Family nursing and life-threatening illness. In M. Leahey & L. M. Wright (Eds.), *Families and life-threatening illness* (pp. 2-25). Springhouse, PA: Springhouse.

Chesla, C. (1989). Mental illness and the family. In C. Gilliss, B. Highley, B. Roberts, & I. Martinson (Eds.), Toward a science of family nursing (pp. 374-393). Menlo Park, CA: Addison-Wesley.

Cleveland, M. (1989). Family adaptation to traumatic spinal cord injury—response to crisis. In R. H. Moos (Ed.), *Coping with physical illness: Vol. 2. New perspectives* (2nd ed., pp. 159-171). New York: Plenum. (Reprinted from *Family Relations*, 1980, *29*(4), 558-565)

Dunst, C. J., Trivette, C. M., & Deal, A. G. (1988). *Enabling and empowering families: Principles and guidelines for practice.* Cambridge, MA: Brookline.

Easterbrook, G. (1987, Jan. 26). The revolution. *Newsweek*, pp. 40-74.

Ferrari, M., Matthews, W. S., & Barabas, G. (1985). The family and the child with epilepsy. In D. H. Olson (Ed.), *Family studies: Review yearbook* (Vol. 3, pp. 63-69). Beverly Hills, CA: Sage. (Reprinted from *Family Process*, 1983, *22*, 53-59)

Figley, C. (1983). Catastrophes: An overview of family reactions. In C. Figley & H. I. McCubbin (Eds.), *Stress and the family: Vol. 2. Coping with catastrophe* (pp. 3-20). New York: Brunner/Mazel.

Flannery, J. (1990). Guilt: A crisis within. *Journal of Neuroscience Nursing, 22*(2), 92-99.

Fradkin, L., & Liberti, M. (1987). Caregiving. In P. Doress & D. Siegal (Eds.), *Ourselves growing older* (pp. 198-212). New York: Simon & Schuster.

Gaynor, S. E. (1990). The long haul: The effects of home care on caregivers. *Image: Journal of Nursing Scholarship, 22*(4), 208-212.

Gerhardt, U. E. (1985). Stress and stigma: Explanation of illness. In U. E. Gerhardt & M. E. Wadsworth (Eds.), *Stress and stigma: Explanation and evidence in the sociology of crime and illness* (pp. 161-204). New York: St. Martin's.

Hennen, B. K. (1987). The family and stress. In D. B. Shires, B. K. Hennen, & D. I. Rice (Eds.), *Family medicine: A guidebook for practitioners of the art* (2nd ed., pp. 37-41). New York: McGraw-Hill.

Hennen, B. K., Seitz, M., & Seitz, B. (1987). The chronically disabled child and the family. In D. B. Shires, B. K. Hennen, & D. I. Rice (Eds.), *Family medicine: A guidebook for practitioners of the art* (2nd ed., pp. 42-50). New York: McGraw-Hill.

Hirsch, L. L. (1988). Problem differentiation. In R. B. Taylor (Ed.), *Family medicine* (3rd ed., pp. 58-65). New York: Springer-Verlag.

Johnson, S. B. (1985). The family and the child with chronic illness. In D. C. Turk & R. D. Kerns (Eds.), *Health, illness, and families: A life span perspective* (pp. 220-254). New York: John Wiley & Sons.

Kahn, A. M. (1990). Coping with fear and grieving. In I. M. Lubkin (Ed.), *Chronic illness: Impact and interventions* (2nd ed., pp. 65-85). Boston: Jones & Bartlett.

Kaplan, D. M., Smith, A., Grobstein, R., & Fischman, S. E. (1977). Family mediation of stress. In R. H. Moos (Ed.), *Coping with physical illness* (pp. 81-96). New York: Plenum. (Reprinted from *Social Work*, 1973, *18*, 60-69)

King, B., & Mishel, M. (1986, April). *Uncertainty appraisal and management in chronic illness.* Paper presented at the Nineteenth Communicating Nursing Research Conference, Western Society for Research in Nursing, Portland, Oregon.

Kosten, T. R., Jacob, S. C., & Kasl, S. V. (1985). Terminal illness, bereavement, and the family. In D. C. Turk & R. D. Kerns (Eds.), *Health, illness, and families* (pp. 311-337). New York: John Wiley & Sons.

Larkin, J. (1987). Factors influencing one's ability to adapt to chronic illness. In V. A. Lambert & C. E. Lambert (Eds.), *Adaptation to chronic illness: Nursing Clinics of North America, 22*(3), 335-342.

Leavitt, M. B. (1989). Transition to illness: The family in the hospital. In C. Gilliss, B. Highley, B. Roberts, & I. Martin (Eds.), *Toward a science of family nursing* (pp. 262-283). Menlo Park, CA: Addison-Wesley.

Leventhal, H., Leventhal, E. A., & Van Nguyen, T. (1985). Reactions of families to illness: Theoretical models and perspectives. In D. C. Turk & R. D. Kerns (Eds.), *Health, illness, and families* (pp. 108-145). New York: John Wiley & Sons.

Lipman-Blumen, J. (1975). A crisis framework applied to macrosociological family changes: Marriage, divorce, occupational trends associated with World War II. *Journal of Marriage and the Family, 3,* 889-902.

Lovejoy, N. (1986). Family response to cancer hospitalization. *Oncology Nursing Forum, 13*(2), 33-37.

McCubbin, H. I., & McCubbin, M. A. (1987). Family assessment in health care. In H. I. McCubbin & A. I. Thompson (Eds.), *Family assessment: Interventions for research and practice* (pp. 53-78). Madison, WI: University of Wisconsin–Madison Press.

McCubbin, H. I., & Thompson, A. I. (1987). Family typologies and family assessment. In H. I. McCubbin & A. I. Thompson (Eds.), *Family assessment: Interventions for research and practice* (pp. 35-49). Madison, WI: University of Wisconsin–Madison Press.

McCubbin, M. A., & McCubbin, H. I. (1987). Family stress theory and assessment: the T-Double ABCX model of family adjustment and adaptation. In H. I. McCubbin & A. I. Thompson (Eds.), *Family assessment: Interventions for research and practice* (pp. 3-32). Madison, WI: University of Wisconsin–Madison Press.

McCubbin, M. A., & McCubbin, H. I. (1989). Theoretical orientations to family stress and coping. In C. Figley (Ed.), *Treating stress in families* (pp. 3-43). New York: Brunner/Mazel.

Mercer, R. T., May, K. A., Ferketich, S., & DeJoseph, J. (1986). Theoretical models for studying the effect of antepartum stress on the family. *Nursing Research, 35*(6), 339-346.

Mishel, M. H. (1988, April). Coping with uncertainty in illness situations. *Proceedings of Conference: Stress, coping process, and health outcomes: New directions in theory development and research* (pp. 51-84). Rochester: Sigma Theta Tau International, Epsilon Xi chapter, University of Rochester.

Mishel, M. H. (1990). Reconceptualization of the uncertainty in illness theory. *Image: Journal of Nursing Scholarship, 22*(4), 256-262.

Mishel, M. H., & Murdaugh, C. L. (1987). Family experiences with heart transplantation: Redesigning the dream. *Nursing Research, 36*(6), 332-338.

Montgomery, J. (1982). *Family crisis as process: Persistence and change.* Washington, DC: University Press.

Murray, R. B., & Zenter, J. P. (1985). *Nursing concepts for health promotion.* Englewood Cliffs, NJ: Prentice-Hall.

Musto, D. (1987, April 28). Aids and panic: Enemies within. *Wall Street Journal*, 7.

Olson, D., McCubbin, H. I., Barnes, H., Larsen, A., Muxen, M., & Wilson, M. (1989). *Families: What makes them work* (2nd ed.). Newbury Park, CA: Sage.

Pearlmutter, D. R., Locke, A., Bourdon, S., Gaffey, G., & Tyrrell, R. (1984). Models of family-centered care in one acute care institution. *Nursing Clinics of North America, 19*(1), 173-188.

Priestman, T. J. (1986). Impact of diagnosis on the patient. In B. A. Stoll (Ed.), *Coping with cancer stress* (pp. 21-27). Boston: Martinus Nijhoff.

Rainsford, G. L., & Schuman, S. H. (1981). The family in crisis—A case study of overwhelming illness and stress. *Journal of the American Medical Association, 246*(1), 60-63.

Reiss, D., & De-Noir, A. K. (1989). The family and medical team: a transactional and developmental perspective. In C. N. Ramsey (Ed.), *Family systems in medicine* (pp. 435-444). New York: Guilford.

Rowat, K. M., & Knafe, K. A. (1985). Living with chronic pain: The spouse's perspective. *Pain, 3*, 259-271.

Seyle, H. (1956). *Stress of life.* New York: McGraw-Hill.

Steinbauer, J. R. (1989). Spinal injury: Impact and implications for family medicine research. In C. N. Ramsey (Ed.), *Family systems in medicine* (pp. 458-468). New York: Guilford.

Stone, R., Cafferata, G. L., & Sangl, J. (1987). Caregivers of the fragile elderly: A national profile. *Gerontologist, 28*(5), 616-626.

Turk, D. C., & Kerns, R. D. (1985). The family in health and illness. In D. C. Turk & R. D. Kerns (Eds.), *Health, illness, and families* (pp. 108-145). New York: John Wiley & Sons.

Turnbull, H. R., & Turnbull, A. P. (1985). *Parents speak out: Then and now* (2nd ed.). Columbus, OH: Charles E. Merrill.

Voydanoff, P., & Donnelly, B. W. (1988). Economic distress, family coping and quality of family life. In P. Voydanoff & L. Majka (Eds.), *Families and economic distress: Coping strategies and social policy* (pp. 97-115). Newbury Park, CA: Sage.

Walker, C. (1988). Stress and coping in siblings of childhood cancer patients. *Nursing Research, 37*(4), 208-212.

Walker, L. A. (1987, June 21). What comforts AIDS families. *New York Times Magazine*, 16-22, 63, 78.

Wright, L. M., & Leahey, M. (1987). Families and life-threatening illness: assumptions, assessment, and intervention. In M. Leahey & L. M. Wright (Eds.), *Families and life-threatening illness.* Springhouse, PA: Springhouse.

Wyszewianski, L. (1986). Families with catastrophic health expenditures. *Health Services Research, 21*(5), 617-632.

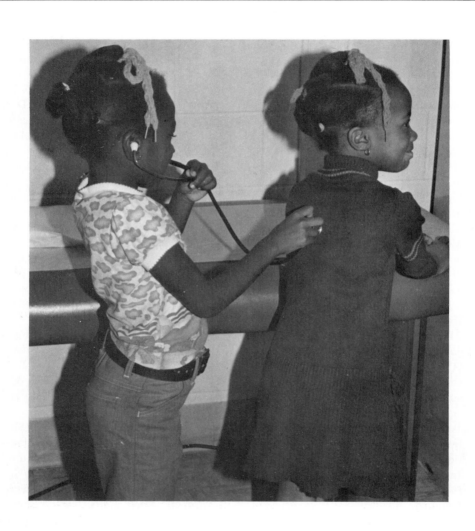

5

Family Coping with Health and Illness: A Critical Link

✦

CHAPTER GOALS

✦ To review the literature that establishes the link between adaptive and maladaptive coping with health and illness

✦ To describe characteristics of family functioning that are important for successful coping during health and illness

✦ To discuss the potentially negative effects of family vulnerability and maladaptive coping characteristics on the course of an illness

✦ To examine some cultural, ethnic, and racial variations in family coping styles and their impact on health and illness

OVERVIEW

THIS chapter first reviews pertinent literature that establishes the link between adaptive and maladaptive family coping with health and illness, and then describes characteristics of family functioning that are important for successful coping with health and illness. Included are family vulnerabilities and potentially negative effects that maladaptive family coping can have on the course of an illness. Also examined are some of the cultural, ethnic, and racial variations in family coping styles that influence health-seeking and illness behaviors. Identifying these different coping behaviors helps health-care professionals understand patient behaviors and heightens their awareness of situations with potentially positive and negative effects on the course of the illness. Within the framework of the Resiliency Model of Family Stress, Adjustment, and Adaptation, this chapter focuses on the adaptation phase of the model (Fig. 5-1).

✦ ADAPTIVE FAMILY CHARACTERISTICS

The family's health is partially defined by the family's effectiveness in meeting family and individual needs. Some characteristics of family functioning that are important for successful coping with health and illness are drawn from societal sources and some are unique to the family. A variety of behaviors can be used for successful coping.

Sedgwick (1981) identifies the healthy role of the family as significant for successful coping with specific behaviors. She describes the role of the family as information gatherer. The family makes and implements decisions; it resolves conflict and provides for the individual growth and development of its members. The family creates an emotional context that fosters self-disclosure, trust, cooperation, and acceptance among its members. Finally, it engages in productive and adaptive activities with regard to internal needs and societal expectations. These are essential activities for effective family functioning and can be applied universally to families as role criteria for health.

Friedman (1986) also describes a number of coping strategies that include both internal and external mechanisms. The successful family knows how to use the coping mechanism most appropriate for the problem presented. Finally, DeChesney and Magnuson (1988) describe open communication, mutual respect and support, differentiation (the balance between intellectual and emotional systems), shared problem solving, shared decision making, flexibility, and enhancement of personal growth as characteristic of healthy family actions.

Additional characteristics for adaptive family coping with illness have been identified by Kennedy (1982) and can also be summarized from the following discussion on differentiation of self. Kennedy points out that families that deal constructively with illness or hospitalization are those that rally around to support the ill member through the illness experience. They are nurturing, attentive, and characterized by "thereness." This behavioral response may facilitate the patient's acceptance of dependency and regression as integral to the sick role. If this behavior is carried to excess

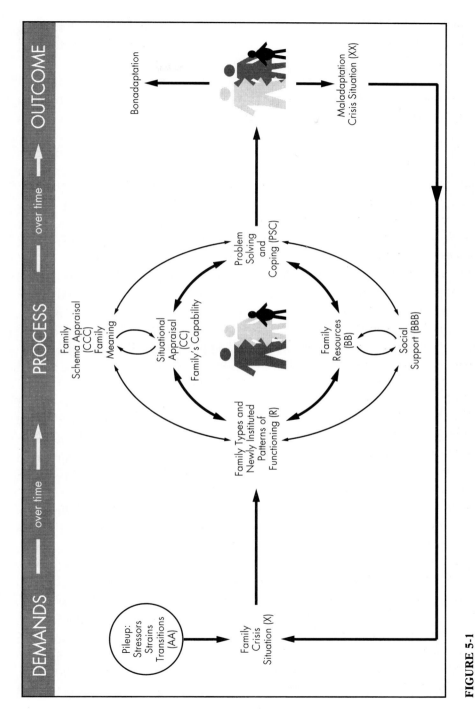

FIGURE 5-1

Adaptation Phase of the Resiliency Model of Family Stress, Adjustment, and Adaptation. This chapter focuses on the family's coping capabilities that involve all components of the Adaptation Phase of the Resiliency Model.

the family's support may interfere with the patient's movement toward health, especially if family members fail to encourage efforts toward independence.

Bowen (1978) identified characteristics of adaptive family coping with illness. These characteristics demonstrate a high level of differentiation within and between members; that is, there is a balance between emotionalism and intellectualism in the family system. The family has a low level of anxiety overall. It is flexible, spontaneous, and goal-directed in its decisions. Finally, role structures are not rigid. Hansen's (1981) research findings with normal families validate the characteristics of well-differentiated persons. She found that families that functioned better operated on a more spontaneous basis. Parents were clearly in charge, yet flexible. These families were more involved in community affairs and friendships.

People with a good level of differentiation balance emotional and intellectual systems and are less anxious. They are flexible and make good decisions. Structural aspects of family life, such as parental roles, are not rigid. They relax, enjoy life, and have a sense of humor, yet care deeply enough about changes in relationships to challenge them. Children in these families are treated as unique individuals and are given support and leadership in achieving their full potential.

People with high levels of differentiation are rare. They enjoy rich emotional lives, appreciate the unique personalities of others, and freely engage them in shared pursuits. Children in these families are given much freedom to develop their own personalities. Even so, well-differentiated persons can potentially function poorly during stress, especially if residual chronic anxiety surfaces.

A study of 60 couples conducted by Richards (1989) supports Bowen's theory that the functioning of the family system is directly related to the functioning of the individual and that the married couple must be compatible for effective family functioning. When using Bowen's theory of the family system, Heiney (1988) suggests it is crucial to assess family conflict coping styles, the place of the child in the family framework, levels of dependence and self-esteem, and rigid relationships within the family.

The Resiliency Model of Family Stress, Adjustment, and Adaptation further delineates the differences in family capability to cope with the impact of a stressor such as illness (McCubbin & McCubbin, Chapter 2). Based on research with healthy families, the Resiliency Model has as its goal the description of the variability of family adaptation following change or crisis (Mercier, 1989). The Resiliency Model depicts adaptive family characteristics as the family's resources (strengths, capabilities, and social support), the family's appraisals (situational and schema), the family's typology and its resiliency, the presence of pileup, and the family's problem-solving capabilities.

According to this model as described in Chapter 2, families that adapt successfully to an illness situation have the following characteristics:

1. Resources that meet the demands of the illness
2. Form a positive appraisal of the stressor event
3. Typologies (such as balanced or regenerative families) with characteristics that successfully meet demands of the specific illness
4. Low in vulnerability, pileup, and life cycle stressors
5. Good problem-solving capabilities

The Resiliency Model highlights family typologies as determinants of predictable family patterns of behavior (McCubbin & McCubbin, Chapter 2). These patterns explain how the family system functions and behaves. These patterns can change as a family matures or adaptation is needed. However, the patterns are particularly evident at times of crisis and can help health-care professionals understand family behavior. The patterns also can predict areas wherein the family will have problems in coping.

Family typologies highlight those family characteristics that provide more successful adjustment and adaptation to stress. Olson, Russell, and Sprenkle (1983) described 16 family typologies. In their scheme, depicted in Fig. 5-2, families with moderate amounts of cohesiveness and adaptability (balanced families) are more successful in adjusting to stressors.

In the typologies developed by McCubbin and McCubbin (1989), families high in hardiness, coherence, flexibility, and bonding, as well as those that value and participate in family time and routines, were considered stronger and more capable of enduring stress. Additionally, such families recover more easily from the impact of stressors and reestablish family patterns of predictability and stability. The *regenerative*, the *resilient*, and the *rhythmic* family typologies are depicted in Fig. 5-3.

During a health crisis the family struggles to balance its demands and resources at both the individual-family and the family-community levels of family functioning. Consider the Roberts family as an example. Suppose Bob Roberts sustains a knee injury while playing tennis and the prescribed

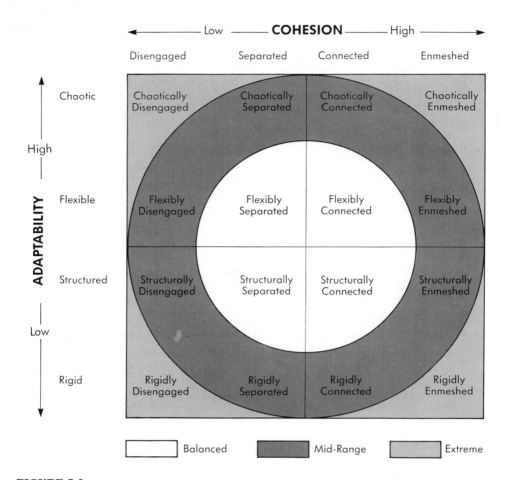

FIGURE 5-2
Circumplex Model of 16 family typologies.
(From Olson, D.H., Russell, C.S., and Sprenkle D.H. (1983). Circumplex model VI: Theoretical update. *Family Process*, *22*, 69-83.)

treatment is surgery followed by 6 weeks of no weight-bearing on the affected leg. Bob is the primary breadwinner for the family. He has paid sick leave for 2 weeks; therefore the family will be without his income for 4 weeks. To prevent a crisis or disruption during Bob's illness, the Roberts must first seek a balance between individual family members' needs and those of the family itself. The Roberts need to respond to a temporary change in roles and must find an alternative source of income.

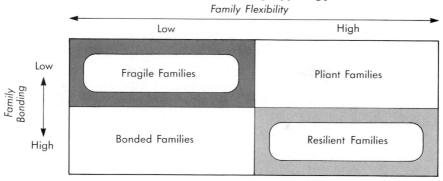

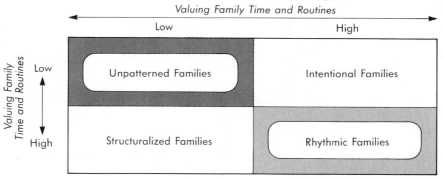

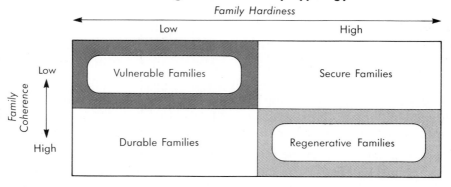

FIGURE 5-3
Three family typologies.
(From McCubbin, H.I., McCubbin, M.A. (1989). Theoretical orientations to family stress and coping. In C.R. Figley (Ed.), *Treating stress in families*. New York: Brunner/Mazel.)

To meet these demands, Nancy gets a job and Bob supervises the children, who participate more in meal preparation and house chores and become more independent. On a second level, a balance must be sought between the Roberts family and the community. The family and the work community may compete for family members' time and involvement. The fact that Nancy will be working outside the home may precipitate an imbalance if family demands increase. The new arrangement may make it difficult to provide adequate child care. In-laws may voice disapproval of Nancy working outside the home. Nancy and Bob may feel guilty or dissatisfied with this arrangement. The children may feel neglected by their mother, and Bob may be bored at home with his limited activity.

While the Roberts attempt to balance demands and resources on the family and community levels, other factors may come into play. Bob's reaction to and coping with his illness must be considered. If the stress effect of his injury brings the family together to gather resources, the experience will be a constructive and positive one for the Roberts. Although some reactions to illness, such as denial, secondary gains, anger, rejection of the sick role, bargaining, depression, regression, and depersonalization, may be negative, they are also normal as long as they are temporary. If Bob reacts in any of these ways, more time will be needed for the family to balance demands and resources.

The family's perception of Bob's health crisis affects everyone. The family's previous experience and education about the injury influences them. Bob's status as the identified patient in the family system is important. If the Roberts object to the 6-week recovery time or react in an overprotective manner, the result may impede Bob's recovery and impair the coping ability of the entire family. To cope successfully the Roberts must differentiate fact from feeling and examine other attitudes, beliefs, and values about the illness. They need to balance their perceptions of fear and anxiety with facts and planning so that the crisis can be resolved in the best way possible. Although theorists may differ in the specificity of their ideas about family health, most believe that it is the outcome of many interacting factors; it is the result of the interaction between individual members and the family unit, between the family unit and the larger social system, and between sociocultural subsystems and individual family members. To assess the health of a family it is necessary to judge it in the context of this multifaceted framework.

✦ FAMILY VULNERABILITIES AND MALADAPTIVE CHARACTERISTICS
Pileup

In a study of how healthy families deal with stress, McCubbin and McCubbin (1987) identified pileup (AA) and family typology and resiliency (R) as the interpersonal and organizational conditions of the family system. These are the most predictive factors of successful or unsuccessful coping behaviors. The pileup of demands on or within a family unit increases the family's vulnerability to stress. The family's life cycle stage, which includes its various normative demands, can enhance pileup. McCubbin and McCubbin propose that the pileup of family stressors and strains is related to the family's stage of development. The nature of pileup varies with each stage of the family life cycle. The following factors influence the degree of pileup during family adaptation:

1. Prior family strains
2. The illness and its hardships
3. The aftermath of coping over time
4. Social ambiguities about expected family behavior during the illness and its crises (McCubbin and McCubbin, Chapter 2)

Family Typologies

Those family units that are characterized by typologies such as vulnerable, fragile, and unpatterned often adjust poorly to stressors (McCubbin and McCubbin, 1989) (See Fig. 5-3). For example, vulnerable families have low family coherence and hardiness. (Coherence is the degree to which families value loyalty, trust, caring, and shared values in managing life stressors; hardiness is the family's sense of control over life and its sense of adventure in solving problems.) Such a family may get angry and criticize one or more members when stress is high. This family does not feel it has much control over life generally and is prone to attribute good or bad events to luck. These are families that may be seen screaming at one another in waiting rooms of hospitals and blaming everyone for the bad luck that caused the illness event. Such families are not likely to try new behaviors and may divorce if the pileup of stressors becomes too high. The health-care professional working with the vulnerable family needs to be skilled in moderating the emotions in these situations and in not imparting blame.

Often, vulnerable families respond well to the role modeling that comes from participating with other families in a support group.

As Olson et al. (1989) note, the impact of a stressor is likely to be a more serious problem for families in the adolescent or launching stage of the family life cycle because of the accumulation of life changes and the depletion of family interpersonal, social, and economic resources. Also, Olson's circumplex model of 16 family typologies depicts those families that fall into the extreme categories as maladaptive (see Fig. 5-2).

Concerning maladaptive characteristics, the theoretical perspective of the family systems theory supplement McCubbin's ideas. Two model forces within the family predict how members will function: (1) the level of differentiation of self and (2) the level of anxiety. Differentiation refers to the inclination and capacity of a living system to advance progressively to a higher level of complexity and organization. Anxiety corresponds to differentiation of self, in that as differentiation increases, chronic anxiety decreases (Bowen, 1978; Kerr & Bowen, 1988).

Differentiation

Bowen (1978) defines differentiation of self as the degree to which the intellectual and emotional systems are separated, yet integrated, in a person. Bowen has described a continuum of differentiation—low, moderate, good, and high. Few people completely lack or completely possess self-differentiation.

People with low self-differentiation experience life primarily on an emotional basis. Their lives appear chaotic and in constant turmoil. Feelings, repetitive behaviors, and ineffective thoughts predominate. Dreams and fantasies, rather than goals, guide their decision making. Each member of the family is socially, emotionally, or physically ill. Anxiety is chronically high, and intellectual system input is minimal. They can live seemingly normal lives if no stressors intervene to upset them.

People with a moderate level of differentiation are less dominated by the emotional system. They are less repetitive and have some flexibility in behavior. Yet the emotional system still pervades their interpersonal relationships. They gain emotional comfort by pleasing others, avoiding conflict, and giving and receiving affection. If they find a comfortable relationship, they fuse with the other person, thus creating anxiety for both persons. Children in such families are often controlled and not treated with the flexibility that allows for optimal development.

Kerr (1980) developed a multigenerational perspective of physical illness based on Bowen's idea that undifferentiated multigenerational processes can result in emotional, social, or physical illness. Kerr hypothesized that the level of differentiation of the family is the foundation of disease formation.

Anxiety

Kerr (1980) draws on earlier studies to support the theory that many diseases are latent within all people and are activated by the anxiety cycles within families. Warthin (1913) found a high incidence of cancer in some families. The cancer's occurrence, seriousness, and prognosis could be predicted by the family dynamics. Welch-McCaffrey (1985) discusses the fact that anxiety is evident in the family and in the individual with cancer throughout the entire course of the illness. He believes cancer should be considered an illness with both physical and mental components. Woodyatt and Spetz (1942) presented material close in concept to that of Warthin. They found that diabetes runs its course through a family in three to four generations, with more serious diabetes developing at a younger age, as in the families with cancer. Kerr also found indications of this pattern of disease in tuberculosis, leprosy, and rheumatoid arthritis. What connects these several studies is Kerr's interpretation that anxiety is the common thread that triggers the onset of the disease.

Kerr's formulations agree with those of Simonton, Mathews-Simonton, and Creighton (1978), that the symptoms or diagnosis of cancer has a unique psychological meaning for the patient. Kerr's ideas have been applied to patients who had myocardial infarctions (Miller & Winstead-Fry, 1982) to explain differences in recovery. Health-care professionals treating physical illnesses must consider multigenerational processes at work, especially in noncompliant patients. These patients may fail to cooperate in self-care because the family system needs the illness to ignore or cover up other family problems. For example, parental conflict may be projected to a child with diabetes who responds with repeated incidents of acidosis. The family systems theorist views people as active participants in their health status. (Kerr, 1980; Simonton et al., 1978).

Kerr and Bowen (1988) emphasize the stages of self-differentiation and their influence on the amount of independence in relationships within the family. Chronic anxiety, a response to an imagined threat or to what might occur, often exists in a poorly differentiated family. Acute anxiety, a response to a real threat, is usually self-limiting and is successfully dealt with by the individual. Kerr and Bowen (1988) relate anxiety to the level of control individuals have over their emotional functioning. The greater the anxiety is, the less control the individual will have. Families who are undifferentiated will experience insecurity and anxiety to the point of panic when threatening events occur. During such periods of anxiety, differentiation forces become unbearable and physical symptoms of illness may appear.

Potentially negative effects of unsuccessful overall family coping during the course of an illness surface as undifferentiated, dysfunctional, multigenerational processes that result in illness, psychosomatic families, or maladaptive behaviors. Weitzman (1985) made the following generalizations about dysfunctional families:

1. Communication is often negative.
2. The structure of the family often involves problems with role definitions and extreme enmeshment or disengagement.
3. The dynamics of family life involve responding to crisis after crisis with no time or energy left to build positive relationships.

Some examples of undifferentiated multigenerational processes are evident in cancer families and alcoholic families. Warthin (1913) noted a high incidence of reduced fertility in families with cancer. Also, the neoplasm tended to develop at an earlier age in the members of the youngest generations and often showed an increased malignancy.

Kerr (1980) concluded further that the disease was latent within all individuals in the family and had no clear genetic pattern. So the occurrence of the disease depended on the level of family functioning and concurrent anxiety. Simonton and Simonton (1975), in their assessment of personality characteristics of persons prone to or afflicted with cancer, described the interactive processes that result in illness. They found that the diagnosis of cancer was often preceded by a loss or by a cluster of stressful events 6 months previously. The person's response to the loss or to stressors was one of holding-in, internalizing, or rigidity. Eysenck (1988) reported that a number of studies through the years have suggested that cancer is associated with a personality in which the individual lacked emotional expression and responded to stressors with feelings of helplessness or hopelessness. Rather than seek solutions to the problem or mourn the loss, the person continued to flounder. Interaction and support among family members was minimal or nonexistent. Often, this response to stressful events was characteristic of the person and the family since early in their development. After a review of relevant contemporary literature, Thomas (1988) concluded that consideration of the personality as it predisposes an individual to mental or physical illness must be an important area for future research.

Addiction to alcohol is a complex social problem. It has physiological, psychological, and sociological dimensions, all of which are poorly understood. Developmental theorists propose that psychological components from early experiences in family relationships are responsible for the addiction. Some geneticists believe that some families are genetically susceptible to alcohol addiction. However, most geneticists agree that a combination of genetic predisposing factors and environmental factors such as geographical location and cultural systems must be taken into account to explain alcoholism (Heath, 1989). Social scientists attribute it to high levels of stress in modern life and to social drinking customs.

Gold (1980) described a cycle of behavior that leads to substance abuse. Substance use is reinforced because it gives the family member a sense of power regarding the area of conflict, thus reducing anxiety. The substance-using activity itself creates new sources of conflict that contribute to the family member's already low self-esteem if guilt or fear of discovery is associated with the behavior. Eventually the substance abuse itself perpetuates the need to continue.

Several theorists have identified family traits that predispose to drug abuse. Chein (1980) described a family that was too overwhelmed to treat children as persons, lacked a male role model, had no stability, distrusted society, and had no expectations for its children. Stanton (1980) described the usual family interaction picture as that of overinvolvement of the opposite-sex parent while the same-sex parent is punitive, distant, or absent. According to Pasquali, Arnold, and DeBasio (1989), family members who are enmeshed in the family structure have the potential for becoming drug abusers. The substance abuse facilitates assertive behavior that is lacking, but ultimately the individual becomes more dependent and enmeshed in the family. The families of substance users have characteristics that distinguish them from other types of families with disruptive behavior. Stanton (1980) notes the following characteristics:

1. A history of multigenerational addictive behaviors, including nonsubstance-related activities, such as gambling and television watching
2. An aggressive and direct expression of conflict
3. The abuser's great dependence on others with an expectation to be shielded from stress
4. Use of any conflict to justify drinking
5. The harboring of an illusion of independence from the addiction through membership in a peer group
6. A higher level of mother-child symbiosis
7. Death themes and untimely deaths within the family
8. Immigrant parents, possibly resulting in a cultural disparity between parents and children.

According to Frawley (1988), addictive behavior involves an interplay of chemical and emotional components that trigger a neuronal reward center. When this center is not satisfied, emotions such as anxiety, anger, and panic are experienced, leading to the use of the addictive substance. The consequences of addiction are damaging to the central components of self-esteem, which are successes, feedback from others, physical health, a sense of being in control of oneself, and a feeling of going toward the things one values. Nuckols and Greeson (1989) discuss the breakdown of the family unit in recent decades and the emergence of a narcissistic movement as contributing to addiction. Cravings for feelings of belonging and positive self-esteem are satisfied biochemically by drugs. Frawley (1988) describes addiction as a family disease and advises families to cope with the problem as they would with any other chronic disease.

Although some maladaptive behaviors in response to the illness itself can be seen in family interactive styles over several generations, these are often temporary and limited to the illness situation that arises. The longer these behaviors continue the more destructive they can be to the ill person and to the family situation. Some of these maladaptive behaviors are noncompliance with relapse, overprotectiveness and enmeshment, rigidity and avoidance of conflict, and encouragement of dependence. Captain (1989) further supports this idea and advocates therapeutic intervention as a way to effect changes in family structure and function.

Family interventions can be enhanced and families supported by a

diagnostic and evaluation process that examines the strengths and defi-
ciencies in the family system. Family functioning can be enhanced by
interventions that target both the vulnerabilities and dysfunctional patterns
of the family unit and the family's interpersonal capabilities and strengths,
which, if addressed, can serve as a catalyst for other family-system,
wellness-promoting properties. Families have an inner resistance and
adaptive abilities that can be strengthened with outside help, even after the
family unit has moved toward a state of dysfunction. These resources can
play a critical role in successful adaptation.

✦ CULTURAL, ETHNIC, AND RACIAL DIFFERENCES: IMPACT ON HEALTH AND ILLNESS

Cultural, ethnic, and racial differences may distinguish a family from
the community. These differences can be strengths and can enhance the
family's ability to balance demands and resources. Theorists and health
professionals sometimes show bias toward families who do not share their
own personal values and views of effective family functioning. When
differences in viewpoint exist between provider and patient, health-care
practices may not be based on the patient's needs (Tripp-Reimer & Afifi,
1989; Sue & Sue, 1990). Health professionals must accept cultural
differences and not impose personal ideologies. Ethnicity is a powerful
influence on our daily lives; it provides us with a sense of belonging and
guides family life.

Too little is known about the influence of culture on health care. Also,
difficulties abound when generalizing from generation to generation or
from group to group. Martin and Belcher (1990) researched the impact of
nurses' cultural backgrounds on their attitudes toward caregiving. Midwest
American, African English, and African Zulu hospital oncology nurses
participated in a study about different approaches to caring for cancer
patients. Midwest American and Zulu nurses showed the greatest difference
in attitudes. Midwest American and African English shared Anglo-Saxon
cultural heritage; Zulu and African English had African roots in common.

Individuals within groups also may have different beliefs and practices.
Tripp-Reimer and Afifi (1989) state that health behavior is a result of the
patterns of our cultural background and that the behaviors of the
health-care provider and the patient may differ. A careful assessment of

beliefs, values, and practices is needed to establish the cultural identity of the patient. The health-care professional needs to be open to and ever-curious about the variety of cultural differences among families. Families must not be stereotyped on the basis of cultural background. Friedman (1986) emphasizes the importance of understanding cultural influences within the family as a key to understanding the family's behavior and values.

Families are unique with regard to age, sex, education, and the generation of immigration. Their health values, beliefs, and customs are influenced by their cultures, but are not necessarily transmitted to every generation. Health-seeking behaviors are determined by their customs, folk remedies, and beliefs. What families view as health, illness, and crisis and what resources they deem important to make use of all can vary according to cultural, ethnic, and racial differences.

Stereotypes of certain cultures have not been supported by research. For example, research has not supported the cultural stereotype that black and Chinese elders are reverend. Professionals who planned interventions based on the stereotype probably underestimated the needs of these elders. It is thought that serious erosion of the cultural patterns of kinship and community in the urban United States is the cause of the decline in elder reverence (Jackson, 1970, 1971; Kalish & Yuen, 1971; Carp & Kataoka, 1976).

Results of a study conducted by Sugarek, Deyo, and Holmes (1988) among whites, blacks, and Mexican-Americans reveal that Mexican-Americans are more likely to believe that control of their health is a matter of chance or the responsibility of other people such as doctors or nurses. Professionals may assume that this fatalistic attitude is typical of Mexican-Americans. However, it is also possible that they lack knowledge, money, and experience, thereby feeling in less control of themselves in a health-care situation.

Tripp-Reimer's (1983) study of urban Greek immigrants found that ethnic groups have members who are more or less acculturated to the dominant society. Traditional health beliefs and behaviors of the Greek community were integrated politically, economically, and geographically into the larger metropolitan community, yet remained culturally distinct. The retention of beliefs and practices concerning the "evil eye" varied dramatically among generations, thus limiting generalizations concerning the prevalence of this belief.

In her study of northern rural blacks and whites, Leininger (1985) not only found differences in these two groups' care and health values, beliefs, and attitudes, but also noted differences between rural and urban groups. Touch was perceived as an essential part of caring for blacks of all ages, yet it was difficult for white nurses to convey their caring through touch, especially to black teenagers and adults.

Although sensitivity to cultural differences in families is essential, ethnic affiliation provides only a clue to the health professional's assessment and intervention. Each family is unique and varies in its customs and beliefs. The health-care professional must not overgeneralize or stereotype individuals on the basis of cultural or ethnic affiliation.

Sue and Sue (1990) believe health-care providers should become culturally aware of their own values, biases, and assumptions about human behavior especially as it pertains to the definition of family. Also, it is important to learn the worldview of the culturally different family and how that family views the definition, role, and function of the family and the illness. Sue and Sue suggest the use of a framework that helps to understand differences in communication styles and structural alliances in the family and at the same time helps to pinpoint cultural differences that exist within a particular family.

Sue and Sue (1990) outline some general principles that may be helpful and practical. First, they propose the use of a value-orientation framework that compares the worldviews of middle-class white Americans and ethnic minorities. Whether groups value a lineal, collateral, or individualistic orientation has major implications for their definitions of the family and what they consider to be appropriate goals and strategies in family health care. Other value preferences, such as time dimension, relationships to nature, and so forth are equally important and influential. For example, Western culture advocates a direct approach to defining and solving a family problem. Asian cultures tend to accommodate or deal with problems indirectly. In contrast to American values, ethnic minorities or subgroups that view people as harmonious with nature or believe in the overwhelming power of nature (acts of God) may find the health-care providers' mastery-over-nature approach inconsistent with or antagonistic to their worldview. Indeed, attempts to change family patterns and relationships may be perceived as the problem itself because it may potentially upset the family's preestablished harmony. A second example concerns time dimension variations. Both American Indians and black Americans tend to value a present-time orientation, whereas Asian Americans and Hispanic Americans focus on a combination of past and present. Asian societies have valued the past, as reflected in ancestor worship and in equating age with wisdom and respectability. This contrasts with U.S. culture in which youth is valued over the elderly.

Second, Sue and Sue believe an effective cross-cultured family health-care provider needs to be especially attentive to traditional cultural family structure and extended family ties. Understanding husband-wife relationships, parent-child relationships, and sibling relationships from different cultural perspectives is crucial. Asian Americans and Hispanics have a more patriarchal spousal relationship, whereas this relationship among white and black Americans is based on equality. For example, equal division of labor in the home between husband and wife or creating a more equal relationship may violate Hispanic cultural norms. Ho (1987) contrasts with white Western norms the view of most minority families that the wifely role is less important than the motherly role. Health-care providers should not judge the health of a family on the basis of the American ideal of equality of the sexes.

Third, Sue and Sue advise health-care professionals to use the natural help-giving networks and structures that already exist in the minority culture and community. It is important to recognize the many forms of assistance available. Atkinson, Morten, and Sue (1989) discuss some of these roles in detail such as consultant, ombudsman, change-agent, facilitator of indigenous support systems, and outreach role. Health-care professionals may attempt to serve as resource persons in developing programs that would improve life conditions through prevention and remediation. Health professionals need to see and work with the family in its natural environment and avoid the intimidating atmosphere of large, informal and unfamiliar health-care institutions.

A final recommendation for the family-oriented health-care provider is the need to be creative in developing appropriate intervention techniques when working with minority populations. With traditional Asian Americans, subtlety and indirectness may be called for rather than direct confrontation and interpretation. Formality in addressing members of the family may be more appropriate. Cultural, racial, and system factors determine approaches, so the more the health professional understands about these factors, the more effective he or she will be with families.

REFERENCES

Atkinson, D., Morten, G., & Sue, D. W. (1989). Future directions in minority group/cross-cultural counseling. In D. Atkinson, G. Morten, D. W. Sue (Eds.), *Counseling American minorities: A cross-cultural perspective* (3rd ed., pp. 271-296). Dubuque, IA: W. C. Brown.

Bowen, M. (1978). *Family therapy in clinical practice.* New York: Jason Aronson.

Burr, W. R. (1973). *Theory construction and the sociology of the family.* New York: John Wiley & Sons.

Captain, C. (1989). Family recovery from alcoholism: Mediating family factors. *Nursing Clinics of North America, 24*(1), 55-67.

Carp, F., & Kataoka, E. (1976). Health care problems of the elderly of San Francisco's Chinatown. *Gerontologist, 16*, 30-38.

Chein, I. (1980). Psychological, social, and epidemological factors in juvenile drug abuse. In D. J. Lettieri, M. Sayers, & H. W. Pearson (Eds.), Theories on drug abuse: selected contemporary perspectives, *NIDA Research Monograph 30*, (pp. 76-82). Rockville, MD: National Institute on Drug Abuse.

DeChesnay, M., & Magnuson, N. (1988). How healthy families cope with stress. *AAOHN Journal, 36*(9), 361-365.

Eysenck, H. J. (1988). Personality and stress as causal factors in cancer and coronary heart diseases. In M. P. Janisse (Ed.), *Individual differences, stress, and health psychology* (pp. 129-145). New York: Springer-Verlag.

Frawley, P. J. (1988). Neurobehavioral model of addiction: Addiction as a primary disease. In S. Peele (Ed.), *Visions of addiction: Major contemporary perspectives on addiction and alcoholism* (pp. 25-43). Lexington, MA: Heath.

Friedman, M. M. (1986). *Family nursing: Theory and assessment.* Norwalk, CT: Appleton-Century-Crofts.

Gold, S. R. (1980). The CAP control theory of drug abuse. In D. J. Lettieri, M. Sayers, & H. W. Pearson (Eds.), Theories on drug abuse: Selected contemporary perspectives, *NIDA Research Monograph 30* (pp. 8-11). Rockville, MD: National Institute on Drug Abuse.

Hansen, C. (1981). Living with normal families. *Family Process, 20*, 53-75.

Heath, D. B. (1989). Environmental factors in alcohol use and its outcomes. In H. W. Goedde & D. P. Agarwal (Eds.), *Alcoholism: Biomedical and genetic aspects* (pp. 312-324). New York: Pergamon Press.

Heiney, S. P. (1988). Assessing and intervening with dysfunctional families. *Oncology Nursing Forum, 15*(5), 585-590.

Ho, M. K. (1987). *Family therapy with ethnic minorities.* Newbury Park, CA: Sage.

Jackson, J. (1970). Aged Negroes, their culture departures from statistical stereotypes and rural-urban differences. *Gerontologist, 10*, 140-145.

Jackson, J. (1971). Negro aged: Toward needed research and social gerontology. *Gerontologist, 11* (suppl.), 52-57.

Kalish, R., and Yuen, S. (1971). Americans of East Asian ancestry: Aging and the aged. *Gerontologist, 11* (suppl.), 36-47.

Kennedy, M. J. (1982). Impact of illness and hospitalization. In J. Haber, A. M. Leach, S. M. Schudy, & B. F. Sidelau (Eds.), *Comprehensive psychiatric nursing* (pp. 677-692). New York: McGraw-Hill.

Kerr, M. (1980). Emotional factors in physical illness. *The Family, 7,* 59.

Kerr, M. E., & Bowen, M. (1988). *Family evaluation: An approach based on Bowen theory.* New York: W. W. Norton.

Leininger, M. (1985). Southern rural black and white American lifeways with focus on care and health phenomena. In M. Leininger (Ed.), *Qualitative research methods* (pp. 195-216). Orlando, FL: Grune & Stratton.

Martin, B. A., & Belcher, J. V. (1990). Influences of cultural background on nurses' attitudes and care of the oncology patient. In C. R. Ash & J. F. Jenkins (Eds.), *Enhancing the role of cancer nursing* (pp. 277-296). New York: Raven.

McCubbin, H. I. & McCubbin, M. A. (1987). Family stress theory and assessment: The T-Double ABCX model of family adjustment and adaptation. In H. I. McCubbin and A. Thompson (Eds.), *Family assessment inventories for research and practice* (pp. 3-32). Madison, WI: University of Wisconsin–Madison.

McCubbin, M. A., & McCubbin, H. I. (1989). Theoretical orientations to family stress and coping. In C. R. Figley (Ed.), *Treating stress in families* (pp. 3-43). New York: Brunner/Mazel.

Mercier, R. T. (1989). Theoretical perspectives on the family. In C. L. Gilliss, B. L. Highley, B. M. Roberts, & I. M. Martinson (Eds.), *Toward a science of family nursing* (pp. 9-36). Menlo Park, CA: Addison-Wesley.

Miller, S., & Winstead-Fry, P. (1982). *Family systems theory in nursing practice.* Reston, VA: Reston.

Nuckols, C. C., & Greeson, J. (1989). Cocaine addiction: Assessment and intervention. *Nursing Clinics of North America 24*(1), 33-43.

Olson, D., McCubbin, H. I., Barnes, H., Larsen, A., Muxen, M., & Wilson, M. (1989). Families—What makes them work (2nd ed.). Newbury Park, CA: Sage.

Olson, D. H., Russell, C. S., & Sprenkle, D. H. (1983). Circumplex model VI: Theoretical update. *Family Process, 22,* 69-83.

Pasquali, E. A., Arnold, H. M., & DeBasio, N. (1989). *Mental health nursing: A holistic approach* (3rd ed). St. Louis: Mosby–Year Book.

Richards, E. (1989). Self-reports of differentiation of self and marital compatibility as related to family functioning in the 3rd and 4th stages of the family life cycle. *Scholarly Inquiry for Nursing Practice, 3*(3), 163-175.

Sedgwick, R. (1981). *Family mental health: Theory and research.* St. Louis: Mosby–Year Book.

Simonton, O. C., Mathews-Simonton, S., & Creighton, J. (1978). *Getting well again.* New York: Bantam.

Simonton, O. C., & Simonton, S. S. (1975). Belief systems and management of the emotional aspects of malignancy. *The Journal of Transpersonal Psychology, 1,* 29-47.

Stanton, M. D. (1980). A family theory of drug abuse. In D. J. Lettieri, M. Sayers, & H. W. Pearson (Eds.), Theories on drug abuse: selected contemporary perspectives, *NIDA Research Monograph 30* (pp. 147-156). Rockville, MD: National Institute on Drug Abuse.

Sue, D. W., & Sue, D. (1990). *Counseling the culturally different: Theory and practice* (2nd ed.). New York: John Wiley & Sons.

Sugarek, N. J., Deyo, R. A., & Holmes, B. C. (1988). Locus of control and beliefs about cancer in a multi-ethnic clinic population. *Oncology Nursing Forum, 15*(4), 481-486.

Thomas, S. P. (1988). Is there a disease-prone personality? Synthesis and evaluation of the theoretical and empirical literature. *Issues in Mental Health, 9,* 339-352.

Tripp-Reimer, T. (1983). Retention of a folk healing practice (Matiaswa) among four generations of urban Greek immigrants. *Nursing Research, 32,* 97-101.

Tripp-Reimer, T., & Afifi, L. A. (1989). Cross-cultural perspectives on patient teaching. *Nursing Clinics of North America, 24*(3), 613-619.

Warthin, A. S. (1913). Heredity with reference to carcinoma. *Archives of International Medicine, 12,* 546-555.

Weitzman, J. (1985). Engaging the severely dysfunctional family in treatment: Basic considerations. *Family Process, 24*(4), 473-485.

Welch-McCaffrey, D. (1985). Cancer, anxiety, and quality of life. *Cancer Nursing, 8*(3), 151-158.

Woodyatt, R. Y., & Spetz, M. (1942). Anticipation of the inheritance of diabetes. *Journal of the American Medical Association, 120,* 602-605.

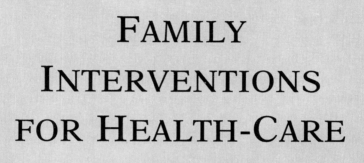

FAMILY
INTERVENTIONS
FOR HEALTH-CARE
DELIVERY

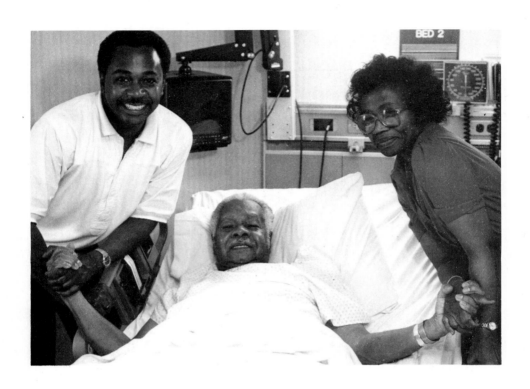

6

Creation of a Health-Care System with a Family Perspective

✦

CHAPTER GOALS

✦ To describe the foundation needed for a family perspective in the health-care system

✦ To identify possible areas in the existing health-care system where family involvement could be improved

✦ To offer pathways to creating a health-care system with a family perspective

OVERVIEW

T HIS chapter describes the foundation needed for a family perspective to exist in the health-care system and identifies possible areas in the existing health-care system where the family perspective and family involvement would improve services. Also identified are obstacles that diminish the ability of the health-care system to establish family-oriented services. We offer possible solutions to overcoming these obstacles with the intent of creating an improved health-care system, one with a stronger family perspective. In terms of the Resiliency Model of Family Stress, Adjustment, and Adaptation, this chapter focuses on social support (BBB), or more specifically, the health-care system as a family resource (Fig. 6-1).

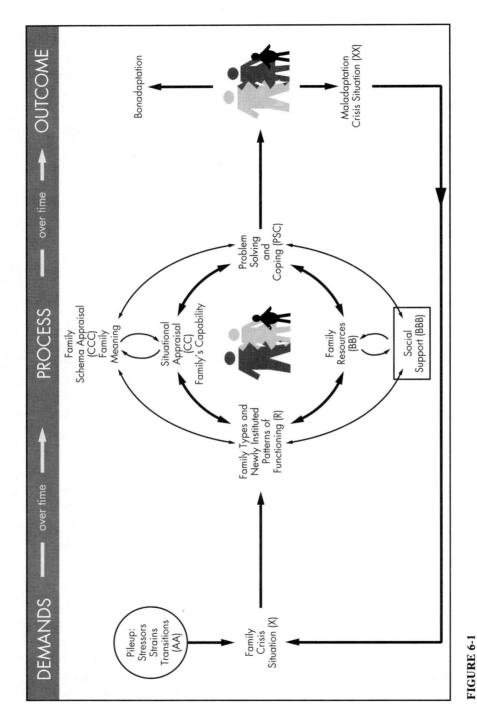

FIGURE 6-1

Adaptation Phase of the Resiliency Model of Family Stress, Adjustment, and Adaptation. This chapter focuses on social support (BBB), or the health-care system as a family resource.

✦ FOUNDATIONS OF A FAMILY PERSPECTIVE

Integrating stronger family involvement into the existing health-care system will take time and effort, but it is not an impossible endeavor. A family perspective in health care includes the involvement and use of families in all aspects of wellness and illness. The family would be highlighted as the critical unit of treatment. Current research and studies have made sufficient strides in demonstrating the value and benefits this approach can bring to the promotion of wellness and the treatment of illness (Anderson & Holder, 1989; Cleveland, 1980/1989; Doherty, 1985; Leventhal, Leventhal, & Van Nuguyen, 1985; McCubbin, Needle, & Wilson, 1985; Reiss & De-Noir, 1989; Schmidt, 1983/1985; Storer, Frate, Johnson, & Greenberg, 1987; Turk & Kerns, 1985).

Researchers also have assisted in developing tools to implement family-oriented services (H. I. McCubbin & M. A. McCubbin, 1987; M. A. McCubbin & H. I. McCubbin, 1987; McCubbin & Thompson, 1987; Morisky, Levine, Green, Shapiro, Russell, & Smith, 1983; Kerns & Turk, 1985). Coupled with these developments are strong public feelings indicating that health needs are not being met and demanding change within the health-care system. Complaints regarding the expense, fragmentation, authoritarianism, inaccessibility, and impersonal nature of the health-care system have been expressed by Starr (1982), Easterbrook (1987), and Anderson and Holder (1989). Many have demanded that health care have a greater impact in "human terms." Since the presence of a family perspective in the health-care system can involve greater impact in "human terms" and more cost-effective services (Doherty, Baird, & Becker, 1987; Huygen and Smits, 1983/1985; Schmidt, 1983/1985), education of the public and health professionals about the advantages of this perspective could propel movement toward the family perspective. In light of these developments, the ingredients necessary to drive forward a movement that can champion family-oriented health care may be present.

Background: The Present Health-Care System and the Family Perspective

The education of health professionals and delivery of health care are focused primarily on the ill individual as the unit of treatment (Baird & Doherty, 1990; Turk & Kerns, 1985). Both the organizational and physical setup of hospitals usually do not lend themselves to family involvement. In the physician's office the realities of tight scheduling and unawareness of the advantages of family-oriented services preclude the pursuit of psycho-social areas vital to a family perspective (Hepworth & Jackson, 1985). Outpatient clinic areas are known for poor family involvement (Bozett, 1987). However, the family perspective is emerging, especially in the areas of pediatrics and maternity. Apparently the presence of a child is the catalyst. In fact, a recent U.S. law protecting handicapped children (PL 99-457) requires family participation on the health-care team (DeGraw et al., 1988).

Since the survival and well-being of a child clearly depends on a functioning family unit, the child's presence overtly demonstrates the need for a family perspective in health-care delivery. Clearly the whole is just as important as the part. A well-functioning family will be more likely to facilitate the child's adjustment or adaptation to an illness. Why should this tendency be any different for the ill adult? Certainly, an ill family member who can no longer participate in roles and tasks within the family affects family functioning. This incapacity necessitates change in family function-ing, potentially causing family difficulties. In fact, the effects on family functioning may be even greater if an adult member is ill, depending on the roles held by that individual. However, since the ill family member is an independent adult as opposed to a dependent child, the implications for family involvement and support in health-care delivery seem less clear. Since the sick role involves feelings of helplessness and dependence similar to those of a child, is it not possible that the needs of the adult are also similar and require a well-functioning family for support?

Verification of the value of a family perspective is evident in recent research on the family's ability to have positive and negative effects on wellness and illness (Becker, Steinbauer, & Doherty, 1985; Morisky et al., 1983; Ramsey, Abell, & Baker, 1986; Storer et al., 1987). These studies underscore the family's capability to enhance or hinder the efforts of health professionals to: (1) produce optimum states of wellness, (2) increase the individual's functioning in illness, and (3) achieve greater compliance with treatment plans. Therefore the family perspective offers health profession-als a tool for promoting wellness, increasing functioning and compliance of the ill individual, and fostering the opportunity for personal and familial growth during health and illness experiences. This approach also may provide the opportunity to prevent family hindrance or resistance in illness situations and health promotion.

A study at McMasters University clearly demonstrates the value of the family perspective (cited in Schmidt, 1983/1985). This study explored the value of convening the family to discuss health issues and the ability of this meeting to decrease the use of health and illness services by individual family members. Two groups of 42 families each were studied. The families in the two groups were matched for health problems and use of health services the year previous to the study. The first group was given opportunities as needed to convene as a family with the health-care professional to discuss emotional or psychosomatic complaints. The second group was not given this opportunity. Over the next year the first group had a 49% decrease in the use of health and illness services, whereas the second group had an increase of 10%. The value to the family was clear in the decreased number of illness experiences. Addressing the primary complaint of many health professionals, that no time is available for this service, the study demonstrated that convening the family saved valuable health and illness service time, since 28% of the families needed only one or two 60-minute meetings. Schmidt (1983/1985), in a paper presented at a conference concerning the family and medicine, commented on this study and judged the dividends as well worth a 60-minute investment. Another study by Huygen and Smits (1983/1985), also done in a primary care office setting, documented a comparative decrease in the use of health and illness services when families received therapy for emotional problems. These studies demonstrate that support and empowerment of the family with information and encouragement to solve its own problems is beneficial to all.

Essential Components of a Family Perspective

The family perspective in health care is a proactive stance that encourages families to reach their full potential by focusing on strengths, capabilities, and acquisition of knowledge and skills. The family would become a collaborative partner with the health professional in promoting wellness and dealing with illness of its individual members. This contrasts with current reactive approaches that correct existing problems (Dunst, Trivette, & Deal, 1988). Positive goals would be targeted instead of treatment of negative outcomes. The family would become the unit of treatment and the vehicle to obtaining positive outcomes.

The patient–family–health professional relationship. Since the family perspective relies on positive relationships between patients and their families, we need to examine and understand more fully patient–family–health professional relationships. Both Ragiel (cited in Leavitt, 1989) and Doherty (1985) explored patient–family–health professional relationships. Figure 6-2, adapted from Doherty's work (1985), demonstrates the triangular nature of these relationships with the solid arrows representing lines of mutual influence between the three principals—health professionals, patient, and family. The broken arrows denote lines of influence from one principal to one of the dyad relationships: (1) patient-family, (2) patient-health professional, and (3) health professional-family. Since equality is difficult to split among three principals, a constant struggle for power exists. The power shifts between the dyads as tension develops within a dyad and a third party is brought in to stabilize the situation. Each principal is capable of supporting or undermining a dyad, so each principal is affected by what takes place within the triangle. Interestingly, Ragiel describes information-hoarding as a method of maintaining power. This concept needs further exploration so that information exchanges especially at the time of diagnosis can be further understood.

This triangular representation of patient–family–health professional interactions demonstrates the family's influence on the patient's behavior and on the patient-health professional's relationship. It points out the importance of dealing with the patient within the context of the family, since that contextual relationship is ever present. Treating patients within the context of the family is especially important during serious illness or health interventions that require changes in life-style. Certain attitudes need to pervade patient–family–health professional relationships so that a family perspective in health care may be implemented successfully.

Mutual respect. Health-care professionals need an awareness of their feelings regarding patients and their families so that they can communicate respect effectively. They need to develop respect for the variety of socially, culturally, physically, religiously, and ethnically different families. Since this respect does not necessarily come naturally, differences in attitudes between health professionals and families may result in approaches and treatment that are not based on family needs or desires (Sue & Sue, 1990; Tripp-Reimer & Afifi, 1989). In regard to the role of the health professional

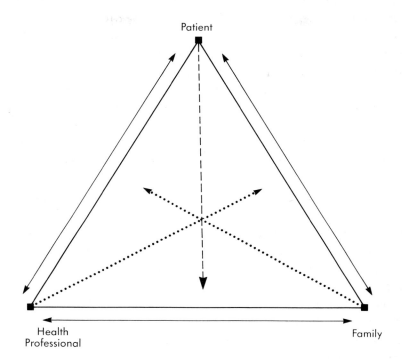

FIGURE 6-2
The Patient–Family – Health Professional relationship.
(Modified from Doherty, W.J. (1985). Family interventions in health care. *Family Relations, 34,* 32.)

as a source of social support, supporting individual and family self-esteem is considered the most important (Olson et al., 1989). Sincere emotional concern, a vehicle to establishing self-esteem support, may be difficult to convey if the health professional lacks respect for the patient or family. Therefore health professionals need to heighten their awareness of their attitudes and prejudice toward different types of families. Self-awareness and value clarification can begin with a broad definition of *family* that encompasses the wide variety of families in our society today (see Chapter 1). Since it may be necessary to deconstruct a lifetime habit of prejudices and values, educational efforts along these lines need to begin early and remain as an educational thread throughout basic educational programs, through postgraduate studies (for example, nurse practitioner programs, internships, residency programs, and the like), and into the posttraining practice setting.

Studies demonstrating the value of sensitizing health-care professionals to their feelings, prejudices, and values are rare. One study done in 1972 by Jacobs, Charles, Jacobs, Weinstein, and Mann (cited in Bloom, 1985) focused on data that demonstrated that patients from the lower socioeconomic class were unlikely to be referred by the physician for insight therapy (therapy that increases self-awareness about how the individual affects others and is affected by others). After some exploration, Jacobs and his colleagues inferred that the doctor had little confidence in the effectiveness of this treatment for these patients. They also discovered a conflict between the patient's and the physician's culturally determined expectations about openness. The difficulties seemed to stem from the social distance between the middle-class doctor and the lower-class patient.

To rectify the situation, Jacobs and his colleagues studied 120 patients. A portion of these patients and their physicians were subject to 15-minute orientation sessions. The doctors were taught that this socioeconomic group had difficulty in exploring feelings, being motivated, and accepting the fact that help was not immediate. In turn, the patients were taught the difference between discussions with the psychiatrist and their family physician. They learned about the need for openness and how to discuss their problems with the different kinds of doctors. Results showed that those in the control group without an orientation were less likely to profit from insight therapy than those in the oriented group. In addition, the orientation helped increase the motivation and ability of both the patient *and* the physician to work together. Even this limited educational procedure was capable of diminishing social distance, thus increasing the respect between the patient and doctor. The potential value of applying similar educational efforts to families and to the training of health professionals is obvious. Practice settings also need to consider offering this kind of continuing education so that their specific patient/family populations can be better understood.

Just as prejudice can hinder patient–family–health professional interactions, feelings surrounding certain illness situations also can interfere. These feelings need to be examined by health professionals in the classroom and clinical setting. Illness situations involving topics such as sex, finances, and death may be difficult for some practitioners to discuss with families. Hepworth and Jackson (1985) found that doctors confronted with terminal illness or death had difficulty coping with their own sense of failure. The physician became awkward and detached from the patient, which increased the loneliness and helplessness of the patient and family. Murray and Zentor (1985) found that health professionals became frustrated, angry, and judgmental when the patient could not or would not get well. Slaby and Glicksman (1985) also note that physicians were reluctant to talk with their patients about feelings related to serious illnesses and death. Practitioners frequently exposed to the acutely or terminally ill patient especially need planned opportunities to explore their feelings and reactions, perhaps in peer-support groups. Sharing with colleagues may assist in preventing the burn-out so common in these practice areas (Beardslee & Demaso, 1982/1989; Slaby & Glicksman, 1985).

All health-care workers at some point will have to manage difficult illness situations, and they also will need to cooperate with families with divergent values or those that inspire negative feelings. Therefore health professionals must become aware of and learn to deal with these problems. They need to understand and recognize their own negative behavior and reactions to certain families and situations (Sue & Sue, 1990). This personal development is essential to dealing with families in distress (which is often the result of illness) and requires that health professionals see themselves as persons with feelings and vulnerabilities (Doherty, 1985). Health professionals need to become detached from the situation, evaluate the dynamics, and find a solution. The responsibility to refrain from labeling the patient (for example, "uncooperative," "disruptive," and so on) and instead, to examine relationships to make changes, lies with the health professional, not the client (Murray & Zenter, 1985). It is only by setting aside their own prejudice that health professionals will be able to see and understand the true meaning an illness has for patient and family. Self-awareness can make health professionals more effective in offering support and in motivating families to follow treatment plans (Hennen, Sietz, & Sietz, 1987). The result is a family–health professional partnership that empowers families, instead of an authoritarian relationship that fosters helplessness (Doherty et al., 1987).

Mutual trust. Health-care professionals expect families to trust them and are often resentful if they do not. Yet, they themselves seldom trust families well enough to allow them "ownership" and responsibility for their illness and its treatment. Instead, health professionals forge plans and expectations as the expert, expecting the nonexpert patient to comply

(Doherty et al., 1987). This implies that the family is somehow inferior. How can mutual trust exist here?

Collaborative relationships between families and health-care professionals reflect application of sociobehavioral principles that foster understanding between partners (Doherty et al., 1987). Collaboration implies sharing information and equal participation in decision-making, work, and assumption of responsibilities (Lancaster, McCance, & Vanderschmidt, 1986). With appropriate knowledge and guidance, families are capable of receiving and sharing information, making decisions, and developing effective plans. As partners, families would be an active, responsible participant in health maintenance activities and illness. These empowered families would likely offer the health professional the assets and expertise they hold to manage illness situations effectively.

The effectiveness of allowing families to "own" the illness situation is clearly demonstrated in a report supported by the Community Control of Hypertension Project (Storer et al., 1987). This report noted that 69% of diagnosed hypertensive individuals did not comply with their treatment regimens. After a number of different trial interventions were tried, the most effective intervention in terms of both health-effectiveness and cost-effectiveness was the extended family–based, self-help group. In these self-help groups the family was allowed to "own" the problem through receiving all the information and skills needed to manage the problem. A family volunteer received specific training and was subsequently tested to be certified as a Hypertension Health Counselor. This person became the family "expert" and added greatly to the knowledge base of the family. The extended family group (including all members with hypertension, even outside the nuclear family) provided a forum where questions could be asked. The "expert" was able to reply knowing the cultural, linguistic, and educational makeup of the individual family members as well as their health belief model. The large number of opportunities for reinforcement of the treatment regimen, both inside the group and outside, provided the hypertensive family members with feelings of motivation and success. The family was able to create an effective plan, a plan the health-care professional might never have chosen as a possible solution.

The extended family groups studied obtained a 90% (N = 258) hypertension control rate. Even church-based groups similarly organized did not meet with the same success (72%, N = 535). This demonstrates that families who are allowed to "own" the illness problem and are given the knowledge can be very capable problem-solvers. The commitment to a strategy developed within the family appears to be stronger than commitment to strategies devised outside of the family. In family relationships lies a powerful resource waiting to be tapped by health-care professionals.

Tools for family intervention

Collaboration. Just as collaboration with the family is important, so is collaboration among health professionals, allied health practitioners, and community resources. A single practitioner cannot be all things to families, nor can a single practitioner handle all the biological, psychological, and social ramifications of the family and the illness situation. To provide the kind of comprehensive services families need, knowledge and expertise are needed from many disciplines.

Collaboration also provides greater continuity of care for families. Hennen (1987a) cited several studies that demonstrated the benefits provided by greater continuity in health-care delivery. Ettlinger and Freeman (1981) found that continuity of care reaped better compliance with treatment regimens. May and Kaelbling (1971) found that less delay in seeking health care occurred in settings with greater continuity. Becker, Drachman, and Kirscht (1974) described greater satisfaction in the patient–health professional relationship and better disclosure of behavioral problems with continuity of care. In comparing costs between fragmented and comprehensive health care, Heagarty, Robertson, and Kosa (1970) reported a decrease in costs related to fewer laboratory tests being performed. It appears that collaboration between health services may reap special benefits for both the family and the health-care professional.

However, professional differences and rivalries often interfere with the collaborative process (Anderson & Holder, 1989; Doherty, 1985; Doherty & McCubbin, 1985; Hepworth & Jackson, 1985). The age of specialization is here. Medicine alone has 63 speciality practice areas (Murray & Zenter, 1985). Horizontal organizational patterns that acknowledge and respect differences and expertise are lacking. Attempts to protect "turf" interfere with collaboration, especially between traditional and nontraditional fields. Moreover, some professionals view collaboration as indicative of limitations in their own practice skills, which makes them uncomfortable (Hepworth & Jackson, 1985). Lack of collaboration fractionates care and decreases opportunities to learn, by example, more about families from other colleagues heavily endowed with specific skills and knowledge that can be used to assist families. "Involved at every level of interprofessional collaboration are issues of identity, economic well-being, and power" (Doherty, 1985 p. 136). These issues need to be faced for successful collaboration.

Collaboration among health colleagues early in their educational programs is a good place to initiate the breakdown of these barriers and to begin fostering the seeds of cooperation. Schools of medicine, nursing, allied health, and medical social work are often in close proximity. Interactive classes and shared clinical experiences would strengthen the professions and encourage mutual respect and collaboration.

For example, the Association of Teachers of Preventive Medicine and the Center for Educational Development in Health came together in 1977 to "plan, develop, and implement a curriculum project to facilitate the teaching of preventive medicine, especially clinical preventive medicine in schools of medicine" (cited in Lancaster et al., 1986 p. 48). In their studies of the situation, it became clear that the physician-nurse combination was a good vehicle for providing comprehensive preventive health care. As a result, programs at *all* educational levels were developed to reflect a collaborative nurse-physician practice. The opportunity to develop mutual respect and collaboration between the two disciplines during training would ensure the use of this model in the actual practice setting. Two disciplines that have a great deal to offer each other would be brought together.

Convening the family. Family interventions need to become more systematic to experience the advantages they can offer the family. Schmidt (1983/1985), Doherty and Baird (1983), and Doherty (1985) have proposed recommendations to accomplish this. First, they suggest that certain medical conditions and treatment regimens almost always cause family problems. Second, specific normative transitions (that is, the family life cycle transitions) and situational stressors (that is, problems of living) also frequently cause family coping difficulties or physical illness in the family. With these facts in mind, Schmidt developed a list that included medical and family situations in which convening the family would be helpful. The list includes: pregnancy, failure to thrive, recurrent childhood poisoning, preschool and school-age behavior problems, adolescent maladjustment, major depression, chronic illness, diabetes, heart disease and surgery, poor adherence to medical regimen, frequent use of health services, terminal illness, and bereavement. Schmidt compiled this list based on supporting research data available at the time (35 sources cited in Schmidt, 1983/ 1985).

Many of the situations on Schmidt's list relate to normal transitions in the family life cycle. This would appear to indicate that planned interventions of a preventive nature would be beneficial at the juncture of the different stages of the family life cycle. Relationships established through these preventive health measures would be invaluable in assisting families dealing with short-term illnesses when time to build relationships is limited. Established health professional–family relations also would make the family more comfortable in seeking advice and expressing worries. The health professional would be creating a resource that could enhance the family's appraisal of its capabilities to face illness.

Schmidt also listed surgery as a situation needing a family meeting. Anticipatory information concerning expectations of the surgical events is needed by the family to plan strategies to cope with the situation. Other situations requiring anticipatory guidance need to be listed too. For example, the family going home with the newborn from the intensive care nursery or the family going home from the rehabilitation center with a severely disabled family member could both use the advantages found in convening the family (see Chapter 11). Each situation involves becoming completely responsible for the continuing care of the "patient," which can be a frightening experience especially without support. The need for life-style changes (for example, diet changes) is another situation that would also benefit from a family meeting. In fact, Doherty and Baird suggest that convening the family produces more successful outcomes when life-style changes are required (cited Anderson & Holder, 1989).

Doherty and Baird (1983) designed an urgency continuum to demonstrate when convening the family was most needed. The continuum begins with minor acute problems and routine, self-limiting problems in which the patient is usually seen alone. It then moves on to regular recurrence of symptoms, treatment failure, and routine preventive/educational care as desirable times to convene the family. Finally, the continuum culminates with chronic illness, serious acute illness, psychosocial problems, life-style problems, and death as situations essential to having a family conference. Doherty and Baird focus family interventions on four functions: (1) education, (2) support, (3) prevention, and (4) challenge—urging families to make changes or accept referral to a specialist. In 1985 Doherty reiterated the need for this approach to be used as a framework for a more consistent application of family interventions in general practice. Doherty describes the role of the family therapist as handling severe and chronic psychosocial problems at the end of the continuum. Hepworth and Jackson (1985) and

Anderson and Holder (1989) see the roles of the general practitioner and family therapist as more collaborative, running parallel instead of tacked on the end of a continuum.

Doherty (1985), Schmidt (1983/1985), and Hennen (1987b) have described several obstacles to holding family meetings. Doherty infers that these obstacles stem from the belief that only trained family therapists are equipped to deal with families. He counters that notion by pointing out that health practitioners with proper training in family interviewing are capable of dealing with health-related and life-cycle issues, saving the chronic psychological issues for the family therapist. Schmidt (1983/1985) and Rodgers (cited in Hickey, 1990) see the reluctance of health practitioners to meet with families as being related to several issues—lack of time, awkwardness in talking to two or more individuals (is power a question here?), lack of familiarity with theoretical constructs to examine family interactions, and perceived inability to process information for effective recommendations. Hennen (1987b) adds lack of space, payment, and organized, effective family-based records as obstacles to convening the family.

Early and continuing education, experience in family interviewing, professional support groups, and collaboration with colleagues skilled in family interventions can help break down some of these barriers. A systematic approach indicating when to convene the family also would be useful and may offer guidelines to health practitioners that could eradicate other obstacles.

Family assessment and community resources. Practitioners preparing for the primary care of families need to be taught ways of charting a family tree that would include important family features, problems, relationships (both within the family and outside), illnesses with possible triggering life events, and community ties. The Resiliency Model of Family Stress, Adjustment, and Adaptation also may be helpful in organizing family information based on model components. Many family assessment tools have been developed to measure family strain and stress (for example, the Family Stressor Index [FILE], the Family Strain Index [FILE], and the Family Adaptation Checklist [FAC]) and family strengths and weaknesses (for example, the Family Coherence Index [FCOPES], the Family Hardiness Index [FHI], the Family Time and Routine Inventory [FTRI], the Family Bonding Index [FBI], and the Family Flexibility Index [FFI]) (McCubbin & McCubbin, 1989). These assist in evaluating family functioning (McCubbin

& McCubbin, 1989). Use of nursing diagnoses to label family difficulties also may be valuable. Further information on family assessment and family assessment tools are offered in Chapters 7 and 9 and in the Appendix.

Family practitioners evaluating and supporting families also need knowledge and information concerning available community resources and services (Anderson & Holder, 1989). It is essential to update this information as new resources are developed and old ones expanded. The degree to which families use friends and relatives for support can be measured with the Friends and Relatives Support Index (McCubbin & McCubbin, 1989). The Social Support Index also can be used to determine family integration into the community, the family's view of the community as a source of support, and family feelings that emotional, esteem, and network support are available in the community.

Therapeutic communication, teaching, and crisis intervention skills. Therapeutic communication (which can include observing, interviewing, supporting, and listening), teaching, and crisis intervention skills may be particularly useful to the family-oriented practitioner, although they are not specific to family interventions alone. These tools assist in gathering information needed to assess family appraisals and functioning (other specific family assessment tools and therapeutic interventions are covered in Chapter 7) and in offering assistance and support. Since these tools are not specific to family interventions and information concerning them is plentiful elsewhere, they are not discussed here in depth. However, resources will be identified for those wishing to explore further information.

As identified in nursing and medical critiques of health practice, knowledge of therapeutic communication, teaching skills, and crisis intervention skills exists, but the actual skill or confidence in using them is lacking (Hepworth & Jackson, 1985; Lancaster et al., 1986; Leavitt, 1989). This ineptness discourages implementation of the skill in the practice setting. Therefore the importance of more educationally guided practice opportunities related to developing these skills cannot be overstated.

Therapeutic communication. Previous to learning therapeutic communication skills, the health practitioner's verbal and nonverbal responses are usually not helpful and often insensitive (Narrow & Buschle, 1982). Therapeutic communication, a most crucial tool for family interventions, is not natural and must be learned (see Sundeen, Stuart, Rankin, & Cohen, 1989). Since it is impractical and inappropriate to send every patient and family who wishes to express their feelings to the psychiatrist or psychologist, these skills are essential to health-care practice and vital in implementing the family perspective. Therapeutic communication also develops relationships strong in trust and mutual respect, which are essential to the healing process. Health-care practitioners interacting with families need to be skilled in therapeutic communication.

Teaching. Since obtaining information about the illness situation is a high priority for families (Hickey, 1990), developing good teaching skills along with communication skills is also essential to implementing the family perspective in health-care delivery. Teaching techniques that have proven to be the best need to be learned (see Hunter, 1982; How to Teach Patients, 1989; Cummings, 1980). Health professionals would then understand the need to assess learning readiness first and to gather information concerning previous knowledge or experience with illness before teaching. Teaching methods and aids that can enhance the learning process would also be learned. The ability to develop, implement, evaluate, and document a teaching plan could then be cultivated. Health professionals would be aware that single learning sessions are rarely adequate and "dosing" information may be necessary. Procedures learned by families in one setting may not be transferable to another (for example, hospital to home). Research, reported by Joyce and Showers (1980), suggests that only 5% of individuals lectured to will be able to use the information, whereas if there is opportunity to practice, 12% will be able to do so (cited in Thousand, Nevin-Parta, & Fox, 1987). However, of those who listen, practice, and receive coaching and feedback, 83% will be able to use the information and material successfully. The value of applying these teaching skills to patient–family–health professional interactions can be twofold: (1) meeting the family's need for information, thus increasing family coping abilities; and (2) increasing compliance with treatment plans.

Crisis intervention skills. Family crisis often occurs during illness, especially at the time of diagnosis; therefore the ability to apply crisis intervention skills is vital to the family perspective (see Aguilera, 1990). Crisis intervention is not a form of psychotherapy and is indicated in situations where there is sudden inability to cope with life. According to Aguilera (1990), this approach includes determination of the immediate cause of the crisis and focusing on direct encouragement of adaptive behavior that will bring the patient and family back to their previous level of functioning. Its goal is resolution of the immediate crisis. Crisis intervention is a mode of treatment that does not require advanced degrees in psychiatry or psychology and can be learned and implemented by all health practitioners. The importance of families or significant others to the crisis intervention process was recognized by Jacobson, Strickler, and Morely as early as 1968 (cited in Aguilera, 1990). To implement the family perspective, health professionals need confidence when confronting family crisis. Crisis intervention skills can be a useful tool for the nonpsychiatric health professional encountering family crisis.

Tools for change. Since few health professionals enter a health practice with an established family perspective, they need to acquire tools to surmount obstacles to the family perspective. Strategies from organization theory, change theory, and assertiveness training need to be learned and discussed in relation to some of the more common barriers to the family perspective. Opportunities to apply assertiveness, organization, and change theory and skills need to be an integral part of a health-practitioner's curriculum. This will prepare the health professional to initiate the implementation of a family-oriented practice in institutional work settings where it is not present or valued.

Research is another valuable tool in promoting the family perspective. The scientific knowledge base of the family perspective needs to be expanded. The family's relation to health and illness and therapeutic relationships between the health practitioner and the family need to be explored in greater depth. More evidence continues to be needed that clearly demonstrates the value of systematic intervention with families in prevention and treatment of physical and mental illness (Doherty, 1985). With a firmer scientific base, educators, health professionals, policymakers and third-party payers can be further convinced as to the advantages family-oriented services can provide and the directions that need to be taken. Students, practitioners, and educators need encouragement to participate in more research on families and family intervention strategies.

✦ FAMILY NEEDS: GUIDELINES FOR ESTABLISHMENT OF FAMILY INTERVENTIONS IN THE DELIVERY OF HEALTH CARE

The key to developing a family perspective within the health delivery system lies in learning what families need. Studies indicate that actual family priorities differ significantly from what health-care professionals perceive as family priorities (Graves & Ware, 1990; Jacono, Hicks, Antonioni, O'Brien, & Rasi, 1990; O'Neill-Norris & Grove, 1986). Therefore health-care professionals should not rely totally on their intuition or perceptions in determining the needs of families during illness. Most studies prioritizing family needs during illness are focused around the critically ill family member who is usually in intensive care settings. More research on different settings is needed to understand the full range of family needs throughout the health and illness experience.

Family Need for Information

The need for information was listed within the top four priorities of almost every study designed to prioritize family needs during the illness experience (Breu & Dracup, 1978; Daley, 1984; Hampe, 1975; Leske, 1986; Molter, 1979; O'Neill-Norris & Grove, 1986). Families wanted information about the condition, prognosis, progress, and comfort of their ill loved one. They wished to be assured that the best possible care was being given (Leske, 1986; O'Neill-Norris & Grove, 1986). They wanted this information offered at a level they could understand (Leske, 1986; Molter, 1979; O'Neil-Norris & Grove, 1986). Furthermore, they wanted all information imparted with openness to questions, a caring attitude, honesty, acceptance, and respect (Hampe, 1975; Leske, 1986; Molter, 1979; O'Neill-Norris & Grove, 1986). One study indicated that nurses did not realize the family's strong desire for honesty and for acceptance by the health-care professional (O'Neill-Norris & Grove, 1986). Hickey (1990) reviewed studies on family needs and suggested that health-care professionals consider the findings of these studies when imparting information to families.

Families need information to plan realistic coping strategies. Each institutional setting is obliged to look critically at its information-imparting methods and to explore ways of improvement. In-service classes for *all* staff who deal with patients and their families need to be designed to sensitize them to family needs. This could increase tolerance to constant requests by "demanding" families seeking information and encourage a better understanding of family behavior. Ways of imparting information should be taught based on educational theory and practice. Health-care professionals must realize that research shows that 55% of what we say is communicated through our behavior and dress, 35% comes from tone of voice, and only

10% from what we actually say in words (cited in Minnesota Nurses Association, 1988).

Another way to strengthen informational lines to families and decrease family anxiety at the same time is through better coordination of efforts and more effective interdepartmental communication. Rainsford and Schuman's (1981) studied a family with an overwhelming number of illness events and found the lack of continuity and coordination between the physician and supporting services increased stress by reinforcing the family's sense of disorder, as well as perpetuating a lack of understanding. Beardslee and Demaso (1989) pointed out that contradictory recommendations can cause bewilderment. The need for collaboration and coordination between all services helping the family requires a central source through which information can be coordinated. Nursing has experience and success in the role of coordinator, teacher, communicator, and collaborator. These skills need to be put to greater use in collaborative and coordinating efforts.

One successful example of coordination and collaboration in implementing a family intervention was achieved in a waiting-room program designed at the University of Illinois Medical Center (Hoffman & Futterman, 1971/1977). Through collaboration of the departments of pediatrics, psychiatry, occupational therapy, and medical social work, a program was developed for the waiting room of a pediatric oncology outpatient clinic. Patients and their families usually waited from a half-hour to 2 hours to see the physician and receive test results. Using a play program as the focus, a psychologist and occupational therapist made themselves available to both children and parents in the waiting room. Interaction among families was facilitated to encourage a supportive and communicative group atmosphere. When parents reacted negatively toward the physician or the treatment, a conference between the physician and the family was set up with the family's social worker as the mediator. The program goals were: (1) to facilitate anticipatory mourning, (2) to help family members maintain a sense of mastery, (3) to assist the child in maintaining a sense of identity, and (4) to reinforce the integrity, cohesiveness, and openness of family interactions. This program took a silent, tense, depressing, and immobile waiting-room atmosphere and made it come alive with activity from which emerged a wide range of coping activities.

The collaboration and coordination of several different disciplines clearly made a difference for families attending this clinic and can have similar results in other settings. However, the financial, logistical, and potential competitive aspects of this kind of collaboration generally prohibit its frequent use (Hepworth & Jackson, 1985). These barriers need to be overcome.

Family Need for Hope

Returning to the studies on family needs, three studies listed *hope* as the family's most important need (Leske, 1986; Molter, 1979; O'Neill-Norris & Grove, 1986), and two studies listed *relief of anxiety* as the family's greatest need (Breu & Dracup, 1978; Daley, 1984). This apparently indicates that *realistic* hope is what families seek.

Family needs for hope cannot be fulfilled by health-care professionals merely acting as a friend or with charisma (Engel, 1977); it requires *skill* in therapeutic communication and crisis intervention and *knowledge* of family systems, family dynamics, and community resources. Anderson and Holder (1989) describe offering hope to families as one of the most effective interventions for behavioral disorders. Awareness of family strengths, available effective treatments, and community resources are necessary to offering hope. If this knowledge and these skills are not part of the repertoire of health professionals in areas where imparting hope is important, continuing education in these skills and knowledge is needed. As stated earlier, studies have shown that practitioners are often uncomfortable with their abilities to carry out interpersonal skills with families. Therefore the need for continuing education from preservice education into the practice area is evident. New and established health practitioners need support as they continue developing and refining these skills. Also, constant updating of knowledge, skills, and available community resources is necessary in a field that is so newly emerging.

To offer hope and relief of anxiety, it is necessary to understand what the illness means to the patient and family. This is accomplished by convening the family and asking them to share their perceptions of the illness experience. Reactions, behaviors, activities, and feelings surrounding the onset and duration of the illness need to be elicited from the family. Family appraisals and health belief models need to be explored to obtain a better understanding of family behavior. Adaptive family behavior can then be reinforced and problem solving encouraged while convening the family at points throughout the illness. While convened, families can uncover successful coping strategies used in the past and discover possible strategies and solutions applicable to the present and future situations. Compromise then needs to be encouraged in choosing strategies useful to the illness situation. Encouraging mobilization of the family's social support network can help relieve strain and stress (Dunst et al., 1987). Other useful community resources can be identified. It appears that formal or informal support groups comprising patients and families going through similar experiences can be more effective than meeting with a health professional alone in terms of creating hope, buffering stress, and promoting health (Dunst et al., 1987; Halm, 1990). Therefore family meetings including other families going through similar experiences can also help foster hope.

In the family needs studies, opportunities to talk about feelings and the family member's death were ranked very low (Molter, 1979; O'Neill-Norris & Grove, 1986). This may reflect a preference to discuss feelings with friends rather than with the health professional. O'Neill-Norris and Grove conjecture that talking about the anticipated death of a family member also threatens possibilities for hope, a greater need than sharing feelings. This sets up a very difficult situation for health practitioners who are taught to cure, comfort, and get feelings out in the open. They cannot cure. With no hope to give, hope appears false to offer. Therefore comforting is difficult (O'Neill-Norris & Grove, 1986). Reactions to the difficulties of the situation come from all sides of the patient–family–health-care professional relationship.

To find hope where there appears to be none is not easy. Perhaps the answer is to look at ideas used by individuals like Bernie Siegel, a surgeon who has been successful in offering cancer patients hope when there is none. Dr. Siegel was motivated by his own frustrations and feelings of failure when dealing with incurable cancer patients in his practice. In his book, *Love, Medicine, and Miracles* (1986), he asks patients and their families to look at their illness as a gift, as an opportunity for growth. He asks them to uncover their feelings and beliefs about themselves, their illness, and their treatment. By resolving conflicts, the mind can then direct all its energy toward healing, self-healing. He uses mutual support groups, guided imagery, visualization, religion, and meditation as tools to facilitate the healing process. His purpose is to improve the quality of life, even if it is only from minute to minute. He does not offer a cure, but he does provide an opportunity to manage the situation. His success in drawing large numbers of people to his seminars indicates there is reason to consider this approach.

Physical Practice Setting and Family Needs

Although families considered the physical setup of institution waiting areas, such as comfortable furniture, telephones, and bathrooms, as a low priority, certain aspects of physical design can either enhance or hinder family involvement. An office without a conference room big enough to hold a group of people would make it difficult to convene the family. Hospitals with small rooms will find it difficult to accommodate a cot for a family member wishing to spend the night with the patient. It is difficult to talk privately with patients and their families if there is no place to do so. Lack of inexpensive living accommodations near hospitals may make it difficult for families living far away to remain nearby. The message this lack of facilities broadcasts is clear: we do not need families. There is a real need for more versatility in design to accommodate family needs. At this point efforts to change these things are limited but moving forward. Examples like the Ronald McDonald Houses that have been established near hospitals to house patient's families at little or no cost are good beginnings.

Family Need To Be Involved in Physical Care

In O'Neill-Norris and Grove's and Leske's studies on family needs, the desire to participate in the physical care of the patient received a low rating, whereas this desire was rated high (number 2) in Hampe's study. This discrepancy may be explained by the fact that Hampe studied terminally ill hospitalized patients, whereas O'Neill-Norris and Grove and Leske studied patients in an intensive care setting. In certain situations (for example, caring for children and the terminally ill) it appears that involvement in physical care can create feelings of usefulness and caring instead of helplessness. More studies on the need for family involvement in the care of the ill family member in different settings and at various developmental age levels should be undertaken so that the nature of family needs in different illness situations can be better understood.

Other Family Needs

Discrepancy in family needs can be found in several areas. In the intensive care setting the need for financial assistance was listed low (number 31) in Leske's study. However, financial concern may be a greater issue after the experience is over and the bills arrive; this factor was not examined. Families dealing with long-term care situations such as nursing homes, where "confusion of newcomers to governmental systems (Medicare/Medicaid) is legendary" (Reimann, 1986, p. 17), may view financial assistance as a high priority. This also may hold true for families managing long-term home-care (Hennen et al., 1987; Johnson, 1985). Another discrepancy occurs in the low need to express feelings by families studied in intensive care settings (Molter, 1979; O'Neill-Norris & Grove, 1986), as opposed to Cleveland's (1980/1989) study of families caregiving at home, which found great value in airing feelings.

These variations demonstrate the need for more studies on family needs in a variety of practice and illness settings. Research on family needs during chronic illness is always needed, since family involvement in this situation is high. Family studies need to uncover the difficulties families have in outpatient settings, which are considered the least family oriented of all services (Bozett, 1987). Short-term resolvable illnesses need greater attention in family research than presently received. Also, many studies of families and illness consist of author descriptions or views of family needs and often do not reflect the *family's* views of its needs.

This section has analyzed only the major needs expressed by families. The analysis demonstrates how family reports of its needs can be used as a resource to understand and plan family interventions. More often than not, institutional needs are met with little regard for families. Within hospitals and community settings, family-oriented practitioners with the use of family input need to develop philosophies, policies, routines, interventions, and physical designs compatible with family involvement.

✦ PRIMARY OBSTACLES TO A FAMILY PERSPECTIVE IN HEALTH CARE

The major obstacles to a family perspective in health care need to be analyzed to understand areas to overcome in establishing this approach. At the basis of the present health-care system are two main obstacles: the biomedical model and the present reimbursement system. These obstacles are now being questioned as to their ability to deal adequately with the biological, psychological, and social dimensions of illness and wellness. A climate conducive for the creation of a family perspective within the health-care system is beginning to evolve.

Biomedical Model: An Individual Focus

Our present health-care system is based on a biomedical model, one that attempts to define and reduce all illness to biological terms and processes. It is a disease-oriented model that operates on a cause-and-effect basis and focuses on the ill individual. The value this model offers is clearly seen in the technological advances that have been made in relation to diseases and their cures. In fact, this success has given this model its influence and power.

Engel (1977, 1978, 1980, 1987), Antonovsky (1979), and Doherty, Baird, and Becker (1987) have described well the implications and limitations of the biomedical model. According to these authors, the biomedical model is founded on hard science and physical signs and symptoms to legitimize itself. Consequently, gray areas such as social, psychological, and behavioral dimensions of illness are disregarded. Sickness is defined in physical terms; psychosocial issues are considered outside of medicine's responsibility. The body and the mind are viewed as separate, so "problems of living" (social and psychological problems) appear irrelevant. The focus on disease and pathogens fosters a disregard for the patient as a person, and therefore little interest is invested in the patients' and families' view of illness and its treatment. Moreover, the model excludes efforts to treat the total patient in practice areas. Patients and their diseases are evaluated outside of the context of family and community. Human relationships and their effects on promotion or prevention of illness are secondary concerns in the biomedical model. As a result the full potential for healing that can be found in these relationships and in the health professional–patient–family relationships may not be realized. Families may find it difficult within the biomedical model to feel empowered to use all their resources to manage illness.

Sickness encompasses both the physiological component of disease and the psychosocial component of illness; the psychosocial component includes family and community response with cultural and spiritual aspects as well (Neuman, 1989). Current research reflects a growing awareness that both the biological and the psychosocial aspects of sickness should receive equal consideration. In the past, only terms such as *fever, pain*, and *loss of vigor* indicated potential illness (Engel, 1974). Now, such terms as *depression, anxiety, stress,* and *strain* are becoming legitimized as equivalent in indicating potential for illness. Krantz and Manuck (1985) suggest that the cause of atherosclerosis and essential hypertension may lie in an increased responsiveness to the behavioral stimuli of stress. A new discipline called *psychoneuroimmunology* is developing that pinpoints psychosocial stressors such as major life adjustments, job-related stress, family difficulties, and death of a spouse as capable of producing immunological deficits that increase the opportunity for infection and neoplasm (Doherty et al., 1987). It appears that the function of immune system is linked to psychophysiological processes and modulated by the brain (Ader & Cohen, 1985). These findings and developments advance the view of illness to include "human terms" as well as "biological terms." This finally opens the health-care system to approaching sickness in a way that reflects the total patient, a patient *within the family unit.* Those health-care professionals strongly involved in a biomedical approach now may have the cause-effect relationship they need to legitimize broadening their focus to include the family when treating the ill individual.

The health-care system's current emphasis on disease hinders full implementation of the family perspective. In the ancient Oriental societies, doctors were paid only if the patient remained healthy (Craven & Sharp, 1972). Certainly this is a different approach from that of Western society, where efforts are aimed at solving problems of disease instead of exploring the causes and development of health and well-being. The opportunity to *develop* health within families is not always taken by health professionals today. Therefore an interest in a modality like the family perspective that can promote wellness may be lacking. With wellness as an ideal, the roles families take in maintaining wellness, offering support, affecting health decisions, attaching meaning to illness, and dealing with illness would be sought by health professionals for treating their patients. In a system that focuses on wellness, the family perspective would offer many advantages.

Our society is beginning to allocate more thought, energy, and money to determine what makes and keeps people healthy. Health has been taken for granted in the United States (Olson et al., 1989). Health and healthy life-styles are now beginning to be a valued, sought-after commodity, and many families are willing to spend money, time, and effort in these directions. This attitude also is being reflected in the health-care system. Research is identifying factors that keep us healthy (General Mills Family Report cited in Olson, 1989; McCubbin et al., 1985). Modalities are being developed that foster both physical and mental health (Becker, Steinbauer & Doherty, 1985; Kerns & Turk, 1985; Keicolt-Glazer et al., 1985; Morisky et al., 1983). With wellness as an ideal, the system may now be ready to explore ways of attaining that goal; the family perspective is one of those ways.

At the basis of creating and ensuring the establishment of health-care services with a family perspective needs to be a holistic philosophy where the patient would not be viewed as living in a vacuum but as an integral part of a whole—the family. The responsibility of the health-care professional would then go beyond the individual to include the family. Illness would be explored as a human experience as well as a biological entity. Several health models have been proposed as alternatives to the biomedical model. One of those models that could illuminate the family perspective in its proper light is the biopsychosocial model (Fig. 6-3).

The biopsychosocial model was proposed by Engel (1977), who named the model *biopsychosocial* to reflect an encompassment of the biological, psychological, and social dimensions of illness and the patient. This model is based on the works of biologists Paul Weiss (1969) and Ludwig von Bertalanffy (1968), both of whom searched for a more holistic scientific model that could expand the limits of scientific inquiry. With these goals in mind they devised the general systems theory.

Just as the aim of general system theory is to expand the limits of scientific inquiry, the intention of the biopsychosocial model is to expand the limits of medical inquiry (Engel, 1980). The model suggests that patients/persons should be viewed in the context of the systems within which they exist. Each system is an integral part of its higher and lower systems and a part of the whole system. The interaction between the parts and the whole provide a dynamic internal network within which information and material pass. "Nothing exists in isolation" (Engel, 1980 p. 537). Engel places the patient within a hierarchy of systems with the smallest system comprising subatomic particles and the largest system being the biosphere (see Fig. 6-3). The person/patient is "the highest level of the organismic hierarchy and the lowest level of the social hierarchy" (Engel, 1980 p. 537). Within this model each system has its own particular qualities and attributes. Therefore the methods, principles, and criterion to define and study one system may not necessarily apply to other systems or the whole. Each system can be fully characterized and appreciated only when related to the larger system of which it is a part. Engel considers the

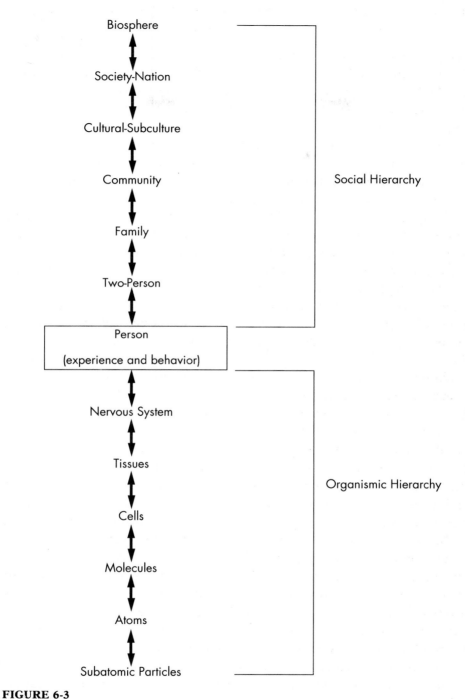

FIGURE 6-3
Hierarchy of natural systems in the biopsychosocial model.
(Modified from Engel, G.L. (1980). The clinical application of the biopsychosocial model. *American Journal of Psychiatry, 137* (5), 537.)

biomedical model as a subset of the biopsychosocial model encompassing the organismic hierarchy and invites health practitioners to be *truly* scientific by including the *human* domain (the social hierarchy) in their medical inquiries (Engel, 1987).

Engel contends that treating patients with systematic disregard for the human side of illness or of other systems in the hierarchy may potentially have dire consequences in health-care delivery. This thought has been reiterated by Doherty, Baird, and Becker (1987). Health and illness behaviors and physical signs and symptoms need to be examined in the context of significant personal relationships, which would also include the context in which the patient is treated—the health professional–patient–family relationship. Both the higher social systems and the lower organismic systems of the person need to be examined with the same aggressiveness and critical inspection. For these reasons Engel believes health-care practitioners who wish to offer optimum health care to their patients need to embrace the biopsychosocial model, since this model encompasses the total person. The biopsychosocial model appears to lend strength and support to proposals for a family perspective in the health-care system. As a foundation in health education and practice this model could bring value to a family approach.

Current Reimbursement Issues

Current reimbursement programs are probably one of the biggest obstacles to the development of a family perspective in health care. In the free-enterprise system of the United States, the potential for reimbursement drives businesses and the medical industry to seek specific directions that acquire payment. The U.S. health-care reimbursement system has few economic incentives to adopt a family perspective (Doherty et al., 1987). The reimbursement system is closely linked with the biomedical model. Mainly, reimbursement is given to those treatment modalities derived from the biological sciences (those in the organismic hierarchy) and related to disease and not health. As a result, few preventive treatment efforts and limited psychosocial aspects of care are reimbursable. This negates the very core of the family perspective as a vehicle to promoting health and enhancing treatment during illness. Those practitioners who adopt a family perspective must ask for out-of-pocket expenses from families or offer free services. This precludes its frequent use and hinders the development of strategies and skills that meet family needs.

For example, Medicare and many private health insurance plans do *not* pay for routine physical examinations, eyeglasses, hearing aids, general dental work, routine foot care, drugs, meals, homemaker, full-time nursing care in the home, or any other service deemed unnecessary (Siegal, 1987). The preventive health measures that would keep the elderly as functioning members of their families and society are missing. The support (for example, financial, physical care respite, emotional) to families providing care for their elders or the disabled in the home is not provided. Psychosocial support measures for families and individuals are limited and often categorized as unnecessary. Furthermore, Kemper and Murtaugh (1989) found that nursing homes can cost families as much as $30,000 per year (cited in Wiener, Hanley, & Harris, 1990). Medicare does not pay for custodial nursing home care, the most needed and most likely to devastate a family's financial resources (Siegal, 1987). It pays well below the actual cost for skilled nursing home services. The burden of nursing home payments can strain or destroy a family's budget and savings. A health-care system that is intended to support people during illness actually strangles families emotionally and financially and sets the stage for family crisis.

Families should be considered part of the health-care system, as providers of health care in the home and members of the collaborative health-care team. It is the family that provides support and can encourage the risk-reduction behavior that keeps family members healthy (Leventhal et al., 1985; McCubbin et al., 1985). In illness, families provide support, monitor or carry out treatments, and at times participate in physical care, especially for the chronically ill. In fact, Levin and Idler described families as the "hidden health care system" (cited in Murray & Zenter, 1985). If they too are health-care providers, financial resources should be present to support and enhance their role. The cost of health care in the "hidden" system has been shown to be less than the formal health-care expenses of a nursing home (Quinn, 1986). With proper support families could more often carry out this role and would not be so strained. Furthermore, patients could be more contented in familiar surroundings. In Dejong, Branch, and Corcoran's (1984) study of 75 spinal cord–injured patients, marriage increased the chances that these individuals were living more independently, a situation that decreases health-care costs. Providing money for emotional and financial support of the spouse could decrease the strain of these situations, thereby preventing possible divorce and increasing the opportunities for a positive outcome.

As families assume the role of caregiver, they will need the proper

---

Essential Equipment for Successful Family Caregiving in the Home

Attainment of necessary physical care skills for home care of their
  ill family member
Assertiveness skills for obtaining necessary information
Physical equipment to implement care
Provisions to physically alter the home as necessary for providing care
Appropriate supervision of care
Respite care to prevent physical and emotional drain
Appropriate emotional support that includes therapy if needed
Finances to do all of the above

"equipment" to be successful (see box above). Current reimbursement programs cover family caregiving "equipment" in a minimal fashion. Assistance may be forthcoming for some equipment, home care, and supervision; however, any supervision by visiting nurses, for example, would be reimbursable only for "medical acts" and not for emotional support so vitally needed or for reinforcement of skills. Respite care is rarely covered by third-party payers.

To move the health-care system toward a family perspective, a reimbursement system must be established to compensate supportive family interventions. Further research is needed to support and explore the potentials of this perspective as well as to develop tools for implementation. This may persuade third-party payers that a family perspective in health care is to their advantage. These are not easy tasks, and the evolution will occur gradually.

✦ ADVOCACY: CREATION OF DEMAND FOR THE FAMILY PERSPECTIVE
Creating Public Awareness

Education of the public, health and allied health professionals, and policymakers in health-care institutions and in the legislatures can initiate strides toward establishing philosophies and policies that complement the family perspective. Policymakers especially need information to formulate and implement plans. These individuals, on both national and local levels, need to realize the value and potential benefits of family-oriented services. Those health professionals and families committed to this approach need to initiate grass-root action to stimulate support for family-oriented attitudes and approaches. Heightened public awareness can be a powerful resource to obtain a goal. Often this resource is neglected by health professionals so strongly entrenched in their own daily practices. Public awareness can establish a demand health-care workers alone may not be able to create.

For example, Children of Aging Parents is a group that originally offered mutual support groups for family caregivers (Fradkin & Liberti, 1987). Eventually, it developed to found an organization that also compiles information on caregiving services and on local and national legislation concerning caregiving. The founders of this organization, Louise Fradkin and Mirca Liberti, sparked support by appearing on national television news shows and interviews with national magazines. They also have appeared before state and federal legislative committees to testify regarding the need for emotional and financial support, as well as respite, for caregivers.

By aligning ourselves with groups espousing similar family-oriented goals, like Children of Aging Parents, and initiating other action groups, health-care professionals and interested families can bring the family perspective to the foreground. This could create a demand for the family perspective and begin to relay information to policymakers. Along with this, health-care workers and individuals interested in the family perspective need to seek policy-making positions within health institutions and legislatures. Through these positions the family perspective can be brought to the forefront and collaboration can take place with persons able to stimulate the formulation of family-oriented policies. This could funnel more detailed information into the policy-making systems and create a conducive atmosphere for implementation of a family perspective in health-care delivery.

Demonstration of the Value of the Family Perspective to Insurers and Policymakers

Demonstrating the cost-effectiveness of a family perspective could help convince third-party payers and those who control the financial resources of Medicaid and Medicare of the value of the family perspective. Policymakers of these financial resources need proof of the following:

1. Keeping the family healthy means keeping the individual healthy. (Doherty et al., 1987; Huygen & Smits, 1983/1985; Schmidt, 1983/1985).
2. Allowing the family to own and take responsibility for treatment plans means better adherence to treatment plans (Storer et al., 1987).
3. Supporting the family through and after the death of a family member means completion of the family grieving tasks and movement back to health (Hepworth & Jackson, 1985; Kosten, Jacobs, & Kasl, 1985).
4. Supporting families through illness experiences, especially those involving caring for the chronically ill and disabled means attaining a level of wellness for both patient and family and needing less institutional care (Cleveland, 1980/1989; Dejong et al., 1984).

If these four tenets were satisfied, then policymakers and the general public could be faced with lower illness costs. The family perspective has the potential of fulfilling these promises and more. Continued research that demonstrates the cost-effectiveness of a family perspective in health care needs to be undertaken to provide further evidence of the value of this approach. This research can then be used to support the need for family-oriented health services.

✦ CONCLUSION

It is hoped that the pressure of current research, the need to contain health-care costs, and public demand will direct health-care institutions and policymakers to implement a family perspective in health care. The increasing number of health-care professionals skilled in implementing family interventions should also help in establishing this perspective. It would be unfortunate to see further delay in implementation of an approach that has so much to offer in promoting wellness, enhancing treatment in illness, and strengthening a fundamental unit of our society — *the family.*

REFERENCES

Ader, R., & Cohen, L. (1985). CNS-immune system interaction: Conditioning phenomena. *Behavioral and Brain Sciences, 3,* 379-394.

Aguilera, D. C. (1990). *Crisis intervention: Theory and methodology* (6th ed.). St. Louis: Mosby–Year Book.

Anderson, C. M., & Holder, D. P. (1989).

Family systems and behavioral disorders: Schizophrenia, depression, and alcoholism. In C. N. Ramsey (Ed.), *Family systems in medicine* (pp. 487-502). New York: Guilford.

Antonovsky, A. (1979). *Health, stress, and coping.* San Francisco: Jossey-Bass.

Baird, M. A., & Doherty, W. J. (1990). Risks and benefits of a family systems approach to medical care. *Family Medicine, 22*(5), 396-403.

Beardslee, W. R., & Demaso, D. R. (1989). A staff group in a pediatric hospital: Content and coping. In R. H. Moos (Ed.), *Coping with physical illness: Vol. 2. New perspectives* (2nd ed., pp. 359-369). New York: Plenum. (Reprinted from *American Journal of Orthopsychiatry*, 1982, *52*, 712-718)

Becker, L., Steinbauer, J., & Doherty, W. J. (1985). A biopsychosocial smoking cessation protocol. *Family Systems Medicine, 3*(1), 103-110.

Bloom, B. (1985). *Stressful life event theory and research: Implications for primary prevention.* Rockville, MD: United States Department of Health and Human Services.

Bozett, F. W. (1987). Family nursing and life-threatening illness. In M. Leahy & L. M. Wright (Eds.), *Families and life-threatening illness* (pp. 2-25). Springhouse, PA: Springhouse.

Breu, C., & Dracup, K. (1978). Helping the spouse of critically ill patients. *American Journal of Nursing, 78*, 50-53.

Cleveland, M. (1989). Family adaptation to traumatic spinal cord injury—response to crisis. In R. H. Moos (Ed.), *Coping with physical illness: Vol. 2. New perspectives* (2nd ed., pp. 159-171). New York: Plenum. (Reprinted from *Family Relations*, 1980, *29*(4), 558-565).

Craven, R., & Sharp, B. (1972). The effects of illness on family function. *Nursing Forum, 11*(2), 187-193.

Cummings, C. (1980). *Teaching makes a difference.* Snohomish, WA: Snohomish Publishing.

Daley, L. (1984). The perceived immediate needs of families with relatives in the intensive care setting. *Heart and Lung, 13*, 231-237.

DeGraw, C., Edell, D., Ellers, B., Hillemeier, M., Liebman, J., Perry, C., & Palfery, J. (1988). Public law 99-457: New opportunities to serve young children with special needs. *Journal of Pediatrics, 113*(6), 971-974.

Dejong, G., Branch, L. G., & Corcoran, P. J. (1984). Independent living outcomes in spinal cord injury: Multivariate analyses. *Archives of Physical Medicine and Rehabilitation, 65*, 66-72.

Doherty, W. J. (1985). Family interventions in health care. *Family Relations, 34*, 129-137.

Doherty, W. J., & Baird, M. A. (1983). *Family therapy and family medicine: Toward the primary care of families.* New York: Guilford.

Doherty, W. J., Baird, M. A., & Becker, L. A. (1987). Family medicine and the biopsychosocial model: The road toward integration. In W. J. Doherty, C. E. Christianson, & M. B. Sussman, (Eds.), *Family medicine: The maturing of a discipline* (pp. 51-68). New York: Haworth.

Doherty, W., & McCubbin, H. I. (1985). Families and health care: An emerging arena of theory, research, and clinical intervention. In W. Doherty & H. I. McCubbin (Eds.), *Family relations* (pp. 5-10). Minneapolis: National Council of Family Relations.

Dunst, C. J., Trivette, C. M., & Deal, A. G. (1988). *Enabling and empowering families: Principles and guidelines for practice.* Cambridge, MA: Brookline.

Easterbrook, G. (1987, Jan. 26). The revolution. *Newsweek*, pp. 40-74.

Engel, G. L. (1974). The psychosomatic approach to individual susceptibility to disease. *Gastroenterology, 64,* 1085-1093.

Engel, G. L. (1977). The need for a new medical model: A challenge for bio-medicine. *Science, 196*(4286), 129-136.

Engel, G. L. (1978). The biopsychosocial model and the education of health professionals. *Annals of the New York Academy of Sciences, 310,* 169-181.

Engel, G. L. (1980). The clinical application of the biopsychosocial model. *American Journal of Psychiatry, 137*(5), 535-544.

Engel, G. L. (1987). Quiet! Scientist at work: The doctor-patient interaction as a scientific procedure. *Family Systems Medicine, 5*(1), 115-120.

Fradkin, L., & Liberti, M. (1987). Caregiving. In P. Doress & D. Siegal (Eds.), *Ourselves growing older* (pp. 198-212). New York: Simon & Schuster.

Graves, J. K., & Ware, M. E. (1990). Parents' and health professionals' perceptions concerning parental stress during a child's hospitalization. *Children's Health Care, 19*(1), 37-42.

Halm, M. (1990). Effects of support groups on anxiety of family members during critical illness. *Heart & Lung, 19*(1), 62-71.

Hampe, S. C. (1975). Needs of the grieving spouse in a hospital setting. *Nursing Research, 24,* 113-120.

Hennen, B. K. (1987a). Continuity of care. In D. B. Shires, B. K. Hennen, & D. I. Rice (Eds.), *Family medicine: A*

guidebook for practitioners of the art (2nd ed., pp. 3-7). New York: McGraw-Hill.

Hennen, B. K. (1987b). The family as the unit of care. In D. B. Shires, B. K. Hennen, & D. I. Rice (Eds.), *Family medicine: A guidebook for practitioners of the art* (2nd ed., pp. 16-24). New York: McGraw-Hill.

Hennen, B. K., Seitz, M., & Seitz, B. (1987). The chronically disabled child and the family. In D. B. Shires, B. K. Hennen, & D. I. Rice (Eds.), *Family medicine: A guidebook for practitioners of the art* (2nd ed., pp. 42-50). New York: McGraw-Hill.

Hepworth, J., & Jackson, M. (1985). Health care of families: Models of collaboration between family therapists and family physicians. *Family Relations, 34,* 123-127.

Hickey, M. (1990). What are the needs of families of critically ill patients? A review of the literature since 1976. *Heart & Lung, 19*(1), 401-415.

Hoffman, I., & Futterman, E. (1977). Coping with waiting: Psychiatric intervention and study in the waiting room of a pediatric oncology clinic. In R. Moos (Ed.), *Coping with physical illness* (pp. 265-279). New York: Plenum. (Reprinted from *Comprehensive Psychiatry, 1971, 12*(1), 67-81).

How to teach patients. (1989). Springhouse, PA: Springhouse.

Hunter, M. (1982). *Mastery teaching.* El Segundo, CA: TIP.

Huygen, F. J. A., & Smits, A. J. A. (1985). Family therapy, family somatics, and family medicine. In D. H. Olson (Ed.), *Family studies review yearbook* (pp. 45-54). Beverly Hills, CA: Sage. (Reprinted from *Family System Medicine, 1983, 1*(1), 23-32)

Jacono, J., Hicks, G., Antonioni, C., O'Brien, K., & Rasi, M. (1990). Comparison of perceived needs of family members between registered nurses and family members of critically ill patients in intensive care and neonatal intensive care units. *Heart & Lung*, *19*(1), 72-78.

Johnson, S. B. (1985). The family and the child with chronic illness. In D. C. Turk & R. D. Kerns (Eds.), *Health, illness, and families: A life span perspective* (pp. 220-254). New York: John Wiley & Sons.

Kerns, R. D., & Turk, D. C. (1985). Behavioral medicine and the family: Historical perspectives and future directions. In D. C. Turk & R. D. Kerns (Eds.), *Health, illness, and families: A life span perspective* (pp. 338-353). New York: John Wiley & Sons.

Kiecolt-Glaser, J. K., Glaser, R., Williger, D., Stout, J., Messick, G., Sheppard, S., Richer, D., Romisher, S. C., Briner, W., Bonnell, G., & Donnerberg, R. (1985). Psychosocial enhancement of immunocompetence in a geriatric population. *Health Psychology*, *4*, 25-41.

Kosten, T. R., Jacobs, S. C., & Kasl, S. V. (1985). Terminal illness, bereavement, and the family. In D. C. Turk & R. D. Kerns (Eds.), *Health, illness, and families* (pp. 311-337). New York: John Wiley & Sons.

Krantz, D. S., & Manuck, S. B. (1985). Measures of acute physiologic reactivity to behavioral stimuli: Assessment and critique. In A. M. Ostfield & E. D. Eaker (Eds.), *Studies of cardiovascular diseases*. United States Department of Health and Human Services, Publication no. 85-2270.

Lancaster, J., McCance, K., & Vander-schmidt, H. (1986). A curriculum project for clinical prevention: The role of the nurse. *Family, Community, and Health*, *8*(4), 48-53.

Leavitt, M. B. (1989). Transition to illness: The family in the hospital. In C. Gilliss, B. Highley, B. Roberts, & I. Martin (Eds.), *Toward the science of family nursing* (pp. 262-283). Menlo Park, CA: Addison-Wesley.

Leske, J. S. (1986). Needs of relatives of critically ill patients: A follow-up. *Heart and Lung*, *15*(2), 189-193.

Leventhal, H., Leventhal, E. A., & Van Nguyen, T. (1985). Reactions of families to illness: Theoretical models and perspectives. In D. C. Turk & R. D. Kerns (Eds.), *Health, illness, and families* (pp. 108-145). New York: John Wiley & Sons.

McCubbin, H. I., & McCubbin, M. A. (1987). Family assessment in health care. In H. I. McCubbin & A. I. Thompson (Eds.), *Family assessment: Interventions for research and practice* (pp. 53-78). Madison, WI: University of Wisconsin–Madison.

McCubbin, H. I., Needle, R. H., & Wilson, M. (1985). Adolescent health risk behaviors: family stress and adolescent coping as critical factors. *Family Relations*, *34*, 51-62.

McCubbin, H. I., & Thompson, A. I. (1987). Family typologies and family assessment. In H. I. McCubbin & A. I. Thompson (Eds.), *Family assessment: Interventions for research and practice* (pp. 35-49). Madison, WI: University of Wisconsin–Madison.

McCubbin, M. A., & McCubbin, H. I. (1987). Family stress theory and assessment: the T-double ABCX model of family adjustment and adaptation. In H. I. McCubbin & A. I. Thompson

(Eds.), *Family assessment: Interventions for research and practice* (pp. 3-32). Madison, WI: University of Wisconsin–Madison.

McCubbin, M. A., & McCubbin, H. I. (1989). Theoretical orientations to family stress and coping. In C. Figley (Ed.), *Treating stress in families* (pp. 3-43). New York: Brunner/Mazel.

Minnesota Nurses Association (1988). *Tips on giving presentations to school children.* St. Paul: Minnesota Nurses Association.

Molter, N. C. (1979). Needs of relatives of critically ill patients: a descriptive study. *Heart and Lung, 8*, 32-39.

Morisky, D. E., Levine, D. M., Green, L. W., Shapiro, S., Russell, R. P., & Smith, G. R. (1983). Five-year blood pressure control and mortality following health education for hypertensive patients. *American Journal of Public Health, 73*, 153-162.

Murray, R. B., & Zenter, J. P. (1985). *Nursing concepts for health promotion.* Englewood Cliffs, NJ: Prentice-Hall.

Narrow, B., & Buschle, K. (1982). *Fundamentals of nursing practice.* New York: John Wiley & Sons.

Neuman, B. (1989). *The Neuman systems model* (2nd ed.). Norwalk, CT: Appleton & Lange.

Olson, D., McCubbin, H. I., Barnes, H., Larsen, A., Muxen, M., & Wilson, M. (1989). *Families: What makes them work* (2nd ed.). Newbury Park, CA: Saga.

O'Neill-Norris, L., & Grove, S. K. (1986). Investigation of selected psychosocial needs of family members of critically ill adult patients. *Heart and Lung, 15*(2), 194-199.

Quinn, J. (1986). Seeking quality alternatives in the community. *Business and Health, 3*(8), 21-24.

Rainsford, G. L., & Schuman, S. H. (1981). The family in crisis—a case study of overwhelming illness and stress. *Journal of the American Medical Association, 246*(1), 603-605.

Ramsey, C. N., Abell, T. D., & Baker, L. C. (1986). The relationship between family functioning, life events, family structure, and the outcome of a pregnancy. *Journal of Family Practice, 22*, 521-527.

Reimann, M. (1986). A gift to concerned family members: Management's role in reduction of admission stress. *Nursing Homes, 35*(2), 17-18.

Reiss, D., & De-Noir, A. K. (1989). The family and medical team: a transactional and developmental perspective. In C. N. Ramsey (Ed.), *Family systems in medicine* (pp. 435-444). New York: Guilford.

Schmidt, D. (1985). When is it helpful to convene the family? In D. H. Olson (Ed.), *Family studies review yearbook* (pp. 45-54). Beverly Hills, CA: Sage. (Reprinted from *Journal of Family Practice*, 1983, *16*(5), 967-973).

Siegal, D. (1987). Problems in the medical care system. In P. Doress & D. Siegal (Eds.), *Ourselves growing older* (pp. 213-228). New York: Simon & Schuster.

Siegel, B. (1986). *Love, medicine, and miracles.* New York: Harper & Row.

Slaby, A. E., & Glicksman, A. S. (1985). *Adapting to life-threatening illness.* New York: Praeger.

Starr, P. (1982). *The social transformation of American medicine.* New York: Basic Books.

Storer, J. H., Frate, D. A., Johnson, A., &

Greenberg, A. (1987). When the cure seems worse than the disease: Helping families adapt to hypertension treatment. *Family Relations, 36,* 311-315.

Sue, D. W., & Sue, D. (1990). *Counseling the culturally different: Theory and practice.* New York: John Wiley & Sons.

Sundeen, S. J., Stuart, G. W., Rankin, E. A. D., & Cohen, S. A. (1989). *Nurse-client interaction: Implementing the nursing process* (4th ed.). St. Louis: Mosby–Year Book.

Thousand, J., Nevin-Parta, A., & Fox, W. (1987). Inservice training to support the education of learners with severe handicaps in their local public schools. *Teacher Education and Special Education, 10*(1), 4-13.

Tripp-Reimer, T., & Afifi, L. A. (1989). Cross-cultural perspectives on patient teaching. *Nursing Clinics of North America, 24*(3), 613-619.

Turk, D. C., & Kerns, R. D. (1985). The family in health and illness. In D. C. Turk & R. D. Kerns (Eds.), *Health, illness, and families* (pp. 108-145). New York: John Wiley & Sons.

von Bertalanffy, L. (1968). *General system theory.* New York: John Wiley & Sons.

Walker, L. A. (1987, June 21). What comforts AIDS families. *New York Times Magazine,* 16-22, 63, 78.

Weiss, P. (1969). The living system: Determinism stratified. In A. Koestler & J. R. Smythies (Eds.), *Beyond reductionism: New perspectives in the life sciences* (pp. 3-55). New York: MacMillian.

Wiener, J., Hanley, R., & Harris, K. (1990). Nursing home care: Still a routine catastrophe. *Gerontologist, 30*(3), 417.

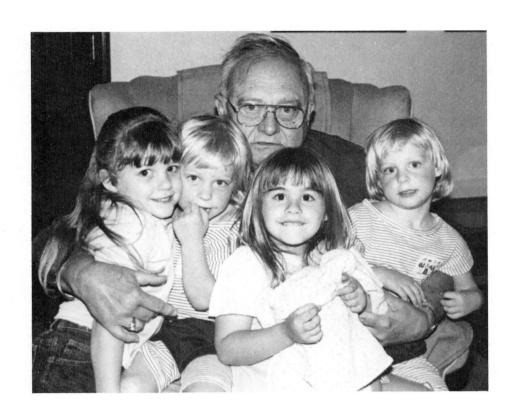

7

Therapeutic Family Interventions

✦

CHAPTER GOALS

✦ To help the health professional differentiate between bonadaptive and maladaptive family functioning prompted by a health crisis

✦ To offer the health professional guidelines for interviewing families

✦ To explain the difference between family therapy and therapeutic family intervention

✦ To describe family behavior requiring referral to a family therapy specialist

✦ To describe therapeutic family interventions that can be implemented by the general health professional

OVERVIEW

H EALTH professionals usually use supportive interventions that target the individual, independent of the family, during actual or potential health crises. Yet sometimes a broader approach is needed. This chapter emphasizes and describes the general health-care professional's ability to interview, assess, and provide therapeutic interventions to families before or during a family health crisis. The chapter explains the difference between family therapy and therapeutic family interventions and describes when it is necessary to refer a family to a family therapy specialist. Aspects of family functioning important to assess during a health crisis are exemplified. The chapter also discusses therapeutic family interventions that can be implemented by the general health-care professional. This chapter identifies those interventions that affect the family as a whole and improve the individual patient's health status within that family. Within the Resiliency Model of Family Stress, Adjustment, and Adaptation, this chapter focuses on social support (BBB), or more specifically, the role the health-care professional can take as a family resource (Fig. 7-1).

✦ BACKGROUND

The general health-care professional has an opportunity to assess and work with family functioning during health crises. The family physician or the community nurse frequently sees families during health examinations, at the onset of an illness, at the initiation of active treatment, and at recovery or death. Family members seek out these professionals for answers to questions, guidance in care, and overall reassurance. Unfortunately, health professionals often do not implement family interventions because their primary focus is the individual patient; they consider the family the focus of the family therapist or family physician. This lack of family focus can be attributed to the education and socialization of the health-care professional.

Family specialists find limited research that correlates the individual's health status to the family system (McCubbin & McCubbin, 1987). Moreover, they debate the merits of the research that does exist, as well as its value to family interventions as a part of health care. According to Burgess (1990) significant nursing research in family phenomena is just emerging. Yet the health-care professionals who have used the family focus in patient intervention are well aware of the positive impact of this approach.

✦ DIFFERENCES IN THERAPEUTIC FAMILY INTERVENTIONS AND FAMILY THERAPY

Family intervention is appropriate for many family members with a variety of problems in various settings. In one sense therapeutic family interventions and family therapy have few perceivable boundaries within

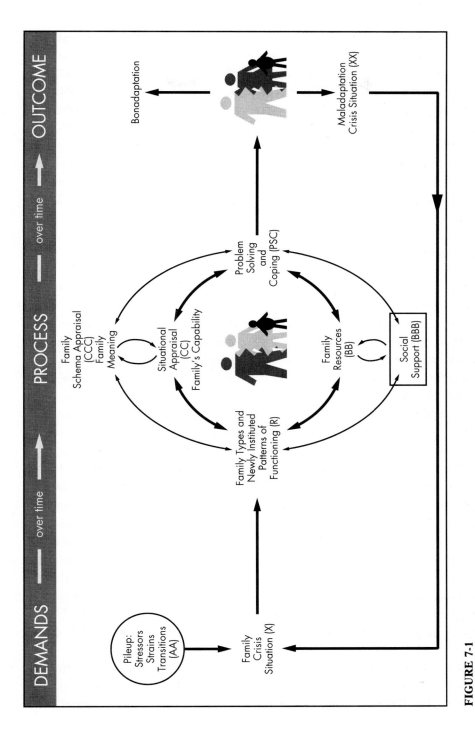

FIGURE 7-1

Adaptation Phase of the Resiliency Model of Family Stress, Adjustment, and Adaptation. This chapter focuses on social support (**BBB**) and the role of the health-care professional as a family resource.

the framework of prevention, treatment, and restoration. Inpatient and outpatient family treatment programs exist for married couples and siblings in traditional family therapy, marital therapy, and intergenerational therapy for single-family units in psychiatric settings (Helm, 1987). Various therapeutic modalities focus on individuals and families who have not received a psychiatric diagnosis but who are in pain or require short-term interventions and support. This therapeutic treatment of families can be useful in many general hospitals, clinics, nursing homes, and industries. Self-help services, which are becoming more widespread, also serve a significant role in helping families and their individual members. These latter approaches need not be led by professionals and are ideally directed by the lay members themselves. (See Chapter 8 for more discussion of self-help and mutual support groups.)

Therapeutic Family Interventions

Health-care professionals will find themselves able to implement therapeutic family interventions in several situations: in emergency rooms, intensive care units, kidney transplant units, preoperative settings, preschool, primary, and secondary schools, nursing homes, and convalescent or rehabilitation facilities. Patients such as unwed mothers and their families, delinquent youths and their parents, and victims of rape and abuse may benefit from therapeutic family interventions.

Therapeutic interventions may be differentiated from family therapy by how greatly emotional stress has pervaded the family's current level of health or illness and by the primary goal of the experience. In family therapy, members' emotional stressors and interactions are of paramount concern; the primary goal is to treat the emotional disturbances manifested in members' thoughts, feelings, and behaviors by encouraging modification in behaviors and family dynamics. In therapeutic family work, emotional stress generally is secondary to some physical illness, normal growth and developmental crisis, or social deviance. In this case the primary objective of the experience is not to change family behavior but to use existing family strengths and resources to initiate prevention, education, and crisis interventions.

Families in crisis can reap many benefits from therapeutic family interventions. Generally, illness in one family member creates a cycle; that is, the illness becomes a stressor for all family members and, in turn, the family-generated stress adds to the stress experienced by the sick member. Because of this cycle, however, what benefits the ill individual also benefits the rest of the family and vice versa. Benefits for the physically ill may include adaptation to hospitalization and illness. The individual's and family's reaction to physical illness and to loss of a limb or visual handicaps is typically a process needing attention. The family member's ability to maintain dignity in light of former self-impressions and capabilities is hampered. A family gathering in which the individual and the rest of the family discuss former and present capabilities is indicated. The family and patient can share frustrations and begin to work through the situational crisis so that the patient can develop a more positive self-perception and be more optimistic about the future. The family and the patient benefit from participation and sharing their concerns and hopes for the future.

For example, a newly diagnosed cancer patient and his or her family benefit from a factual discussion of cancer. This discussion may reduce their anxieties, which are sometimes fostered by misconceptions. It reduces the isolation that is engendered by the possible alterations in body image and life-style and perhaps the prospect of death. Thus therapeutic family interventions can help families cope with the behavioral changes in their loved ones and with the loss they experience. The interventions also can facilitate a more open expression of feelings when the initial denial subsides.

The focus of therapeutic family intervention differs in two respects from that of family therapy. First, the primary emphasis of therapeutic family interventions is working with the "normal," or psychiatrically healthy, family (Wright & Leahy, 1984). These families may be healthy or suffering some form of anticipated or actual health crisis caused by situational or maturational factors such as a sudden illness, chronic disease, accident, or having a baby. Therapeutic family interventions for these crises can include crisis intervention strategies, insight, problem solving, restoration, reeducation, and support. In general, if the family receives support and counseling during this crisis period, it usually does not progress to severe or chronic dysfunction.

Second, therapeutic family intervention is concerned with maintaining the present level of family functioning, preventing further psychological deterioration, and with educating families so that normal adjustment to health crises will ensue or be anticipated. Therapeutic family interventions can be carried out by any health-care provider; advanced education in family therapy is not necessary. Dysfunctional families also can benefit from these therapeutic family interventions.

A major component in implementing therapeutic family intervention is knowing how to talk with families (Wright & Leahy, 1984). Interviewing families can be an exciting and positive experience for health-care professionals who keep a few communication concepts in mind. The professional's essential task is to facilitate open communication with all members and to help the family to help itself. The professional maintains sufficient emotional distance to watch and learn about the dynamics within the family while at the same time maintaining emotional contact with each family member.

The health-care professional should consider some key responsive and active dimensions of communication. The health-care professional's effectiveness depends on his or her openness to learn what works best with each family and the ability and feasibility to reach the family unit. Communication techniques and therapeutic conditions can be individualized to the health-care professional's personality and the needs of the family. Interventions need to contain the key dimensions of genuineness, respect, empathy, concreteness, confrontation, self-disclosure, and catharsis (see box below) (Stuart & Sundeen, 1991).

Genuineness indicates that the health-care professional is an open person who is authentic and honest when relating to family members. *Respect* indicates that the health-care professional regards family members as people of worth and values and accepts them without qualification. *Empathy* is the ability of the professional to understand the family's world from the family's internal frame of reference (family schema). The

---

Key Dimensions of Successful Communication during Interventions

Genuineness	Confrontation
Respect	Self-disclosure
Empathy	Catharsis
Concreteness	

Note. From *Principles and practice of psychiatric nursing* by G. Stuart and S. Sundeen, 1991, St. Louis: Mosby-Year Book.

professional communicates a sensitivity to the family members' feelings. *Concreteness* involves the use of specific layman terminology rather than using abstractions when discussing the family members' feelings, experiences, and behavior or describing the illness and its treatment. *Confrontation* is in the form of statements made by the health professional to expand the family's self-awareness of discrepancies in the family members' behaviors. *Self-disclosure* exists when the health professional reveals information about self, ideas, values, feelings, and attitudes. Self-disclosure is done in a way that makes clear to the family that some statements reflect the professional's personal stance; the family can learn from it but ultimately must choose its own approach. The family is encouraged to talk about the things that disturb it most so that they can vent, examine feelings, and consider options for resolution. Emotional *catharsis* takes place and is of great value during stressful situations.

During initial interviews the professional functions as a participant/observer and temporarily becomes part of the family system by adapting to the rules and manners of the particular family (Helm, 1987). The professional joins the family while still retaining the freedom to encourage, confront, and challenge. The professional may initiate or facilitate convening the family for a meeting or have the opportunity to talk with the family in the health-care setting, community, or home. (Refer to Chapter 6 for further discussion of when to convene the family.) Wherever the meeting occurs the professional can facilitate the communication of each family member and of the family as a unit. It is advisable to meet with the family as a group, rather than to spend time with each family member, and to assist the family to talk to each other as a group. The intent is to increase family communication and encourage its functioning as a unit during problem solving and seeking of resources. The professional may help the family to establish the arrangement and to set rules for the group meetings such as when, where, how often, who attends, no one talks for another, no one interrupts, and so on. Professionals clarify their role with the family as a resource to be used.

Listening and observing are two skills of utmost importance in conducting a family interview. A facial expression that reflects interest and concern can be as effective as a verbal statement. The professional needs to listen both to what is being said and what is not being said. He or she tries to ensure that what is spoken is heard as the sender of the message intended and not as the receiver of the message had either expected or hoped for. In addition, a health-care provider who can match interventions to the family's mood, pace, and communication patterns will help family members clarify and validate their messages to each other (Wright & Leahy, 1984).

The health professional will be more likely to gain entrance into and receive trust from the family if some additional methods of joining the family are tried. One way to show respect for the family's values and hierarchies is to make use of these during family discussions. Suppose that the grandmother is the central communicator for the family. The professional might address all communication through the grandmother at first until the family as a group can be included. Keying in culturally when possible or finding elements of kinship are ways to improve rapport. For example, "I have a grandparent in a nursing home too," may become the basis for discussing concerns a family has about the caretaker role.

The health professional's affirmative attitude toward the family can be powerfully encouraging. Statements such as "You know how to solve this problem" or "You have strength" can confirm the family's sense of self-regard. It also may help to give smaller children toys to play with while talking to older ones or to have parents sit together as they discuss their difficulty with their children.

Eventually the health professional assists the family in obtaining a clear understanding of its problem and the incidents that led up to it. The family's view of responsibility for the problem is then discussed. Does the family perceive the problem as something it needs to change, wants to change, and can change? What resources does the family see affecting the situation? What strengths does the family have to deal with the situation? The health professional helps the family to manage the situation from problem identification to solution to restoration.

Family Therapy

Family therapy is a branch of psychotherapy concerned with the use of family process to treat psychopathological conditions or other dysfunctions in families. The focus is on the process between family members that supports and perpetuates dysfunctional symptoms. The aim of treatment is to modify personality attributes of family members and alter long-standing interactional dysfunction (Beck, Rawlins, & Williams, 1988; Glick, Clarkin,

& Kessler, 1987; Helm, 1987; Minuchin, 1974; Shealy, 1988; Wilson & Kneisl, 1983; Winstead-Fry, 1982).

Family therapy is practiced by clinicians from a variety of backgrounds, including psychology, nursing, social work, and psychiatry. Family therapists are strongly committed to a belief in the importance of the family. Graduate programs provide both theory and supervised clinical practice in this specialty. Psychotherapy for families may vary from intensive analytical therapy based on a psychoanalytical approach to therapy founded on communications and interpersonal transaction in the here and now. The emphasis of a particular family therapy format depends on the skills and interests of the therapist, the specific treatment aims for the clients, and the strengths and limitations of the members of the family, as well as the particular treatment philosophy of the agency in which the therapy is to be conducted. Therapy may shift in emphasis from support to insight with the goal of personality reconstruction. Thus family therapy interventions can overlap with and be supportive of therapeutic family interventions.

✦ REFERRAL FOR FAMILY THERAPY

The general health-care professional may wonder when the family should be referred to a family therapist for in-depth intervention. Generally speaking, referral is warranted when family dysfunction is not resolved by short- or long-term preventive, supportive, and educative interventions. Family therapy is recognized as a primary intervention in treating individual dysfunction when individual therapy is ineffective and the disorder is possibly linked to family dynamics. Thus referral is important when family communication or an individual within the family needs internal and external restructuring because of the specific psychopathological condition, which can be the result of many factors including physical illness.

As to when family therapy is appropriate, or especially indicated over individual or group therapy, can be unclear and controversial. This decision is dictated partially by the availability of resources; many settings do not have a trained family therapist on staff. Even if the resources are available, the therapist's or health-care professional's bias will have an influence in determining the point of referral. Some therapists believe family therapy is the treatment of choice for any problem or symptom. They make no distinction of severity because they conceptualize all emotional problems as within the family framework. Other family therapists recommend certain guidelines in determining which problems should be treated in family therapy.

Helm (1987) has outlined some general situations when family therapy may be indicated. First, the presenting health problem appears in relation to the family system; for example, severe sibling conflicts, marital conflicts, or cross-generational conflicts with partners vs. offspring or parents vs. grandparents. Second, the various types of difficulty and conflict arise between the identified patient and other family members. Third, in addition to the health crisis, the family is in a transitional stage of the family life cycle, such as beginning a family, marriage, birth of the first child, entrance of children into adolescence, the first child leaving home, retirement, or the death of one's spouse. Fourth, individual therapy with one family member results in development of symptoms in another family member. Fifth, there is no improvement with adequate individual therapy, and enlarging the conceptual field to include the family may produce therapeutic benefits. Sixth, the individual in treatment seems unsuitable for intrapsychic or interpretive individual therapy but primarily uses therapy sessions to discuss another family member.

Shealy (1988) outlines some situations in which family therapy is used. A marital problem or sibling conflict is best resolved by family therapy. Enough stress may be generated in changing family situations (for example, birth and death events) that family therapy may be needed to resolve the issue. When a child is being used as a scapegoat or when family members are too closely enmeshed to perceive their problems, family therapy may also be indicated.

Pasquali, Arnold, and DeBasio (1989) describe stressors that may cause dysfunction depending on the family's perception and interpretation of the situation. Family therapy may be indicated when family composition changes, when discrimination or economic difficulties arise, when family members change and grow, and when family relationships are dysfunctional.

Because family therapy is practiced in a variety of settings and involves families at all levels of functioning, the general health professional is exposed to it in many areas of medical practice. Understanding theoretical models used with families and collaborating with family therapists benefit the health-care professional beyond mere knowledge of when to refer the family. As discussed in Chapters 3, 4 and 5, just as the functioning of the family as a whole is affected by the illness of one of its members, so too the family's method of coping with a member's illness can affect the outcome of the illness. Knowledge of family dynamics helps the health-care professional make more acute observations and identify problems more readily within family systems. Such knowledge also assists in selecting effective interventions and in evaluating the accuracy of assessment by the interactional or functional change evident in the family. The remainder of this chapter focuses on those family therapeutic interventions that the general health professional can implement.

✦ ASSESSMENT IN THERAPEUTIC FAMILY INTERVENTIONS

The first intervention the health-care professional needs to consider is to assess whether family behavior during a health crisis is bonadaptive or maladaptive, noting whether the family typology, appraisal, resources, and problem-solving abilities can meet the demands of the illness situation. The professional attempts to gain a holistic perspective in this assessment by viewing the health of the family in the context of the following multifaceted framework: the result of the interaction between individual members and the family unit, between the family unit and the larger social system, and between sociocultural subsystems and individual members (Fig. 7-2).

While observing and interviewing the family the health professional determines whether the family is successfully executing activities to meet family and individual needs and at the same time satisfying societal expectations. If the data gained from the professional's observations and interview affirm the above, then the family is considered generally healthy and adaptive. Overall, a well-functioning family is a flexible one that can shift roles, levels of responsibilities, and patterns of interaction as it passes through periods of varying stressful life changes. However, a well-functioning family may, under acute or prolonged stress, have a member with symptoms of stress, but it is able to rebalance so that functions of all members are restored and symptoms resolve. Therefore the health-care professional observes the family for evidence of this rebalancing.

Many family assessment tools are available to assist practitioners in assessing families. These tools should be reviewed by practitioners to

Questions

- Is family flexible in regard to roles?
- How high is anxiety?
- Are individual members' needs being met?
- Is family as a unit participating?
- What is the family type and pattern of functioning?

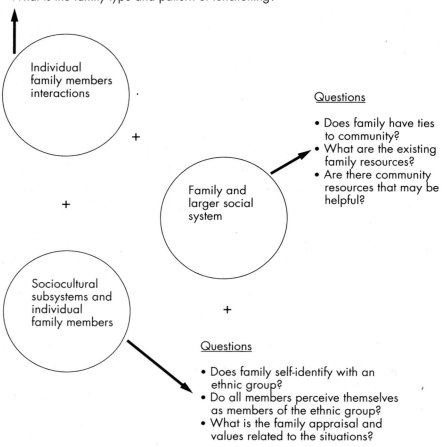

FIGURE 7-2
Multifaceted assessment framework.

determine which tool fits best with their area of practice. Some tools derived from the T-Double ABCX theory, which can be used to assess parameters of the Resiliency Model of Family Stress, Adjustment, and Adaptation are presented in the Appendix. Some examples of the information gained through the use of these assessment tools are presented below.

In measuring family vulnerability (V) both pileup and the family's life cycle stage must be considered. Pileup and life cycle changes can be evaluated by the Family Change assessment tool (see Appendix). This tool assesses the number of stressors and strains in the family and indicate the degree of family vulnerability. This information can then be supplemented by a family interview.

Family typology (T) can be assessed by tools that measure the characteristics of various family typologies (see Figs. 5-2 and 5-3 for family typologies and their characteristics). For example, the Family Bonding and Family Flexibility assessment tools (see Appendix) measure family bonding and family flexibility and can be used to assess the resilient typology (McCubbin & McCubbin, 1989).

A profile of the family's resiliency or ability to withstand stressors can be determined by the combination of assessment tools found in the Appendix. Family changes, coherence, flexibility, bonding, and available social support are measured by these assessment tools. The combination of scores from these tools provide a picture of the family's resiliency by indicating family strengths and weaknesses.

For nurses who use the nursing process, the overall diagnosis of Family Pattern Alterations is the one focused upon during the assessment phase. Diagnoses such as "Coping, ineffective family compromised," "Coping, ineffective family disabling," "Family process, alterations in," or "Parenting, alterations in, actual or potential" may indicate the need for a referral to a family therapist (Townsend, 1988).

Additional characteristics of functional families have been identified by Fogarty (1976), Minuchin (1974), Sedgwick (1981), Gillies (1987), and Taylor (1990). Some of these were discussed in Chapter 5. The health-care professional assesses whether the family behavior reflects the following characteristics and roles:

1. Flexibility is maintained and the family adapts to change during transitional stages of life and periods of stress.
2. Emotional problems are viewed as partially a function of each person, rather than as residing entirely in one family member.
3. Emotional contact is maintained across generations and between family members without blurring necessary levels of authority.
4. Overcloseness or fusion is avoided, and distance is not used to solve problems.
5. Each twosome is expected to resolve the problems between

themselves; bringing a third person in to settle disputes or to take sides is discouraged.

6. Differences between family members are encouraged to promote personal growth and creativity.

7. Children are expected to assume age-appropriate responsibility and to enjoy age-appropriate privileges negotiated with their parents.

8. The preservation of a positive emotional climate is more highly valued than doing what "should" be done or what is "right."

9. Within each spouse there is a balance of affective expression, careful, rational thought, relationship focus, caretaking, and object orientation, and each spouse can selectively function in the respective models and roles.

Overall, the family creates an emotional context that fosters self-disclosure, trust, cooperation, and acceptance among its members. The family reaches a balance by engaging in productive and adaptive activities aimed toward fulfilling internal needs and external societal expectations.

Examples of Implementing Therapeutic Family Interventions

After or concurrently with family assessment the health-care professional can readily implement the therapeutic interventions of support, insight, problem solving, restoration, and reeducation for a family in a health crisis. The professional supports the family by working with existing ego structures in a reassuring manner rather than trying to change basic personalities. Insight is implemented by providing families with increased awareness about how they affect others, how they are affected by others, and by providing information relevant to the specific problem. Problem solving is activated by discussing and encouraging constructive options and alternative solutions to the problems being experienced. Restoration and reeducation are implemented by providing skill and knowledge to families so that they can function more effectively.

Examples of situations in which a health-care professional implements these therapeutic interventions are numerous. For example, if a family member is diagnosed as having a regulative problem such as diabetes, the family's and member's initial reaction might be one of shock or denial. Eventually the family expresses anger and grief, leading to acceptance of the diagnosis. The professional acknowledges the pain involved in accepting the diagnosis and provides the emotional support necessary. Once the diagnosis is accepted, the professional educates family members and the patient about diet, exercise, and medications. The family would learn to respect the limitations imposed by the illness. During family insight and problem-solving sessions, discussions of feelings and behaviors is encouraged so that all members could increase their awareness of the effect of their behavior on others and determine the need, if any, for change. For instance, the patient's refusal to give himself insulin injections, now left to one of the family members, would warrant discussion. Problem solving would focus on what family members and the patient wished to do about the situation. This could be in the form of self-care activities, changes in roles caused by the illness, or honest confrontation between family members.

A newly diagnosed cancer patient's and his or her family's anxieties can be greatly reduced by early interventions. The diagnosis of cancer is often equated with death even though cures are becoming more common. Since the type of cancer, prognosis, and specific treatment are so varied, families benefit from education that clarifies and eliminates misconceptions. Once a definite treatment protocol has been decided and agreed on, the family can be helped to face alterations in body image and changes in life-style and roles, whether temporary or long term. Recurrence and the fear of dying are common reactions. These could be discussed in a trusting and supportive family atmosphere. The health-care professional would help the family and the patient to implement health-oriented behaviors while acknowledging the seriousness of the illness and the difficulty of recovery.

✦ DYSFUNCTIONAL FAMILIES AND THERAPEUTIC FAMILY INTERVENTIONS

Dysfunctional families lack one or more of the previously discussed characteristics of healthy families (see Chapter 5 and earlier discussion in this chapter). All health professionals, regardless of their area of expertise or practice setting, encounter dysfunctional families that are dissatisfied and have overt or covert problems. Some of the more common dysfunctional family patterns include the overprotective mother and the distant father with a timid, whiny child or a destructive, acting-out teenager; the overfunctioning superwife or superhusband and the underfunctioning passive, dependent, and compliant spouse; the spouse who maintains peace at any price and who ignores difficulties in the marriage but who suddenly feels wronged and self-righteous when the mate has legal difficulties or is having an affair; the child who shows evidence of poor peer relationships at school while attempting to parent younger siblings to compensate for ineffective and emotionally overwhelmed parents; the overclose three generations of grandparent, parent, and grandchild in which lines of authority and generational identity are ill-defined and the child is acting-out because of a lack of effective limit-setting by an agreed-on parental figure.

Dysfunctional families in a health crisis can benefit from therapeutic family interventions. Once the health crisis is over and the professional has implemented the interventions, an assessment can be made as to whether the family would benefit from more formal family therapy. In the meantime the health-care professional will encounter family dysfunction either as a temporary reaction to the health crisis or as a long-term way of adapting.

The health-care provider should be aware that poor health or deviancy occurs when any of the following deficits or combination thereof occurs:

1. Psychosocial disruption in individual family members
2. Disturbance in family group process
3. Disruption in the family action in which interdependent relationships between social systems and the family are disturbed
4. Disruptions in family communication, so cultural values are no longer transmitted or reinforced
5. Conditions in which families are out of harmony with the specific characteristics of the locale in which they reside (see box below)

A health crisis that causes one or more of these deficits needs some form of immediate interaction by the health-care professional to restore and

---

Indications of Family Dysfunction or Deficit

Psychosocial disruption in individual family members
Disturbance in family group process
Disruption in the family action in which interdependent relationships between social systems and the family are disturbed
Disruptions in family communication, so cultural values are no longer transmitted or reinforced
Conditions in which families are out of harmony with the specific characteristics of the locale in which they reside

promote health and prevent illness. The health-care professional can offer the family immediate help through crisis intervention with the goal of reestablishing equilibrium. The health-care professional takes the family through the four phases of crisis interaction (assessment, planning, implementation, and evaluation) and helps the family to focus on solving the immediate problem.

For example, consider the potential conflicts inherent in a situation where highly religious parents hold values different from those of the social system. They have refused medical treatment for their diabetic daughter, which reflects a disruption in interdependent social systems and a potential cultural conflict. Since this family's values also conflict with those of the health-care professional, the professional will first have to confirm this conflict and realize that the purpose of family intervention is not to impose one's views on another; the purpose of family intervention is to support and educate the family as thoroughly as possible so that they can make the best informed choices. It is obvious that this family's religious values outweigh the values of the medical profession. The health-care provider must acknowledge this and discuss it with the family in an open and nonjudgmental way. He or she must also educate the family about diabetes, discussing standard treatment, self-help, impending danger signs, health risks, and other complications. This family may have to choose between the health of their daughter and adherence to their religious beliefs. They must acknowledge their emotional reactions to the discovery of the diabetes. The family's resistance to medical advice should not be met with resistance, dismissal, anger, or coercion. Insight will be important. Education about the consequences of diabetes and family discussions will show the family how their decisions will affect their daughter. Members of their religion might support their decision, but the social system in general would not. Perhaps a compromise in treating the diabetes could be reached. Visits with other families who have cared for a diabetic child also may help this family. After supplying support, insight, education, and help with problem solving, the health-care provider must allow the family to make a decision that considers the legal implications if the child dies.

A more complicated example involves the interplay between disruption of a family member's health, a family group process, and a sociocultural value conflict. A distressed spouse brings his wife for evaluation and treatment because she is losing weight and seems depressed. The health-care professional learns that the wife has a previous diagnosis of dysthymic personality and that the couple has a long history of marital discord centering around the education of their handicapped child. The husband wants the child to remain home or be sent to India to live with the paternal grandmother. The wife wishes to take the advice of a social worker and send the child to a special school, but she cannot do so without the husband's permission. This family would receive long- and short-term benefits from family therapy because the conflict is longstanding and an essential part of the family system. Before the health-care provider makes the referral it is important to gain the family's cooperation. The provider should make an assessment and share it with the family. The health-care provider must avoid taking sides and should present the assessment as a way for the family to gain insight. The present conflict about their handicapped child could be explained in terms of longstanding differences. The wife's present weight loss and depression would also be evaluated. Judgments about an individual member's role are avoided. Conflict is discussed as a way some families cope with difficulties. Learning new, less conflictual ways of coping is emphasized and encouraged. The family's reactions to its situation must be acknowledged, discussed, and processed so that it can receive support during this struggle. All options for the child are explored and listed. Visits might be made to educational centers so that the parents can gain a broader view of available facilities. Referral for family therapy would go beyond the immediate crisis to managing the longstanding marital discord in this family.

To ignore any one of the above deficits that arise in families is to approach the family's health needs in an incomplete fashion. The health-care provider could choose to work with the family's individual health problems and the symptoms of the identified patient, but this would not be working with the family as an entity. The health-care professional must acknowledge each family's group process and the sociocultural values that have a significant impact on it.

✦ OBSTACLES TO FAMILY INTERVENTIONS

Some obstacles inherent in attempting to implement therapeutic family interventions originate in the health-care professional's beliefs and in the family's ideas about itself. Health-care professionals may be uncomfortable facing an entire family; they may not know what to say or how to listen to different viewpoints within the family. They may consider families complainers who undermine the patient-professional bond. Professionals interested in prevention, in addition to caring for illness, need to overcome these obstacles within themselves and then within others. The professional skill in involving the whole family and knowing when to refer the family to a specialist develops over time. Family members may have to be convinced of the importance of family intervention. Moreover, third-party payers usually do not cover family-oriented services. Families may not want to, or be able to, afford additional health-care expenses.

A major task of the health-care provider is to overcome some of these common obstacles to intervention. Families may resist intervention initially, since the consumer is used to a focus on the individual patient. Some resistance is typical in the first phase of most therapeutic relationships. Families will insist that they are managing well in spite of the health crisis. They may value their privacy above all else and believe their closeness should not be disturbed by outsiders. The health-care provider can work with these common attitudes by gaining trust through consistent follow-through and acknowledgment of the family's wariness.

As the relationship with the family develops, some members may become anxious about sharing feelings that might be objectionable to other members. Although the professional encourages openness and honesty, he or she helps members reveal themselves at their own pace. The health-care provider can also educate the family about illness and health as family systems issues. Flexibility is the key to success. The times and places for the family sessions should be convenient for the family. The provider may need to initiate the sessions with subgroups in the family if all its members are initially unwilling to meet as a group. The subgroup may encourage other members to participate. The health-care professional must avoid some common barriers to the development of a working relationship with the family and display empathy without becoming overly attached to the family or one of its members. The professional may unintentionally identify with a family member of the same age and sex or to an individual with an illness similar to one of a recently deceased member of the professional's family. Or the member could have an illness that the professional fears acquiring. However, the professional must maintain a balance in encouraging the family's coping skills so as to prevent or disrupt destructive alliances while reducing excessive stress within the family. Sometimes intervention must focus on an anticipatory problem such as engaging the family in grief work in the event of a terminal illness. Family members may view this as unnecessary and prefer to deny the inevitable until it actually occurs.

Some obstacles are external to the family and unrelated to its ability to cope or function. These include limitations on time, place, and finances. Time can be worked out by scheduling sessions that will not increase stress on the family. The place must be accessible to all family members. The professional's office should be spacious enough for patients in wheelchairs and have suitable facilities. The professional may consider making home visits to a bedridden patient. Finances are important to discuss. If insurance does not cover the fees for family intervention, perhaps other arrangements can be made. The family might be able to pay the additional costs, or perhaps the health-care provider will lower the fee. Failure to attend family sessions may not be because of a member's resistance. It is important to expect absences when a member is hospitalized. A member may have an illness, such as organic brain syndrome, that inhibits their participation in the family sessions. The professional may have to continue without this ill member. Other obstacles to family therapeutic interventions are discussed in Chapter 6.

REFERENCES

Beck, C. K., Rawlins, R. P., & Williams, S. R. (1988). *Mental health-psychiatric nursing: A holistic life-cycle approach* (2nd ed.). St. Louis: Mosby–Year Book.

Burgess, A. W. (1990). *Psychiatric nursing in the hospital and the community*. Norwalk, CT: Appleton & Lange.

Fogarty, T. (1976). System concepts and dimensions of self. In P. Guerin (Ed.), *Family therapy theory and practice* (pp. 144-153). New York: Gardiner.

Gillies, D. A. (1987). Family assessment and counseling by the rehabilitation nurse. *Rehabilitation Nursing, 12*(2), 65-69.

Glick, I. D., Clarkin, J. F., & Kessler, D. R. (1987). *Marital and family therapy* (3rd ed.). Orlando, FL: Grune & Stratton.

Helm, P. E. (1987). Family therapy. In G. W. Stuart & S. J. Sundeen (Eds.), *Principles and practice of psychiatric nursing* (pp. 725-751). St. Louis: Mosby–Year Book.

McCubbin, H. I., & McCubbin, M. A. (1987). Family system assessment in health care. In H. I. McCubbin & A. Thompson (Eds.), *Family assessment inventories for research and practice* (pp. 3-32). Madison, WI: University of Wisconsin–Madison.

McCubbin, M. A., & McCubbin, H. I. (1989). Theoretical orientations to family stress and coping. In C. Figley (Ed.), *Treating stress in families* (pp. 3-43). New York: Brunner/Mazel.

Minuchin, S. (1974). *Families and family therapy*. Cambridge, MA: Howard University.

Pasquali, E. A., Arnold, H. M., & DeBasio, N. (1989). *Mental health nursing: A holistic approach* (3rd ed.). St. Louis: Mosby–Year Book.

Sedgwick, R. (1981). *Family mental health: theory and practice.* St. Louis: Mosby–Year Book.

Shealy, A. H. (1988). Family therapy. In C. K. Beck, R. P. Rawlins, & S. R. Williams (Eds.), *Mental health-psychiatric nursing: A holistic life-cycle approach* (2nd ed., pp. 543-558). St. Louis: Mosby–Year Book.

Stuart, G. W., & Sundeen, S. J. (1991). *Principles and practice of psychiatric nursing* (4th ed.). St. Louis: Mosby–Year Book.

Taylor, C. M. (1990). *Mereness' essentials of psychiatric nursing* (13th ed.). St. Louis: Mosby–Year Book.

Townsend, M. C. (1988). *Nursing diagnosis in psychiatric nursing.* Philadelphia: F. A. Davis.

Wilson, H. S., & Kneisl, C. R. (1983). *Psychiatric nursing* (2nd ed.). Menlo Park, CA: Addison-Wesley.

Winstead-Fry, P. (1982). Family theory and application. In J. Haber, A. M. Leach, S. M. Schudy, & B. F. Sideleau (Eds.), *Comprehensive psychiatric nursing.* (2nd ed., pp. 321-339). New York: McGraw-Hill.

Wright, L. M., & Leahey, M. (1984). *Families and psychosocial problems.* Springhouse, PA: Springhouse.

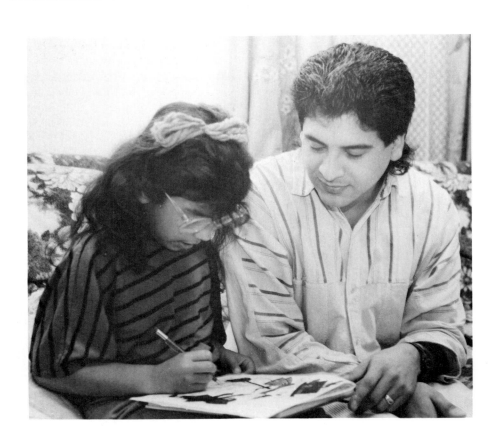

8

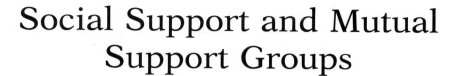

Social Support and Mutual Support Groups

✦

CHAPTER GOALS

✦ To introduce the role of social support in the resolution of health problems

✦ To present the basic principles involved in creating mutual support groups

✦ To illustrate the use of social support groups in family-oriented interventions

✦ To discuss the role of health-care providers in the formation and maintenance of mutual support groups for families coping with a health problem

✦ To examine obstacles that may be encountered in establishing a mutual support group

OVERVIEW

THE purpose of this chapter is to introduce the use of social support and mutual support groups as strategies to facilitate coping by families in crisis. Research that explores positive and negative effects of social support is presented. The indications for the development of a mutual support group are examined along with the steps in establishing a group. The role of professionals as founders of such a group is discussed. In relation to the

Resiliency Model of Family Stress, Adjustment, and Adaptation, this chapter focuses on social support (BBB) (Fig. 8-1).

✦ SOCIAL SUPPORT

Considerable interest exists in the role of social support as a mediator of family stress during illness crises. In Chapter 2 McCubbin and McCubbin characterize social support as "one of the primary buffers or mediators between stress and health breakdown." Gottlieb (1983) coined the phrase *health protection mechanism* in relation to social support. These views reflect the interest in social support shown by consumers and health-care providers alike.

Definition

In Chapter 2 McCubbin and McCubbin elaborate on the ideas of Cobb (1976) and present a definition of social support that involves meaningful contact with people through a mutually supportive communication exchange. Social support can be a source of information, affection, affirmation, or tangible support such as money, physical help, or materials. The McCubbins (see Chapter 2) have proposed five dimensions of social support (see box on p. 216).

Research has demonstrated that social support is generally beneficial for individuals facing crisis. A few studies that focused on social support for husbands and wives found that this support does not always have a positive effect. A critical variable seems to be the cause of the stress. If the stress is caused by financial problems and the husband is the primary breadwinner, then the wife who seeks social support from friends or relatives may escalate stress within the family (Dressler, 1985; Pittman & Lloyd, 1988; Robertson, Elder, Skinner, & Conger, 1991). From the perspective proposed by the Resiliency Model, these research findings are understandable, since according to the model anything can be a stressor. So the wife who is perceived as unloyal because she tells friends and families that her husband is having financial difficulties may add stress to the family. Also, seeking social support may add to pileup if attending a mutual support group meeting disrupts the family schedule or stresses the budget.

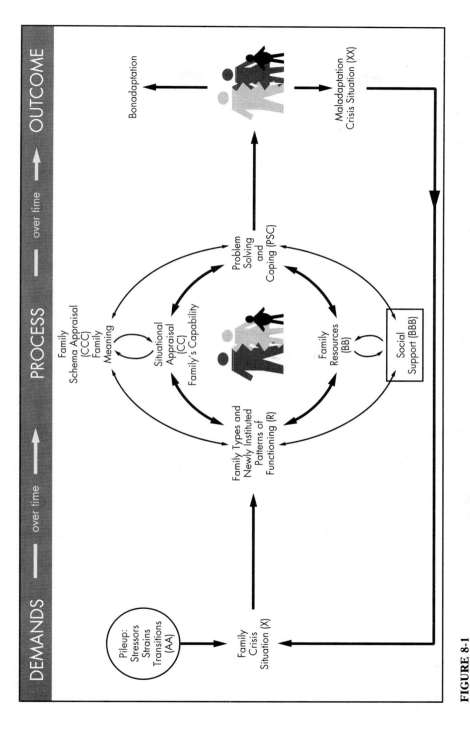

FIGURE 8-1

Adaptation Phase of the Resiliency Model of Family Stress, Adjustment, and Adaptation. This chapter focuses on social support (BBB) and the use of social support groups as a family resource.

McCubbins' Five Dimensions of Social Support

1. *Emotional support*   Confirmation that love and care exist in the relationship
2. *Esteem support*   Confirmation that one is esteemed and valued
3. *Network support*   Confirmation that an understanding communication network exists
4. *Appraisal support*   Feedback that allows one to evaluate how well tasks are being managed
5. *Altruistic support*   Good will from others received in return for having given something of one's self.

Generally, despite the caution contained in the research just cited, the support sought by one family member potentially benefits the entire family (Lin & Ensel, 1989; Reis, Barbera-Stein, & Bennett, 1986; Stevens, 1988). Again, from the perspective advanced by the Resiliency Model, social support sought by one family member could enhance the problem-solving skills of the family, could bring resources that might decrease pileup, or could change the family appraisal of the situation to one that is more positive and advantageous.

Theoretical Background

Nuckolls, Cassel, and Kaplan (1972) demonstrated that women who were highly stressed but who also possessed high psychosocial assets had complications with pregnancy 33% of the time. Highly stressed women without psychosocial assets had a pregnancy complication rate of 91%. Building on these findings, researchers have consistently demonstrated a positive relationship between social support and a desirable pregnancy outcome including fewer maternal and infant complications (Norbeck & Tilden, 1983), enhanced maternal role attainment (Mercer, Hackley, & Bostrom, 1983, 1984), and successful adaptation to parenthood by both parents (Cronenwett, 1985a, 1985b).

Other researchers have demonstrated a relationship between social support and decreased mortality in heart disease. When risk factors such as smoking are controlled for, socially supported individuals are less likely to die from heart disease than isolated, healthy persons (Berkman, 1986). In a study of unhealthy men who survived myocardial infarcts, Ruberman,

Weinblatt, Goldberg, and Chaudhary (1984) found more total deaths and more sudden deaths in isolated men than in supported men.

Social support has been studied in regard to many health and illness phenomena. Cohen (1988) and Norbeck (1988) present comprehensive overviews of the topic for those that wish to explore the many studies involving social support. McCubbin and McCubbin (1989) propose that health-care professionals can offer esteem and appraisal support. On the other hand, professionals also can be sources of demands and conflict. Health-care professionals need awareness of this ability to increase demands and instead must try to be a source of support.

Mechanisms of Social Support

In terms of the goals of this chapter the question of how social support "works" is important. The mechanism(s) by which it exerts its benefits are not well understood. For our purposes three mechanisms will be explored: behavioral, psychological, and physiological (Ganster & Victor, 1988). These mechanisms are then discussed as they relate to the theoretical model of this book.

Behavioral mechanisms. Social support may initiate changes in behavior that decrease stress, facilitates recovery from a stressful event, or prevents stressful episodes from occurring (Ganster & Victor, 1988; Wills, 1985). Socially supported individuals may receive more information about how to avoid or manage stressors. For example, to observe a determined former smoker persuading colleagues to quit smoking brings an appreciation of the strength of social support in decreasing the health risk of smoking.

Persons who have a social network may get advice on health promotion or stress avoidance. Friends and co-workers may offer ideas that allow a person to avoid stressful situations or to mitigate their effects. Likewise, friends and family may provide tangible resources such as money, transportation to health-care facilities, or help with chores that reduce the burden of a stressful situation. Friends may offer direct advice on how to contact psychotherapists or other professional helpers.

In contrast, isolated persons who are stressed have to find resources on their own. They may lack the energy or the skills to do so effectively. As Wills (1985) points out, these behaviors cited above (for example, offering advice, providing resources) do not totally account for how social support influences health because the perception of the support and the resulting psychological responses must also be considered. For example, if the support is perceived as a put-down or insinuates that the receiver is a "loser," the subsequent emotional response would be negative and would probably not reduce stress.

Psychological mechanisms. Social support may enhance self-esteem, self-identity, and bring a sense of control over life (Gottlieb, 1983; Wills, 1985). These positive personal states can decrease the impact of a stressor or facilitate recovery from the stressor. Positive interactions with family, friends, and community members lead to a sense of efficaciousness and being in control. These interactions also lead to a sense of reciprocity.

Persons in a supportive social situation experience less anomie and loneliness. Loneliness is associated with emotional distress in that it denies one a sense of social integration and the opportunity for emotional intimacy (Peplau & Perlman, 1982; Rook, 1984). A primary benefit of social support may be that it overcomes loneliness.

Physiological mechanisms. The literature on stress suggests two ways stress can negatively influence bodily functions. One way is by increasing neuroendocrine responses, which leads to elevated blood pressure, elevated catecholamine levels, increased gastric acidity, and other manifestations of the fight-or-flight response. The second deleterious physiological response to stress is suppression of the immune system. The growing field of psycho-neuroimmunology is exploring the relationships between personality variables, immune response, and neuroendocrine reactivity (Locke & Colligan, 1986). Currently, we can conclude that a more positive emotional state is related to a decreased fight-or-flight response and to increased immune functioning. Social support may help foster a more positive emotional state.

From the perspective of the theoretical model guiding this book, all three explanations of how social support works can be accommodated. The model assumes that a person is a holistic combination of psychological and physiological attributes that communicates within the family and with the larger community.

The psychological explanation of how social support works helps to elucidate the Resiliency Model. People who feel in control of life and who have higher self-esteem probably have fewer pileup demands, since they would handle ongoing life stressors more successfully. Families with higher self-esteem are more likely to have capabilities and strengths to manage crises, as well as a family schema that is positive about managing stress.

Behavioral explanations of the efficacy of social support are also compatible with the Resiliency Model. Social support is mentioned by McCubbin and McCubbin as one of the resources that facilitates crisis management in the adaptation phase. This resource can produce better and more coping strategies and allow the family to uncover alternative solutions to a problem. For example, social support that encourages a behavioral family change by suggesting that all family members need to help with chores when they are not can enhance family problem solving and decrease the impact of some stressors.

The Resiliency Model can also encompass the physiological mechanism of social support. The Resiliency Model identifies the contribution the physical well-being of family members brings to family functioning and management of stressors. Families with abundant social support may find their members healthier due to less suppression of the immune system and decreased fight-or-flight response. Therefore family members may be more available to buffer against stressors and to contribute to overall family well-being and functioning.

In our society the most prevalent and organized manifestations of social support are the self-help and mutual support groups. Mutual support groups preceded the research interest in social support; the primary mechanism underlying their success is the support members give one another in confronting a specific life problem.

✦ MUTUAL SUPPORT GROUPS

Mutual support groups usually comprise individuals or families who share a similar life problem. Within the Resiliency Model, mutual support groups provide networking support. The success of support groups in dealing with crises, enhancing health behaviors, and improving the lives of members is impressive. The success of these groups results from sharing experiences about a problem and discovering a bond with others with similar experiences. The groups also validate the normalcy of certain feelings. The effectiveness of the mutual support group also is derived from the expectation that those who are helped will become those who help others, which enhances self-esteem (Silverman, 1980).

Other findings indicate how mutual support groups work and demonstrate the extent of their effectiveness. Reissman and Gartner (1987) describe a "self-help ethos" that includes self-determination, empowerment of members, mutuality, bottom-up organizational structure, a noncommodity approach to help, and the integration of egoism and altruism. These characteristics transcend all of the groups and give them a common worldview. The dimensions of the self-help ethos are further defined as anti-big, reaffirming of traditional values, use of new age psychology, and as a democratization of everyday life.

A mutual support group may be the linkage a person needs to function in a community. Such groups become powerful influences because they teach members new skills, grounded in experience, that may be generalized to other areas of life. When people help themselves and others, they feel empowered. Empowerment is important for a sense of mastery and control, which enhances self-esteem.

According to Gilbey (1989), the processes by which self-help groups empower their members include kinship, validation, support, role models, knowledge, family support, and the opportunity to help. Because the people who make up the group have lived with the problem, a kinship of common experiences and needs exists. People no longer feel alone. The face-to-face interaction that characterizes mutual support group meetings provides validation of the feelings and concerns associated with the problem. For some people, the support and acceptance they feel in the group is a new experience. The caring environment is therapeutic. The presence of role models who have successfully dealt with, or are dealing with, the same problem that seems hopeless to a new member can be inspiring. Groups also have a reservoir of knowledge and skills about how to manage particular problems. Family members benefit from the fellowship and from knowledge about how to help their kin. Finally, the helper-therapy principle comes into play—people who help others are helped themselves. By constantly moving from help-receiver to helper, the therapeutic benefits of helping affect the person.

Controversy in the literature exists over whether health-care providers, hospitals, and other agencies are part of social support. Gottlieb (1983) states they are not because the relationship is not mutually reciprocal. McCubbin and McCubbin (1989) state that formal organizations can provide social support. Recent work with parents of children with special needs documents that the informal support of friends, family, and social groups is superior to formal support in enhancing family cohesion and in fostering positive behavior by the child (Trivette & Dunst, 1987).

Politically the self-help movement is attractive because it reaches groups traditional services miss, either because the target population does not seek service or because the service provider does not pursue the client. Self-help also is cost-effective because the help is usually free.

Former Surgeon General C. Everett Koop held a conference in 1988 on self-help and public health, an event that may herald the government's involvement in the self-help movement. How "big" government bureaucracies will interact with the "anti-big" self-help movement may raise new challenges for both (Reissman & Gartner, 1987).

Mutual Support Groups and Families

Many examples in the literature support the usefulness of mutual support groups for families in critical care settings (Fournet & Schaubhut, 1986; Mauss-Clum & Ryan, 1981; Pearlmutter, Locke, Bourdon, Gaffey, & Tyrrell, 1984), although most of these studies are not based on research, which limits their usefulness. Of the few research articles published, two support the idea that structured, preoperative teaching in groups decreases anxiety in the spouses of patients undergoing major surgery (Kathol, 1984; Silva, 1979). Similarly, Halm (1990) found a significant decrease in anxiety in family members who attended a support group during the critical phase of a kin's illness.

Mutual support groups for families with a chronically ill schizophrenic member has received considerable attention. Anderson, Reiss, and Hogarty (1986) and West et al. (1985) recommend educational approaches designed to decrease guilt and blame, to present theories about the causes of schizophrenia, to offer effective ways for family members to relate to the schizophrenic person, and to encourage interactions with the community. The authors are convinced that family members can be involved in dealing constructively with their schizophrenic relative. This education supplements other therapeutic endeavors.

Many mutual support groups are national or even international in scope. For example, the National Alliance for Genetic Support Groups is very effective in providing support for families with a genetic illness. Perhaps one of the most frightening diagnoses a family can receive is a genetic disorder (Black & Weiss, 1988). For the individual, a genetic disorder shakes the basic sense that one is a whole, functional person. For the family, it can initiate guilt and fear. Genetic support groups offer educational, supportive, and social services. Professionals often serve as consultants, guest lecturers, or advisory board members. The amount of misinformation and blaming among families can be very destructive with these illnesses, especially if previous demands pileup. A genetic mutual support group can offer parents comfort and information about how to deal with the day-to-day management of a chronic, and perhaps life-threatening, illness.

The National Alliance of Genetic Support Groups tries to encourage "parent-professional collaboration" (Black & Weiss, 1988). Parents need the knowledge professionals have about the disease, and professionals need to know the day-to-day strategies for raising a child with a special need. When such alliances are successful, everyone benefits. When this alliance does not work, it is sometimes because the family will not share problems because they are afraid of the professional's response. Other times it is because professionals will not admit not knowing all the answers, or the professional is using the group to recruit patients.

The parent-professional partnership is one of the contributions genetic support groups have made to the mutual support movement. Ideally, parents would be paid for their participation in conferences and treated as colleagues. This does not happen regularly now, but fund-raising organizations such as the March of Dimes Birth Defects Foundation are willing to consider parental expenses and fees as legitimate parts of budget requests.

The Candlelighters Childhood Cancer Foundation offers support to families of children with cancer. The positive effects of the psychosocial support are documented in research (Adams-Greely, 1986; Blotcky, 1986; Koocher, 1986). Candlelighters offer self-help services from the practical (funds for wigs and prostheses) to the spiritual. This group tries to empower families, not only to cope with cancer, but also to grow as responsible, knowledgeable, and caring individuals.

In a thorough review of the mutual support literature Chesler and Barbarin (1987) found parents with sick children who participated in support groups have a more positive attitude toward medical staff than parents who do not participate. They also found that participating parents did not spread misinformation, nor were they more emotionally burdened than nonparticipants. Some professionals do not value support groups because they believe the groups spread misinformation or increase the emotional burden on the family. Chesler and Barbarin's findings are reassuring for professionals.

The Family as a Mutual Support Group

Usually the family is the primary social support of its members. During times of crisis this function may be limited because of the overwhelming nature of the stressor event. Referral to a mutual support group may not be indicated for short-term crises. However, families facing a short-term crisis should be encouraged to attend those natural, common family events such as church picnics, Little League games, and school functions that can be sources of social support. Such activities provide informal support for family identity and give a shared experience of family life. Moreover, they help families in the midst of crisis maintain a sense of relatedness with their community.

✦ CREATION OF A MUTUAL SUPPORT GROUP

The success of mutual support groups in handling crises, enhancing health behaviors, and improving the lives of members is prompting health-care providers to establish such groups for their intervention activities. The steps in establishing a mutual support group are provided in the following discussion, using mothers of twins as an example.

Step 1: Identification of the Target Population

The first step in establishing a mutual support group is to identify the population in need. Essentially, this is the most important step because if the target population is not accurately defined and recruited the group will fail (Nichols & Jenkinson, 1991; Wheeler & Limbo, 1990). Sometimes a group of clients identifies itself to a health-care provider. For example, a group of mothers, each of whom gave birth to twins, began to talk with one another and realized they had some unique needs. This group may approach a health-care provider for help, or a health-care provider, for example a nurse on the obstetrics unit, may realize many mothers of twins are calling in with unique questions. The nurse then may set out to establish a mutual support group for mothers with twins.

The health-care provider may find few articles on managing twins. For example, how to manage feeding two babies who are hungry at the same time is learned by trial and error. The mothers often feel they are neglecting one or the other. In terms of defining the support group, the health-care provider will have to decide if fathers are to be included and must be clear about the goal. If the goal is to support mothers who are full-time homemakers with educational and emotional techniques, fathers would not be included. This is not to suggest that fathers may not need support, but to include fathers may make an unwed mother uncomfortable or may change the nature of the group to include marital conflicts around child care.

Including the father may also require meeting in the evening, which may be unattractive to the professional or to the members. For purposes of illustration, the group will be composed solely of mothers of twins with the primary goal being education and support.

Step 2: Recruitment of Group Members

Recruitment is the next step in establishing a mutual support group. The organizer has to decide the ideal number of group members. If a small group of 8 to 10 mothers is desired, the organizer would not advertise too widely. Conversely, wider advertising would be indicated if a larger group is desired. For the mothers of twins group, pediatricians, family practitioners, and agencies serving children would be likely sources for names of potential members. The organizer could place advertisements in community papers, put signs up in laundromats or grocery stores, and pass news along by word of mouth to generate participants.

Step 3: Recruitment of Collaborators

The organizer needs to address the question of collaborators. On the one hand, the leader does not want every agency involved with parents to sponsor the group because too much time would be spent reconciling philosophies and coordinating the groups. On the other hand, successful groups usually have been guided by sponsors with expertise and resources (Leventhal, Maton, & Madara, 1988). Many states have clearinghouses that list and provide networking services to mutual support groups. It would be well to call the clearinghouse to ascertain if a mothers of twins group exists. If such a group is already meeting, it would be logical to join with it. If there is no such group, the clearinghouse can be informed that one is starting.

For the purposes of illustrating the process of starting a mothers of twins group, assume that no such group exists, so collaborators must be found. Perhaps a pediatric nurse or a child psychologist who is the parent of twins lives nearby. Such a person would be a valuable collaborator, since they have theoretical and empirical knowledge about raising twins. Also, since space costs can be high, a church or social agency that would provide free space may be another valuable collaborator. The goal is to find collaborators who can provide support (knowledge, space, or other resources) for the fledgling group to get started.

Step 4: Determination of the Professional Role

Before organizing the group the health-care professional needs to determine his or her role. Obviously, if the group is to be a *mutual* support group, the professional cannot be the therapist or the leader. The professional, however, can fill several other roles (Gilbey, 1989; Wheeler & Limbo, 1990).

The professional may be a *resource person* who can provide accurate information about an illness and about the workings of the health-care system. For the mothers of twins group, a resource professional may provide a reading list on twins or may share personal experiences as the parent of twins. The professional may serve as the *convener, or organizer,* of the group. In this role the professional may perform steps one through three cited in this discussion. The professional may serve as a *trainer* of group leaders. If the women who want to start a mothers of twins group have little knowledge of group dynamics or of how to organize a group meeting, the professional may train them to assume these functions. The professional may serve as a *recruiter* for the group. A professional often has access to other professionals and groups who can refer members to the new group.

There is no one correct role for the professional. What is critical is that professionals be clear about their roles so that the members can form accurate expectations. A professional who convenes a group and leaves it in a couple of months has a different commitment than one who will serve as a resource person for an extended period. Role clarity is also important for the professional. Sometimes health-care professionals are reluctant to become involved in starting a group because of the time they think will be required. If the professional clearly decides that the role is one of convener, then a short time commitment is all that is expected.

If the professional follows these steps, a successful mutual support group can be established. Nonprofessionals also can use the first three steps to form a group. Step 4 for a nonprofessional organizer would involve deciding what role, if any, professionals might have in the group.

✦ OBSTACLES TO CREATION AND MAINTENANCE OF A MUTUAL SUPPORT GROUP

Three general obstacles block the success of mutual support groups: (1) use of a deficit approach, (2) ownership issues, and (3) issues of entry and exit from the group (Nichols & Jenkinson, 1991; Silverman, 1980).

The deficit approach refers to the tendency by some professionals (men and women) to be paternalistic in their approach to clients. Part of becoming a professional is learning a body of knowledge that is unique to the profession of which one is a member. That unique knowledge base can create an image of superiority that nonprofessionals may view with contempt. Generally the nonprofessional is made to feel inferior in some way. If the professional is perceived as preaching, as using technical jargon without explanation, or as implying that something is wrong with a person who needs to be in a group, a deficit approach is operating.

People seeking mutual support are vulnerable. To persuade them to feel deficient so that they can participate in a group further detracts from self-esteem. This approach also ignores the mutuality of a support group, which conveys that the members help one another. To avoid a deficit approach, the problem is treated as a distinct entity, not as part of the person's essential self. Genuine caring and respect for group members also decreases deficit feelings.

The second problem that can hamper the success of a group is ownership. If a professional organized the group, he or she may be too involved and find it difficult to relinquish control to the members (Nichols & Jenkinson, 1991). For a mutual support group to grow and become a cohesive entity, it needs to make its own decisions. The members may make wrong decisions or not act fast enough, but if the group is to prosper, the members must run it and feel they own it. Professionals who want to be involved with mutual support groups need to develop a sense of when to participate and when to withdraw. If the professional does not allow the group to become autonomous, two outcomes are possible. First, the group may become a therapy group. If this occurs, the professional will begin to feel angry because he or she is not being paid for professional services. Second, people will no longer participate. Members will quickly sense that their needs are not the most important items.

Issues of entry and exit are another obstacle that can hinder group formation and maintenance. Who is a member? Who cannot be a member? In the mothers of twins example, fathers were excluded. Was this a wise decision or not? Only time will tell.

Some groups have screening procedures for new members or for group leaders. These are usually groups with sufficient economic resources to maintain a staff that can perform the screening activities. Minimally, one would expect members to have some ability to listen to the experiences of others with compassion, to discuss their personal experiences candidly; to desire to help others; to be capable of confidentiality with other members' experiences; to look for answers rather than to preach to other members; and to have experience with the problem that is the focus of the group. As one matures within the group and assumes more leadership, the person would be expected to have adjusted to the problem and to serve as a role model for new members (Nichols & Jenkinson, 1991).

How long the group will last also needs to be decided, as this influences membership. A group such as Alcoholics Anonymous meets for the duration of a recovering alcoholic's life. This group believes that recovery is a day-to-day activity that requires continual support. Other groups have planned beginnings and endings. For example, a group of students meet for mutual support to cope with a particularly demanding course. The group may meet only one semester and then disband; or the group may decide that meeting was so helpful that it will continue for the duration of the educational experience. There is no right length of time for a mutual support group. What is important is that the length meet the members' needs.

✦ CONCLUSION

Social support is a positive buffer for families and their members in coping with stress. When social support is organized into a mutual support group, the benefits of group participation enhance the support offered to individual members. Whether the support is formal (as with a mutual support group) or informal (friends and family), it can be a powerful positive force for managing crises. More professional attention is being directed toward this inexpensive and beneficial method of enhancing well-being.

REFERENCES

Adams-Greely, M. (1986). Psychological staging of pediatric cancer patients and their families. *Cancer, 58*, 449-453.

Anderson, C., Reiss, D., & Hogarty, G. (1986). *Schizophrenia and the family.* New York: Guilford.

Berkman, L. F. (1986). Social network,

support, and health: Taking the next step forward. *American Journal of Epidemiology, 123,* 559-562.

Black, R. B., & Weiss, J. O. (1988). A professional partnership with genetic support groups. *American Journal of Medical Genetics, 29,* 21-33.

Blotcky, A. D. (1986). Helping adolescents with cancer cope with their disease. *Seminars in Oncological Nursing, 2,* 117-122.

Chesler, M., & Barbarin, O. (1987). *Childhood cancer and the family.* New York: Brunner/Mazel.

Cobb, S. (1976). Social support as a moderator of life stress. *Psychosomatic Medicine, 38,* 300-314.

Cohen, S. (1988). Psychosocial models of the role of social support in the etiology of physical disease. *Health Psychology, 7*(3), 269-297.

Cronenwett, L. R. (1985a). Network structure, social support, and psychological outcomes of pregnancy. *Nursing Research, 34,* 93-99.

Cronenwett, L. R. (1985b). Parental network structure and perceived support after birth of first child. *Nursing Research, 34,* 347-352.

Dressler, W. (1985). Extended family relationships, social support, and mental health in a southern black community. *Journal of Health and Social Behavior, 26,* 39-48.

Fournet, K., & Schaubhut, R. (1986). What about the spouses? *Focus Critical Care, 13*(1), 14-18.

Ganster, D. C., & Victor, B. (1988). The impact of social support on mental and physical health. *British Journal of Medical Psychology, 61,* 17-36.

Gilbey, V. J. (1989). Will the health professional meet the challenge? *Canadian Journal of Public Health, 80,* 373-374.

Gottlieb, B. H. (1983). *Social support strategies.* Beverly Hills, CA: Sage.

Halm, M. A. (1990). Effects of support groups on anxiety of family members during critical illness. *Heart and Lung, 19*(1), 62-71.

Kathol, D. (1984). Anxiety in surgical patients' families. *American Operating Room Nurse Journal, 40,* 131-137.

Koocher, G. P. (1986). Psychosocial issues during the acute treatment of pediatric cancer. *Cancer, 58,* 468-472.

Leventhal, G. S., Maton, K. I., & Madara, E. J. (1988). Systematic organizational support for self-help groups. *American Journal of Orthopsychiatry, 58*(4), 592-603.

Lin, N., & Ensel, W. M. (1989). Life stress and health: Stressors and resources. *American Sociological Review, 54,* 382-399.

Locke, S., & Colligan, D. (1986). *The healer within.* New York: Academic.

Mauss-Clum, N., & Ryan, M. (1981). Brain injury and the family. *Journal of Neurosurgical Nursing, 13,* 165-169.

McCubbin, M. A., & McCubbin, H. I. (1989). Theoretical orientations to family stress and coping. In C. R. Figley (Ed.), *Treating stress in families* (pp. 3-43). New York: Brunner/Mazel.

Mercer, R. T., Hackley, K. C., & Bostrom, A. (1983). Relationship of psychosocial and perinatal variables to perception of childbirth. *Nursing Research, 32,* 202-207.

Mercer, R. T., Hackley, K. C., & Bostrom, A. (1984). Social support of teenage mothers. In K. E. Barnard, P. A. Brandt, B. S. Raff, & P. Carroll (Eds.), *Social support and families of vulnerable infants* (pp. 245-272). White Plains, NY: March of Dimes Birth Defects Foundation.

Nichols, K., & Jenkinson, J. (1991). *Lead-*

ing a support group. New York: Chapman & Hall.

Norbeck, J. S. (1988). Social support. *Review of Nursing Research, 6,* 85-109.

Norbeck, J. S., & Tilden, V. (1983). Life stress, social support, and emotional disequilibrium in complications of pregnancy: A prospective, multivariate study. *Journal of Health and Social Behavior, 24,* 30-46.

Nuckolls, K. B., Cassel, J., & Kaplan, B. H. (1972). Psychological assets, life crisis, and the prognosis of pregnancy. *American Journal of Epidemiology, 95,* 431-441.

Pearlmutter, D., Locke, A., Bourdon, S., Gaffey, G., & Tyrrell, R. (1984). Models of family-centered care in one acute care institution. *Nursing Clinics of North America, 19,* 173-188.

Peplau, L. A., & Perlman, D. (1982). Perspectives on loneliness. In L. A. Peplau & D. Perlman (Eds.), *Loneliness: A sourcebook of current theory, research, and therapy* (pp. 1-18). New York: John Wiley & Sons.

Pittman, J. F., & Lloyd, S. A. (1988). Quality of family, social support, and stress. *Journal of Marriage and the Family, 50,* 53-67.

Reis, J., Barbera-Stein, L., & Bennett, S. (1986). Ecological determinants of parenting. *Family Relations, 35,* 547-554.

Reissman, F., & Gartner, A. (1987). The surgeon general and the self-help ethos. *Social Policy, 18*(2), 23-25.

Robertson, E. B., Elder, G. H., Skinner, M. L., & Conger, R. D. (1991). The costs and benefits of social support in families. *Journal of Marriage and the Family, 53,* 403-416.

Rook, K. S. (1984). Promoting social bonding strategies for helping the lonely and socially isolated. *American Psychologist, 39,* 1389-1407.

Ruberman, W., Weinblatt, E., Goldberg, J. D., & Chaudhary, B. S. (1984). Psychosocial influences on mortality after myocardial infarction. *New England Journal of Medicine, 311,* 552-559.

Silva, M. (1979). Effects of orientation information on spouses' anxieties and attitudes toward hospitalization and surgery. *Research in Nursing and Health, 2,* 127-136.

Silverman, P. R. (1980). *Mutual help groups: Organization and development.* Beverly Hills, CA: Sage.

Stevens, J. H. (1988). Social support, locus of control, and parenting in three low-income groups of mothers: Black teenagers, black adults, and white adults. *Child Development, 59,* 635-642.

Trivette, C. M., & Dunst, C. J. (1987). *Caregiver styles of interaction: Child, parent, family, and extrafamily influences.* Unpublished manuscript, Family Infant Pre-School Program. Morganton, NC: Western Carolina Center.

West, K., Cozolino, L., Malin, B., McVey, G., Lansky, M., & Bley, C. (1985). Involving families in treating schizophrenia. In M. Lansky (Ed.), *Family approaches to major psychiatric disorders* (pp. 185-195). Washington, D.C.: American Psychiatric Press.

Wheeler, S. R., & Limbo, R. K. (1990). Blueprint for a perinatal bereavement support group. *Pediatric Nursing, 16*(4), 341-344.

Wills, T. A. (1985). Supportive function of interpersonal relationships. In S. Cohen & S. L. Syme (Eds.), *Social support and health* (pp. 61-82). New York: Academic.

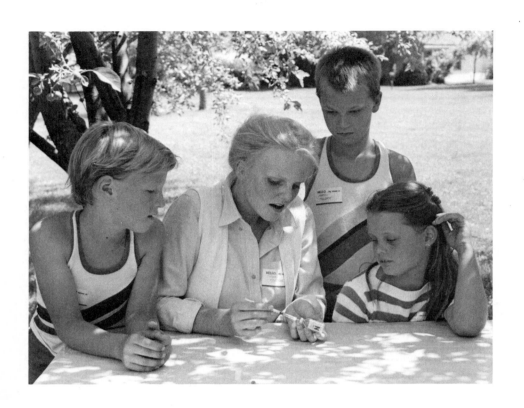

9

The Family as a Resource for Wellness Promotion

♦

CHAPTER GOALS

✦ To emphasize the need for health-care professionals to change their perspective in providing care by focusing on health and prevention instead of illness and by placing the responsibility for health with the family unit

✦ To illustrate the development of interventions that create resources for wellness promotion by directly involving families within their communities

OVERVIEW

M ost health-care professionals today do not participate in wellness promotion and community health education aimed at families. They are preoccupied with treating illness and reducing its residual biological effects. This chapter emphasizes the need for professionals to change their perspective in providing care by focusing on health and prevention of illness and by placing the responsibility for health care with the family. It illustrates the development of interventions that create resources for wellness promotion by directly involving families within their communities. It discusses how the family approach to health promotion is a more fruitful strategy in terms of material resources and human needs. Obstacles to implementing wellness promotion with a family focus are also described throughout. In relation to the Resiliency Model of Family Stress, Adjustment, and Adaptation, this chapter focuses on social support (BBB), or more specifically, the support health professionals can provide for family health promotion in the community (Fig. 9-1).

✦ ILLNESS PREVENTION VS. TREATMENT

The best option for better health is preventive health care. Throughout the twentieth century, medicine has advanced primarily by improving curative care: intensive care units, bypass and transplant surgery, antibiotics, and chemotherapy. But curative care has its limits. To maintain a high level of fitness we must prevent physical decline, not repair it. Open-heart surgery, even at its most effective, will never be as valuable as preventing the need for surgery. For the major killers of American society—heart disease and cancer—the most effective preventive measures involve changes in life-style (National Center for Health Statistics, 1989).

The World Health Organization (WHO) suggests that good health cannot be attained by simply trying to cure diseases or eliminate symptoms. The WHO proposes health promotion be used as a way to mobilize in the public a broader health interest and to stimulate development of resources (WHO, 1985). Such preventive care involves implementing the education needed to evaluate personal health behaviors and to determine what changes are needed. Refocusing our health-care system to emphasize prevention rather than treatment needs to become the goal. For health education to be effective, it must provide us not only with facts by which we can evaluate our options, but also with the opportunities to choose options for enhanced health. Health behaviors, even if rewarding, are often less pleasant and more difficult than other choices. For example, having information about drug abuse or sexually transmitted diseases may not be as important in decision making for a teenager as the possible ridicule from friends if one chooses not to get high or not to have sexual intercourse.

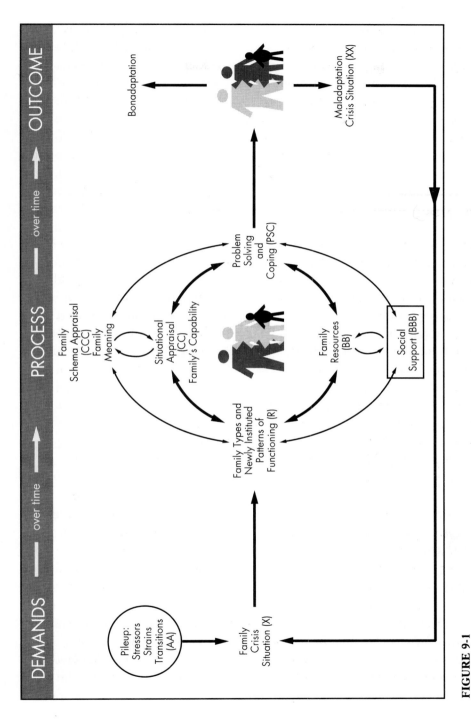

FIGURE 9-1

Adaptation Phase of the Resiliency Model of Family Stress, Adjustment, and Adaptation. This chapter focuses on social support (BBB).

We can refocus our health-care delivery system in several ways. First, emphasis can be changed from treating illnesses after they occur to preventing them. The method of using strategies for health promotion is not new, yet the practice of the total community encouraging health promotion is not widely employed (Allen, 1981; Hipp, 1984). Second, individuals and their families can take an active and more holistic approach to health problems. We can focus on the totality of our lives, including biological, psychological, social, environmental, and spiritual factors, rather than on a single apparent cause of an illness. We can shift from episodic, crisis-oriented medical care to continuous health behaviors. The WHO (1986) suggests that communities create readily available alternatives for citizens willing to practice better health habits. Individuals and families can be encouraged to investigate alternative forms of treatment such as biofeedback, acupuncture, herbs, exercise, massage, diet therapy, and mutual help groups. In addition to this holistic approach, health care can be delivered more humanistically. Such an approach recognizes both provider and patient as equal partners in advocating, establishing, and maintaining health. Individuals and their families need to accept personal responsibility. For too long, health has been seen as the prowess and responsibility of the physician. Finally, the health-care system could make better use of the skills of all health professionals. It must also be recognized that health care can be provided in many settings, not only in medical facilities.

✦ FAMILY FOCUS IN WELLNESS PROMOTION
Rationale

A threefold rationale exists for directly involving the family in creating interventions for wellness promotion. First, the family is the most strategic social unit (Bolman, 1982). Clement-Stone, Eigsti, and McGuire (1987) agree that the family acts as the major socializing unit and teaches cultural behaviors related to health. Families are responsible for controlling health behaviors and resources. Furthermore the authors agree with Friedman (1986) that families have the ability to act in their own best interest. Therefore preventive health services need a family orientation.

Second, a family focus in wellness promotion is less expensive than traditional health care in terms of material resources. In 1989 the U. S. Department of Commerce reported more than $604.1 billion was spent in the health-care industry, or 11.6% of the gross national product (U.S.

Department of Commerce, Bureau of Census, 1991). Physicians' fees have increased at an annual average of 11% (U.S. Department of Commerce, Bureau of Census, 1989); hospital inpatient revenues per day have increased about twice as fast as the overall consumer price index (The Universal Health Care Almanac, 1992). Economists point out two of the factors contributing to the high cost of health care are the lack of resources devoted to primary or preventive care and the lack of knowledge about available forms of health care. Consumers are handicapped in making intelligent purchasing decisions (Palmer, 1979; U.S. Department of Commerce, 1989).

Third, the level of tension is increasing as family members struggle to keep pace with the everchanging, mobile world outside the home. Both men and women are employed in jobs that may not end at 5 PM. The stresses from the workday continue as people carry projects and problems home. A job requiring travel poses additional responsibilities for the spouse who stays at home. The average American now moves at least five times across state lines and changes occupations three times. One of the consequences of this mobility has been a breakdown of the primary community where families are involved and integrated into the community. These social changes create stress for families. One of the most significant protective buffers against stress, the strength of community, social support, may be lacking. Therefore families are the primary group not only for promoting health, but also for managing stress and preventing illness caused by stress. The following sections provide specific examples of the need for family health-promotion programs for dieting and smoking cessation.

Needed Family Health-Promotion Programs

Dieting.   Consider for purposes of illustration the subject of dieting. The relative futility of individually focused programs to reduce weight is now being recognized. Weight reduction is now implemented through group situations in which peer pressure and support play a part. Yet one third of the population of the United States is overweight (Stuart & Sundeen, 1991). Familial tendencies toward obesity and overweight have been identified and are now believed to be related more to sociocultural dietary patterns than to heredity alone. Gutierrez and May (1989) note that a complex combination of social, cultural, economic, physiological, and psychological factors influence our diet.

Obesity is clearly a major public health problem that is a significant risk factor for the development of other serious health problems and chronic disease, including heart disease, hypertension, some forms of cancer, and diabetes mellitus (Katch & McArdle, 1988; Powers, 1980). Rather than allowing obesity to develop and then encouraging people to take part in weight-reduction programs, education about preventing this problem should be implemented and funded by health insurance. Education would include facts and information, evaluation of present behaviors, and ways to process and change old habits affecting weight. These educational programs could take place in schools, churches, fairs, and mall exhibits. The family would be educated about the impact of nutrition during pregnancy, infancy, adolescence, and aging. Economical ways to shop and still purchase quality foods could be taught. Families would adopt and practice healthful nutrition early in life and expect similar practices of their members. The pressure from within a family to adhere to accepted nutritional practices can be a powerful influence on its members.

Smoking cessation. The cost of cigarettes and the sequelae of cancer, emphysema, and other lung-related disorders are significant disadvantages of smoking. Preventing or stopping cigarette smoking is another situation in which the family's influence in prevention is critical and perhaps more crucial than the development of smoking cessation programs for individuals. Health practices such as not smoking should come under the influence of the family unit. Philips (1989) stresses the fact that parental smoking adversely affects whether the child will smoke or not. It appears that parents who smoke exert a greater influence on the likelihood that the adolescent will smoke than pressure from a peer group. The family is also strategically located to provide a more consistent and influential unit in dealing with the smoker who needs support and encouragement to stop. In sum, Gilliss (1989) notes that the family has a complex relationship in which each member is a contributor to, and a reference for, health-care practices.

✦ WELLNESS-PROMOTION PROGRAM DESIGNED FOR FAMILIES

The following is a wellness-promotion program of interventions designed for families (Fig. 9-2). The steps in this intervention process include: (1) eliciting the family's definition of health, (2) assessing family functioning, and (3) educating the family about desired health behaviors. It needs to be implemented as part of health-care services in which families

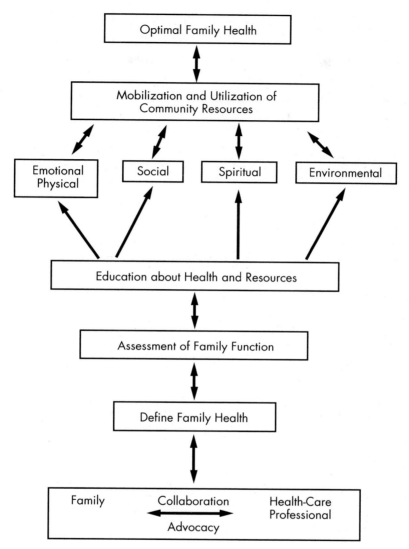

FIGURE 9-2
Wellness-promotion program of interventions.

form a partnership with health-care professionals. Ideally the program is comprehensive and activated at several levels in the community to reach the family early. It can be integrated into church, work, or community settings in which families routinely gather. The integration of the programs into the community setting would involve community participation and thus community ownership of the programs, which would facilitate their effectiveness. These interventions can be used for an individual family or groups of families. The following discussion outlines the steps involved in developing wellness programs with a family focus.

The Family's Definition of Health

Health professionals in partnership with families in their community will implement this wellness-promotion program by following several interventions. They will first decipher the family's intimate definition of health through discussion, exploration, value clarification, introspection, and examination of positive growth experiences. This intervention helps the family to become aware of its health practices and beliefs. It also enables the health professional to gain a clear understanding of where the family stands in its view of health promotion as contrasted to its view of health care during illness. Understanding the family's health beliefs can then be the basis for intervention.

Several considerations play a part in the dynamic character of a family's view health. Age-related considerations are important because families are composed of several generations. Healthy functioning for the adolescent is quite different from that for the middle-aged or elderly person. Also, a family's view of health will change in the different stages of the family life cycle. For example, the health focus for a family with young children will differ from that of a family in later life. Desires, expectations, and capabilities to attain a healthy life-style vary with the accumulation of life experiences and the maturational process.

Family organization and cultural background are key influences in defining what is desirable or essential to healthy functioning. Social groups and occupational demands also greatly affect the family's idea of good health (Sue & Sue, 1990). Satisfying work, love, and recreation are considered essential to a fulfilling life-style. The family discusses its idea of health with the health care professional and evaluates strengths and weaknesses. These discussions can be the basis for the health professional to understand family health behaviors.

Assessment of Family Function

Assessment of the family's function is an important part of the health-promotion program. The family's health may be assessed in a variety of ways. Bross (1983) gathers data on demographic, substantive, and interactional information. Compton and Galaway (1979) offer a more extensive assessment by considering such factors as the family as a social system, roles of family members, family rules, developmental stage of the family, physical and emotional needs, goals, values, aspirations, and socioeconomic aspects. Clement-Stone et al. (1987) offer a detailed family assessment plan involving parameters concerned with both family structure and family process. Other family theorists use family genealogy, time lines, and life chronology (Satir, 1983; Toman, 1976; Watzlawick, 1966).

Several family assessment instruments are available including the Family APGAR, FCOPES, FACES III, the Feetham Family Functioning Survey, and Hymovich's tool (Friedman, 1986). Health practitioners using the Resiliency Model to assess families may wish to use the assessment tools found in the Appendix, as well as other tools such as the Family Hardiness Index, Family Adaptability and Cohesion Evaluation Scales, and the Family Time and Routine Tool. A single assessment tool or a combination of these family assessment tools can offer data for understanding family behavior and for planning family interventions that meet the individual family's needs. To illustrate use of a family scale, let us consider the assessment tool called the Family APGAR.

The Family APGAR can be used by families and health professionals to assess the family for a number of healthy behaviors. These behaviors are adaptation, partnership, growth, affection, and resolve (Smilkstein, 1978). According to Pernice and Kaufman (1985), the APGAR's open-ended questions give the user a qualitative view of the individual family member's satisfaction with the previously described items. Adaptation is measured by determining how resources have been shared in the family and to what degree a member is satisfied with the assistance received when family resources are needed.

Partnership is determined by assessing how decisions are shared and by the members' satisfaction with the material covered in family communication and problem solving. Growth is measured by asking the family how nurturing is shared and how satisfied members are with the freedom available within the family to change sides and retain physical and emotional growth or maturation. Affection is measured by noting how emotional experiences are shared and the members' satisfaction with the intimacy and emotional interaction that exists. Resolve is measured by determining how time, space, and money are shared and what the members' satisfaction is with the time, space, or money commitment that has been made to the family by its members.

The Family APGAR, like other assessment tools, is a vehicle for the family and health professional to determine family resources, attributes, and health needs. Once responses to the scale are reviewed by the family and the professional, they can work together to plan activities that support existing strengths and increase desirable family attributes. Resources can be allocated to fulfill health needs within the economic situation of the family.

Family Education about Health

Considering the Family APGAR score and the family's needs and desires, the family is educated about dimensions affecting health: such as the physical, the emotional, the social, the environment, and the spiritual. (Reed-Flora & Lang, 1982). This helps the family to gain a holistic view of health and to accept responsibility for their health. The family can now be knowledgeable about health expectations, conditions, and actions for each of their members, consistent with the present developmental stage.

Health is seen as an integrated method of functioning. Health functioning is oriented toward increasing the potential of the family and its members within its environment. The family may never achieve a 100% level of health, since today's desires, abilities, and goals may be different from those of the future. Ideally the family's efforts are directed toward an ever higher level of functioning.

When health professionals carry out health promotion education with families, they need to account for family differences. Consider how two families' health needs and expectations differ according to the five dimensions of health (physical, emotional, social, environmental, and spiritual).

✦ ✦ ✦ ✦ ✦

Two families both live in a small suburban Vermont town of 5000 residents. The first family consists of Aretha, an 18-year-old black woman who is a single parent to Cyrus, a 12-month old boy. Physically and emotionally this family needs to meet the needs of this toddler. Cyrus receives health care from a local physician who supervises immunizations and intervenes during illnesses. Cyrus is beginning to talk and has a close relationship with his mother.

Aretha recently moved out of her mother's house to a city 500 miles away.

She is focusing on becoming independent from her family of origin. She is presently intimately involved with a man who frequently stays in the household. Aretha hopes to attend college as soon as Cyrus can be placed in day-care. Physical health concerns for her are yearly checkups including Papanicolauo smears, breast examinations, and birth control. Socially she has limited her contacts to her son and boyfriend. She does not have friends in her community, which is primarily composed of white, two-parent families. Some of her needs include making contacts within this community so that she will have support and find other single parents to relate with. She began attending the local Baptist church for fraternization. Kenneth (1989) concurs that nonfamily relationships are important sources of support for those rearing children.

The second family consists of Ellie and John. They are in their sixties and of French-Canadian descent. The last of their five children recently left home to take a job in another part of the state. They attend the local Catholic church and often volunteer to lead or participate in its discussion groups or prayer meetings. They are respected people in their community and church. They have enjoyed raising their children and are now combating some loneliness and boredom. They spend winters in Florida. Both are relatively healthy but are on diets for high blood pressure and weight reduction. They see health professionals yearly or more frequently for dental, vision, and general body functioning.

These two families obviously differ in terms of their needs for physical, emotional, social, and spiritual health. Overall the health professional and each family work jointly to seek ways to increase self-esteem, self-confidence, and interpersonal relationships. Each family's knowledge about health and the five factors is expanded. Feelings are elicited and then processed into resolutions. All family members will be involved in regular physical exercise, anticipating guidance for life changes and expected developments. Decision making is taught and reinforced, and recreation is provided in the form of stimulating and challenging involvements. Spirituality is a valued aspect of life.

✦ COMMUNITY RESOURCES FOR HEALTH EDUCATION AND ADVOCACY

Alternatives to the present health-care delivery system are being debated today. Chapter 6 details the obstacles to a family-focused care system.

Health maintenance organizations, prepaid group practices, health system agencies, and other alternatives to hospital care are emerging. The purpose behind these attempts is to reallocate the distribution of health-care providers and expenditures in the health-care system to make the system more sensitive to community needs.

The ideally organized health-care system provides comprehensive health care at all levels, avoids duplication of services, keeps physicians and allied personnel working at their appropriate levels of skill and training, and reduces costs. Whether insurance covers the costs or not, family health care needs to be available for both health and illness. Except for immunizations and health screening for certain diseases, people usually wait until they are ill, sometimes terminally, before seeing a health-care professional. Preventive health care and health promotion could decrease this behavior.

Prevention services are less profitable for skilled fee-for-service personnel. Curative care is much more prestigious and rewarding than preventive care, since it is difficult to appreciate the illness that did not happen. Health insurance covers few preventive services, and many people choose not to pay for services whose value is not immediately apparent. Yet there is a point beyond which money cannot improve health. Improvement after this point depends on life-style, diet, and environment. People can alter these factors to improve health. However, some conditions leading to poor health require community effort and cannot be solved one case at a time. For instance, it is difficult to improve nutrition without first reducing poverty and unemployment. Likewise, it is difficult to control infectious diseases without first improving housing and education.

Development of Community Health Education Resources

Families would benefit from learning the effect life-style has on health. Health-care professionals can function as life-style experts and wellness advisors. They would assist families in assessing time, money, energy, freedom, security, and rights, and responsibilities and how to manage these activities. Life-style is a major contributor to chronic illness conditions such as heart and lung disease, cancer, and obesity. With this in mind, families need to adopt life-styles that include a concern for recognizing health problems and risks as early as possible, for educating themselves about signs that need medical attention, and for learning the limitations of self-prescribed, over-the-counter drugs. Families' value orientations about health would be elicited, acknowledged, and assessed in view of health promotion. The health-care professional facilitates this value clarification process. Families would be helped to choose between conflicting value orientations that affect health. Advances in medicine and the social sciences now allow families to assume more control over how these factors affect them. A community-based resource could be developed to help families investigate options related to life-style and choose the most productive combinations for them.

When health is defined to include social and spiritual aspects, it is affected by many factors including heredity, environment, the health-care system, life-style, and value orientations toward health. Community-based resources for health promotion in families would target these factors. Resources would be allocated for a safe environment, adequate medical care, optimal nutrition, exercise, satisfying work, recreation, rest and sleep, life-space, freedom, privacy, challenges, risks, and commitments.

Health Advocacy and Mobilization of Resources

The atmosphere in which to develop community resources for health is one wherein health professionals and family groups combine ideas and design interventions based on the needs and desires of the family and community. Health professionals and families need to combine forces to advocate for health on the local, state, regional, national, and international levels. Health advocacy would be sought in political, financial, and legislative arenas (see Chapter 6 for examples). The types of resources for each community will vary according to the mutually identified needs. Families would be able to use these resources in ways and settings convenient for them. Media sources such as radio, television, and newspapers might feature health education. School, church, social, and work settings in which families routinely function could offer face-to-face opportunities for processing health information, considering options, and changing present behaviors.

Advocacy activities might focus on preventing some disorders. For example, geneticists are able to document genetic causes of a number of diseases and have developed methods for identifying potential carriers of such diseases. Genetic counseling would be available to all parents with family histories of genetically related conditions. Couples could explore their particular situation and assess the risk of delivering an infant with special health-care needs.

Environmental health. Currently, families are involved in legislation to improve sanitation, safety, quality of air, food, and water. Families rely on education about ecology and on personal initiative to pay closer attention to the physical and social environment. Unfortunately, health professionals have not always helped families become educated about or find solutions to environmental health problems. The lack of professional involvement can lead to fragmented efforts and to competition between groups who could otherwise cooperate. For example, leachate not only is a possible carcinogen, but also may be teratogenic. A group concerned with cancer and one concerned with fetal health could join to protest the building of a waste dump if they understood what unites them. Environmental threats are not new; it is only our awareness of them that is new.

A success story of advocacy is the Andersons of Woburn, Massachusetts, whose 3-year-old son, Jimmy, was diagnosed with leukemia in 1972 and died in 1981. Mrs. Anderson noticed that other children in the community were suffering from leukemia. When she questioned whether the water was a source of carcinogens, the board of health screening at that time consisted of a simple screening for bacteria, so no answers were available. The family's doctor paid no attention to her ideas. Mrs. Anderson proceeded to found FACE (For a Clean Environment) and worked with other families in the community to find the source of the problem — an illegal toxic waste dump site. The Andersons succeeded, but at the personal and social expense of being called crazy. They still receive hate mail. Dangers to our health come from the "stuff" of our lives. The challenge is to find a way to integrate this safely back into our lives. We now have environmental agencies such as the Environmental Protection Agency (EPA) and the Department of Environmental Protection (DEP) because of the efforts the Anderson Family and others like them.

With the Anderson's case in mind, community-based education and advocacy for wellness promotion goes beyond educating families about the importance of safe drinking water. The health professional needs to be in the forefront with concerned families to help improve the global environment. Families would be educated and encouraged to make use of the various tests available to detect pollutants; recycling conferences would be scheduled to teach householders as well as our officials how to revamp landfills. Finally, children in the community would be taught about a clean environment and pollutants in schools.

Social health. One major health issue today is improving the quality of our life by applying our existing knowledge about health and by developing new answers for socially and personally destructive behaviors. The community-based resources for health promotion in families would need to target efforts to decrease socially and personally destructive behaviors. Families would be educated about such phenomena as physical, sexual, and emotional abuse and neglect. Information about chronic illnesses such as arthritis, lung cancer, alcoholism, and diabetes that can relate to or be caused by self-destructive behaviors would be disseminated. Families would then be aware of the effects of these behaviors that are self-destructive and of how to decrease or at least detect them early on so that residual illness effects could be treated promptly.

Accidents are the leading cause of death among people under 40 years of age and also cause millions of injuries and permanent disabilities (U.S. Department of Commerce, Bureau of the Census, 1989). Families would be taught safety precautions to reduce accidents involving automobiles, falls, drowning, fires, poisons, firearms, falling objects, electric shocks, planes and trains, and other consumer products.

The abuse of alcohol and other drugs is a major factor in the incidence of accidents, mental illness, suicide, violent crimes, and theft. Much of the physiological damage caused by alcohol and drug abuse can be treated, and increased knowledge of the factors that lead to abuse can help families prevent drug problems. Groups that encourage families to address alcohol and drugs as potential problems would be developed.

Suicide and homicide rank among the four most common causes of death of people 15 to 24 years old (Stuart & Sundeen, 1991). Yet we know how to improve interpersonal relations and self-concept and how to reduce stress. Poor self-concept, stress, and unmet acceptance needs are major contributors to many health problems. Families living in areas lacking necessary biopsychosocial services such as police protection, quality housing, and education in geographical areas such as urban slums, depressed rural areas, immigrant workers' camps, Indian reservations, or housing projects are at risk. Often these families are caught in the cycle of intergenerational poverty. The health professional can assist the family in acquiring basic necessities through community development approaches. Multiple and flexible opportunities for families to attain their desired personal, social, and economic goals must be made available. The development of community approaches originates ideally through schools, churches, social agencies, neighborhood service centers, family life educators, and mental health centers. Some existing examples of antipoverty programs are Headstart, Upward Bound, Job Corps, Mobilization for Youth, and Community Progress.

Families will be at risk for poor health due to a number of stressors. These stressors can include a handicapped parent, loss of a family member, internal imbalance or disorder, role hardships, or vulnerability to normal developmental changes. Death, desertion, chronic hospitalization of a family member, chronic illness, marital discord, birth of a child, school entry, puberty, or retirement also can put the family under stress. The health professional can support families during these stressful times by educating others about the variety of family stresses, thus leading to earlier recognition and intervention. Some examples of community resources for families facing stressors are group meetings for parents of terminally ill children, neighborhood information centers, walk-in clinics for problems of living, homemaker services, public health and visiting nurses, marital counseling, legal aid, reliable day-care centers, and mutual support groups for adoptive or foster parents and children.

Cost containment. Health-care delivery services might be more cost-effective if they were created and controlled by families in their community. Attempts to decrease duplication, fragmentation, expense, and unnecessary interventions and to improve access for all persons may be more successful if solutions came from the community involved. More groups such as the Coalition of Vermont Elders (COVE) need to be encouraged to seek hearings on national health policies. Health-care professionals need to listen to consumers groups' conclusion that the current health-care system needs overhauling. Health-care professionals need to join these consumers in their proposals for change. Health-care professionals and families can be partners in demanding a national health program or in demanding health coverage of all Americans.

Wellness promotion for families needs to be promoted as a cost-effective commodity that can be integrated into traditional health-care settings and expanded into nontraditional consumer markets. The health professional could make use of the marketing concepts of research, product, distribution, price, and communications before making decisions about what to offer families (Echeveste, 1982). Marketing principles can improve cost containment so that one is not priced out of business. For example, research helps to identify product needs, resources, and population markets. With a clearly designed communication mix, one can identify the least productive part so that it either can be improved or eliminated. The marketing concept provides an organized approach with which to plan, implement, and evaluate any given health-care system.

✦ SUMMARY

Health professionals can make more of an impact in the provision of health care if they focus on wellness promotion rather than on illness care. The responsibility for healthy living needs to be placed with the family unit. Families can be directly involved as partners in creating and implementing resources for health promotion. Some aspects of health promotion are deciphering the family's intimate definition of health, assessing the family's present health functions and risks for illness, and educating them about the dimensions of health. Health promotion can be developed through community-based resources that educate and advocate for reducing risks. This proposal entails changing health care's focus from treatment to enhancement, from repair to improvement, and from diminished sickness to increased performance.

The current focus of health-care services on the individual illness is a major obstacle to implementing wellness promotion with a family focus. Cost-effective, consumer-satisfying models of such programs will be a major determinant in adopting this approach universally.

REFERENCES

Allen, R. (1981). *Lifegain*. New York: Appleton-Century-Crofts.

Bolman, W. M. (1982). Preventive psychiatry for the family: Theory, approaches, and programs. In Erickson, G.D., Hogan, T.P. (Eds.), *Family ther-*

apy (pp. 377-401). Monterey, CA: Brooks/Cole.

Bross, A. (1983). *Family therapy*. New York: Guilford.

Clement-Stone, S., Eigsti, D. G., & McGuire, S. L. (1987). *Comprehensive family and community health nursing* (1st ed.). New York: McGraw-Hill.

Compton, B. R., & Galaway, B. (1979). *Social work processes* (2nd ed.). Homewood, IL: Dorsey.

Echeveste, D. W. (1982). Marketing and business. In B. R. Riccardi & E. C. Dayani (Eds.), *The nurse entrepreneur* (pp. 43-62). Reston, VA: Reston.

Friedman, M. M. (1986). *Family nursing theory and assessment.* Norwalk, CT: Appleton-Century-Crofts.

Gilliss, C. L. (1989). Why family health care? In C. L. Gilliss, B. L. Highley, B. Roberts, & I. Martin (Eds.), *Toward the science of family nursing* (pp. 3-8). Menlo Park, CA: Addison-Wesley.

Gutierrez, Y., & May, K. A. (1989). Nutrition and the family. In C. L. Gilliss, B. H. Highley, B. M. Roberts, & I. D. Martinson (Eds.), *Toward a science of family nursing* (pp. 92-112). Menlo Park, CA: Addison-Wesley.

Hipp, E. (1984). Is the wellness movement dying? *Health Values: Achieving High Level Wellness, 8*(5), 10-12.

Katch, F. I., & McArdle, W. D. (1988). *Nutrition, weight control, and exercise.* Philadelphia: Lea & Febiger.

Kenneth, H. Y. (1989). The family and the community mobilizing social support. In C. L. Gilliss, B.H. Highley, B. M. Roberts, & I. D. Martinson (Eds.), *Toward a science of family nursing* (pp. 113-123). Menlo Park, CA: Addison-Wesley.

National Center for Health Statistics (NCHS). (1989). *Health, United States, 1988.* Washington, DC: Government Printing Office.

Palmer, A.K. (1979). Regulation, professional responsibility, and marketing forces in the health care field. *Journal of Medical Education, 54,* 275-283.

Pernice, J., & Kaufman, L. (1985). Family assessment. In S. R. Mott, N. F. Fazekas, & S. R. James, *Nursing care of children and families: A holistic approach.* Menlo Park, CA: Addison-Wesley.

Philips, B. U. (1989). The forgotten family: An untapped resource in cancer prevention. *Family and Community Health, 11*(4), 17-31.

Powers, P.S. (1980). *Obesity: the regulation of weight.* Baltimore: Williams & Wilkins.

Reed-Flora, R., & Lang, T.A. (1982). *Health behaviors.* St. Paul: West.

Satir, V. (1983). *Conjoint family therapy* (3rd ed.). Palo Alto, CA: Science & Behavior.

Smilkstein, G. (1978). The family APGAR: a proposal for a family function test and its use by physicians. *Journal of Family Practice, 6,* 1231-1239.

Stuart, G.W., & Sundeen, S.J. (1991). *Principles and practice of psychiatric nursing* (4th ed.). St. Louis: Mosby–Year Book.

Sue, D. W., & Sue, D. (1990). *Counseling the culturally different: Theory and practice,* (2nd ed.). New York: John Wiley & Sons.

Toman, W. (1976). *Family constellation.* New York: Springer.

United States Department of Commerce Bureau of the Census. (1989). *National data book and guide to sources: Statistical abstract of the United States.* (109th ed.). Washington, DC: U. S. Government Printing Office.

United States Department of Commerce, Bureau of the Census. (1991). *Statistical abstract of the United States: 1991* (111th ed.). Washington, DC: U. S. Government Printing Office.

The universal health care almanac (1992). Phoenix: Silver & Cherner Ltd., compiled and edited by R-L Publications.

Watzlawick, P. (1966). A structured family interview. *Family Process, 5,* 256-271.

World Health Organization (WHO). (1985). *Targets for health for all.* Copenhagen: WHO.

World Health Organization (WHO). (1986). Framework for a health promotion: A discussion document. *Health Promotion, 1*(3), 335-340.

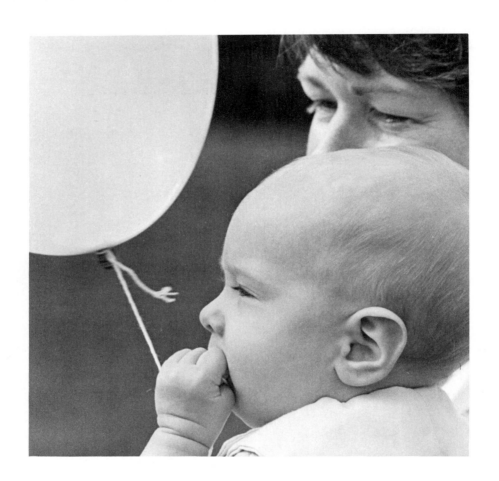

CHAPTER

10

Formal Services Supportive of Family Caregivers

✦

CHAPTER GOALS

✦ To discuss the role of the family as a provider of health-care services

✦ To discuss services that support families coping with the demands of caring for a sick family member

✦ To examine the role of health-care providers in providing supportive services to caregiving families

✦ To examine obstacles in the development and delivery of these supportive services

OVERVIEW

THIS chapter discusses the role of the family in providing care for its members. Services that health-care professionals can offer that directly or indirectly enhance or sustain the caregiving abilities of family members are identified and described. The chapter also describes and illustrates formal services supportive of caregiving functions. A discussion of the obstacles to the development and delivery of supportive services will be undertaken. This chapter focuses on social support (BBB) in the Resiliency Model of Family Stress, Adjustment, and Adaptation, or more specifically,

251

the social support that communities and health-care providers can offer caregiving families (Fig. 10-1).

✦ BACKGROUND

Health-care providers are becoming more aware of the major role families play in providing care to sick members. The family is described as the "hidden health-care system" (Canton, 1983; Robinson, 1989). As the rising cost of health care forces ongoing examination of the strategies for delivering care, family participation becomes an increasingly valuable resource. Services that directly or indirectly improve the family's caregiving functions are being developed and evaluated. Obstacles to the formation and delivery of these services are discussed later in the chapter.

Currently, programs that enhance the family's ability to care either improve caregiving skills or seek to reduce the burden of caregiving. Family caregivers are people who provide health-related services (giving medicines and treatments), personal care (bathing), homemaking services, transportation, shopping, meal preparation, finding services, and other tasks for family members impaired in some way and in need of help with activities of daily living (Parker & Iverson, 1988b). Family caretakers are unpaid and are termed *informal caregivers*. Other informal caregivers are neighbors, friends, and volunteers. This chapter focuses on five areas of family caregiving:

1. Family as provider of health care
2. Demands of family caregiving
3. Services supportive of family caregiving
4. Stress management for family caregivers
5. The role of the health-care provider in support services for family caregiving.

With respect to the theoretical foundations of this book — the Resiliency Model — support for caregivers can be conceptualized as influencing family vulnerability (V) with its pileup and family regenerativity (R) with its newly instituted patterns, as well as maximizing family coping capabilities and resources (B/BB/BBB) (see Fig. 2-1). Support services for family caregiving are important community resources that can enhance family functioning during a crisis. Families may seek these services themselves or be referred by a health-care professional.

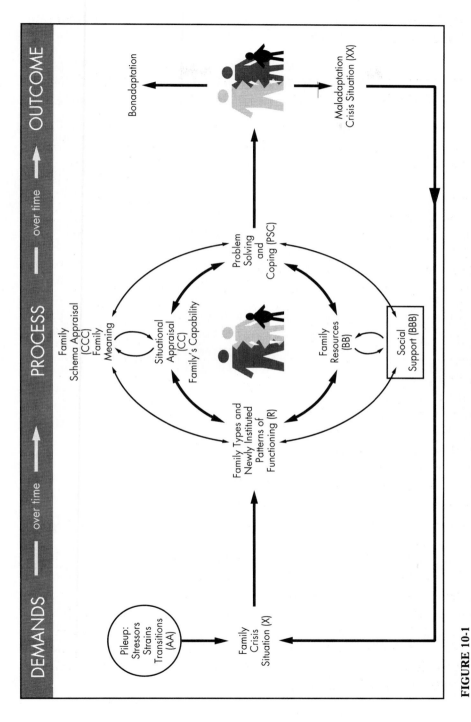

FIGURE 10-1

Adaptation Phase of the Resiliency Model of Family Stress, Adjustment, and Adaptation. This chapter focuses on social support (**BBB**).

✦ THE FAMILY AS PROVIDER OF HEALTH CARE

In general, health care is paid for by the government (40%), private insurance (30%), and the consumer (30%) (Gaynor, 1990). These percentages represent the cash expenses directly related to the illness episode. They do not include such factors as lost income because of less work time, loss of opportunities for advancement, special diets, remodeling a home to accommodate a sick person, and other hidden costs.

Bloom, Knorr, and Evans (1985) studied the cost of caring for children with cancer. In general, the more negative the child's prognosis, the more out-of-pocket expenses the family incurred. More than one third of the family's gross annual income was spent on the illness; the percentage approached 50% (47.9%) for poor families. Only 11% of these expenditures involved medical costs and insurance co-payments. The remainder involved wage loss and other one-time costs related to the disease. The researchers did not include the psychosocial costs, for example, opportunities for promotion that were refused because the family would have to relocate or the loss of future earnings for a sibling who could not go to college because family economic resources were spent on treatment.

With the "graying" of the American population, family involvement in health care has increased. A generation of adults now have caretaking responsibilities for both young children and elderly parents. Approximately 40% of Americans are in this category (Parker & Iverson, 1988a). Most of the care of elderly persons is provided by family members and saves the economy billions of dollars a year (Parker & Iverson, 1988b).

There are some negative consequences to the family's provision of health care that need to be assessed when considering the economic issues. Two concerns are abuse of the elderly and the stress elderly persons experience when cared for by family members.

Elder abuse inflicted by a child is usually associated with drug use or alcohol intoxication and burn-out from caretaking responsibilities. The cost of treatment for abused elders is about $300 million a year (Steinmetz & Amsden, 1983). These costs are probably underestimated because not all cases are reported. Medical and legal costs of treating the abused elder and of seeking legal redress for the abused or punishment of the abuser are high. However, because society does not look at the whole family, the total cost of elder abuse is not known.

The second negative consequence of having families provide health care is the stress the elderly person experiences when cared for by a child.

In our culture parents take care of children until a certain age and then the individual is supposed to be self-sufficient. Research has consistently found that elders prefer help from distant kin and friends (Beckman, 1981; Brody, 1985; Scharlach, 1987). While that finding surprised some, the explanations offered relate to role ambiguity and dependence/independence issues.

Other negative consequences of the adult child as caretaker are coming to light. Cicirelli (1990) and Steinmetz and Amsden (1983) report that some adult-child caregivers were overwhelmingly paternalistic in their approach. The adult-child took control over many areas of the elder's life, believing they were acting in the parent's best interest. Actually, the adult-child's actions diminished the elder's self-esteem and sense of mastery, two factors that are essential to successful aging. Children can successfully function as caregivers if their parent feels confident the child will respect their wishes (Pearlin & Turner, 1987).

Aside from undesirable psychological outcomes of adult-child caregiving, some documented physical health issues must be considered. Some adult-children go to such lengths to hide the fact that they are helping their parent(s) that serious physical symptoms are ignored until a medical crisis arises (Pearlin & Turner, 1987). Parents also may conceal illnesses from the adult-child caregiver so as not to be a "burden."

From the theoretical perspective, undesirable consequences of elder caregiving are not surprising. The family may have a multigenerational transmission of tension about issues of dependence/independence, or family vulnerability may be increased by pileup of caregiving demands. If a multigenerational process is operating, assessment will reveal intense conflict during the children's adolescence. Serious illness involving dependency may strain family relationships, and the role reversal required to care for aging parents will exacerbate the family's discomfort with dependency. It is possible for some families to work these problems through, whereas elder caretaking for some families is emotionally impossible.

The reports just cited and the theoretical explanation highlight the need for a family approach to health care. Literature on the negative effects of family caretaking deal chiefly with the elderly. We need to know if these effects occur in other age groups. As health-care providers we know that delayed treatment results in a more difficult course of treatment at a higher cost. We also know that depression can be a result of loss of control and decreased self-esteem and that a concurrent depression can make other disease processes more difficult to treat. Ways of preventing negative family outcomes and supporting caregivers need to be explored.

✦ DEMANDS OF CAREGIVING ON THE CAREGIVER

Depending on the illness, the physical and emotional energy required for caregiving may be great. For example, caring for a family member who has had a cerebral vascular accident (CVA) with resulting hemiplegia can require the family to provide assistance with all activities of daily living (for example, feeding, dressing, toileting). Health-care activities such as physical therapy, speech therapy, occupational therapy, and medical evaluations may become the responsibility of the family. These activities can be exhausting and time consuming. Participating in them limits a person's availability to other family members and for family functioning. Carrying this kind of responsibility may strain a marital relationship or interfere with effective parenting.

Many studies have explored the demands that caregiving presents to the caregiver. Some of these studies find the caregiver is more depressed, socially isolated, uses more psychotropic drugs, has more stress symptoms, and is less satisfied with life than their noncaregiver peers (Baumgarten, 1989; George & Gwyther, 1986; Robinson, 1989).

Studies also find that wives who are caretakers of infirm husbands are more distressed. It is thought that these wives are in a double jeopardy situation. On the one hand, they are grieving the loss of their husband's former status while he is still physically present but cannot perform the same roles. At the same time, these wives are feeling the strains that accompany the daily chores of caregiving (Barusch & Spaid, 1989; Cantor, 1983). Additionally, these wives often assume the roles and tasks their husbands previously filled. Such a situation can easily lead to pileup of demands.

The literature on caregiving for mentally ill patients attributes family hardship to disruption of domestic routine and to social and leisure life; financial concern; feelings of being trapped; decreased stability of the parents' marriage; emotional overload; and the stresses on the mental and physical health of other family members (Group for Advancement of Psychiatry, 1986).

The literature on the stresses of caregiving is not unanimous in establishing stress as a universal response. One study found that men who were more androgynous, that is, those blending "typical" male and female characteristics in their personalities, enjoyed caregiving responsibilities (Kaye & Applegate, 1990). Orodenker (1990), in a study of 1168 women caregivers, found that employment outside the home buffered the stress of caregiving. She suggests that this is because the women caregivers who were working were healthier and more financially stable. It also may be that employment provides companionship and interests beyond the caretaking role, thereby enhancing self-esteem.

One of the most consistent findings in caregiving research is the caretaker's reluctance to ask for help, even if the burden becomes great. Of importance for practitioners, is the finding that if the caretaker does seek help, it is more likely to be from peers than from their adult children (Barusch & Spaid, 1989; Gnaedinger, 1989). It may be that adult children are critical and interfere with well-established patterns in their parents' lives. On the other hand, if the caretaker turns to an adult child for help, it is usually a same-sex child; that is, mothers turn to daughters and fathers to sons. The implications of these findings are examined in the discussion of obstacles to support services.

Another finding of interest is that respite care and other community services that might decrease caretaker burden are underused. Even if caretakers know of the existence of the respite care center, they may not use them (Warren, Cockerill, Paterson, & Paterson, 1986). Cockerill and Warren (1990) asked the caregivers of patients with multiple sclerosis which respite services they would like. More than half (52%) said the best option was to hire an assistant. The second most acceptable form of relief was to enlist family or friends for periodic relief of caregiving (50%). Only 19% of the respondents favored using hospital admission or day-care centers for respite. Cockerill and Warren suggest that people may feel guilty about seeking relief from caring for a loved one or that the services available may not have a good reputation. Regardless of the cause, these caregivers do not use available respite services and even seem resistant to the idea. The implications of these findings are explored more fully later in the chapter.

Although many caregivers resist seeking relief from caregiving responsibilities, most policymakers are convinced that some relief has to be offered to these unsung heroes of the health-care system. There are many approaches to the question of how to relieve them, as the following sections illustrate.

✦ SERVICES SUPPORTIVE OF FAMILY CAREGIVING
Respite Care

Respite care is one component of the family caregiver support system that provides temporary relief for primary caregivers (Warren & Cohen, 1985). The methods of delivering respite services and the forms of these services vary from region to region. The provision of respite services is controversial. Some fear that providing respite implies that the family is the sole caregiver for the ill person. For example, some families and mental health professionals have opposed the establishment of respite services for families of the mentally ill. They view the programs as a commitment by the state to the idea that the family is the indefinite caretaker of the mentally ill person; moreover, they fear that hospital psychiatric services would be further cut (Zirul, Lieberman, & Rapp, 1989).

Guiding principles for the development of respite services have been proposed by Bader (1985) for caregivers of the elderly, by Warren and Cohen (1985) for caretakers of the developmentally and physically disabled, and by the National Institute of Mental Health (NIMH) (1983) for general community support services. It is generally agreed that respite services can include, but are not limited to, case management, psychoeducational programs, alternative living arrangements, vocational and social rehabilitation programs, crisis intervention, inpatient hospital services, family and patient advocacy, outreach programs, psychotherapy, monitoring of medication use, family support/mutual help groups, and supportive counseling for families. The respite program that a community adopts needs to be flexible enough to meet the varying needs of different families and patients. Respite services can be performed in the home or in a variety of locations outside the home. Given the findings of Cockerill and Warren's study previously mentioned, home-based respite services would be most likely to receive greater acceptance among families.

In 1982, "Dear Abby," Abigail Van Buren, cooperated with the Group for the Advancement of Psychiatry. She used her column to solicit letters from families with a mentally ill member living at home. The respondents' letters described their experiences, needs, and problems. The Group for the Advancement of Psychiatry summarized over 400 responses. These responses are listed in the box on p. 259.

Although this survey dealt with the caretakers of the mentally ill, the idea that families want information, considerate professionals, and help with community services and respite services seems applicable to other groups.

Needs of Caretakers of the Mentally Ill

1. Information about the cause, treatment, and symptoms of the illness
2. Effective strategies for coping with the mentally ill person's behavior and for ensuring the person's compliance with medical regimens
3. Advocates who could help the family deal with courts, regulations, legislators, and financial matters
4. Patient access to short-term hospitalization and other respite services
5. Opportunities to share anger, guilt, and fears
6. Help in accessing community services that might offer housing and employment alternatives for the family and the patient
7. Nonblaming professionals who listen to the family and value the contributions it makes to the care of its ill member

From Group for Advancement of Psychiatry (1986). *Family affairs: Helping families cope with mental illness.* New York: Brunner/Mazel.

Respite programs take many forms from comprehensive ones to neighbor-to-neighbor approaches. Borsuk (1989) reported on a statewide endeavor in New Jersey to maximize caregiver capabilities, to reduce their stress, and to prevent early or inappropriate institutionalization. This program offers a 12-hour course on the needs of the elderly and has been attended by more than 800 persons across the state. A home visitation program involving home health-care agencies also was part of the program. The home visitation program is now run by the In-Home Family Caregiver Project.

On a smaller scale, Pearson and Deitrick (1989) describe the Respite Care Corps, a volunteer program. Volunteers must be in good health, 18 years of age or older, and able to drive. Client families are identified by visiting nurses. The goals of the program are to provide socialization to the homebound elderly person, to provide information, to lend support and contact for caregivers with the community, and to give caregivers relief time.

Another approach is the Extend-a-Family program in Toronto. This program matches families with a handicapped member with host families in the community. The host family contracts for the amount of time they want to be involved each year, up to 30 days. An "Agreement of Service" contract is signed by the two families so that the host family is protected from damage to its home and to ensure commitment by the host family. The primary purpose of the program is to give the caretaker some time off. Other benefits include different social experiences for the handicapped person as he or she interacts with a different environment in the host family home and with members of that family. The community also benefits because host families become spokespersons for the acceptance of the handicapped in the community.

The most common respite care provided in the home of the dependent person is a sitter (if the person is a child) or a companion (if the person is an adult). Services vary widely in the amount of time offered a family and in the training of the sitter/companion. United Cerebral Palsy of Sacramento-Yolo Counties offers 48 hours of free service every 3 months. Families may purchase more time if it is available. The respite workers are primarily college students who receive training. Families are interviewed to develop a care plan for the dependent person and to review the services offered. Parents evaluate the care after each service period.

Homemakers and home health aides are a valuable source of respite care (Cohen & Warren, 1985). The National Home Caring Council develops standards for training workers and for service, provides technical assistance to agencies, and accredits programs. In general, homemakers and home health aides assist with personal care, handle emergencies, and give periodic respite to persons who face intensive caregiving demands.

United Cerebral Palsy of Philadelphia offers a unique approach to respite care with three apartments and one home where dependent persons can receive care (Cohen & Warren, 1985). The facilities are in residential areas and can serve 16 mentally retarded persons at once. There is usually a waiting list for preplanned relief schedules, since emergencies and health-care needs of caregivers take priority.

Adult Day Care

Adult day care is based on the same premises as child day care. Both age groups need socialization, opportunities for learning, and safe care while their primary caretaker is not available, usually because the caretaker is at work. The ill and the elderly also need health and social services. The social service component of the adult day care offers meals, recreation programs, classes, and other services that might be found in senior centers. Some corporations provide child and adult day care as benefits to employees. Combined programs often offer the elderly and the child a chance to interact.

Often, adult day care centers provide a health service component as an extension of the patient rehabilitation services. A person may be able to leave the hospital sooner, and not have to go to a nursing home, if a strong rehabilitation component is part of the day-care center's program. The programs also may offer limited health monitoring on a regular basis. Checking on medication compliance and observing for side effects of medication are frequently offered.

Other Community Services

Home care is defined as the provision of services and equipment to patients in the home with the goal of maintaining or restoring their maximal level of function, comfort, and health (Council on Scientific Affairs, American Medical Association, 1990). The variety of nursing services offered in the home is impressive. The traditional visiting nurse and public health nurse are still providing many services. However, the home care industry has expanded rapidly, driven by the high costs of institutional long-term care, society's aversion to nursing homes, the entrance of women into the workplace, people's preference for home care, and an ever-expanding medical technology. Political debates about finances, policies, and access to home care are ongoing. However, legislators and insurance companies see the need for greater availability of home nursing services. The 18 million members of the American Association of Retired Persons favor home care. At this writing the field is somewhat chaotic with the term *home health* covering almost anything that occurs outside the institutional setting. Many creative programs have been established, some of which are reviewed here.

The Academic Nurse Managed Center is one creative approach that nurse educators have introduced. The centers provide student experience, opportunities for faculty practice, and a commitment to serve an identified population (Higgs, 1989). Some of the services offered include well-child care, health assessment, substance abuse assessment, health education, referrals, and monitoring of chronic conditions (Acree & Gregory, 1989; Barger, 1986). Some receive third-party reimbursement, whereas others are supported by the parent organization.

Although maintaining the elderly in their homes is a positive social goal, it does have disadvantages. For example, if adequate services are not available, the older person may be "incarcerated;" that is, they may be trapped in their own homes and unable to afford more appropriate living conditions. Zink and Bissonnette (1990) studied the grant-funded Living at Home Program of Boston University Medical Center's Home Medical Service. Its goal is to develop community options for physically and emotionally impaired elders who may be disrupted because of health or housing problems. The grant provides the following services:

1. Home repairs and home management
2. Temporary emergency housing for individuals and family members
3. Home-based medical, nursing, mental health, and social services
4. Interpreter services
5. Financial counseling, information, and referral
6. Access to legal, nutritional, and support services

It also offers the more traditional services of education, advocacy, volunteer assistance, case management, and hospice care. At the time Zink and Bissonnette's article was written, about 200 elders in the Boston area were being served, primarily with housing. Either no housing (homelessness), eviction, unsafe housing, or inaccessible housing brought the clients to the program. The success of the program, however, has not guaranteed its continuation after the funding period.

Adapting equipment for home use is a rapidly growing area of medical technology. Virtually any service that can be made portable can be offered in the home. Renal dialysis, intravenous infusions of drugs (including chemotherapy), rehabilitation programs, and other treatment previously requiring hospitalization are now routinely done in the home. So compelling is the home care movement that physicians are beginning to make house calls again. Siwek (1985) conducted a survey of primary care physicians and found that 53% to 82% made house calls.

Although one expects to see a burgeoning of diagnostic and treatment procedures in the home, the provision of supportive services continues to be the main function of home care. For example, programs such as Meals on Wheels provide nutrition to frail elders who would otherwise face malnutrition or institutionalization.

✦ STRESS MANAGEMENT FOR FAMILY CAREGIVERS

Although social institutions can and do provide services that decrease family burden in caregiving, the model that guides this book requires a look at enhancing the personal resources of the caregiver. One way to do that is by teaching caregivers techniques in stress management. Dellasega (1990) examined a two-part program for caregivers of Alzheimer's patients. The first part consisted of understanding the specific stressors affecting caregivers, values clarification, empowerment strategies, and time management. The second part consisted of teaching assertiveness and relaxation techniques. The control group participated in a support group. The caregivers who learned stress management reported no change in the amount of burden they felt but did have less stress. Participants were tested before and after intervention with the Burden Interview (Zarit & Zarit, 1983) and with the Coping Strategies Scale (Beckham & Adams, 1984). It appears that stress management training allowed the caregivers to change their perceptions of the situation, thus decreasing the stress experienced.

It is beyond the scope of this book to present all the techniques of stress management. However, a program tailored to the needs of a caregiver group should enhance the personal resources of the caregiver. The authors believe that everyone should learn some stress management techniques as part of their general education. These techniques are cost effective and can make life more manageable for most people.

Stress management techniques of particular value for caretakers are time management, meditation and visualization, and assertiveness training. These techniques are easily learned.

Douglass and Douglass (1985) offer a comprehensive approach to time management. One of the assumptions they make is that every activity needs to be looked at as if one were being paid for it, since, in effect, we pay for every activity by using up time. For caregivers who are retired (about 55% of them), this philosophy seems particularly useful. One of the "bad habits" many retired persons slip into is to let time drift away. Although this can be a pleasant release from the hectic preoccupation with time during one's working life, if one has specific tasks to accomplish, letting time drift means that tasks either do not get done or are done in a rush. A managed-time approach to caregiving tasks can help create a sense of order in the day and can help caretakers recapture some time for themselves. For nonretired caregivers, time management can help with the integration of family, caretaking, and work responsibilities.

Another group of stress reduction techniques of particular value for caretakers are meditation and visualization (Borysenko, 1987; Ram

Dass, 1990). These techniques are not the same. Meditation involves focusing attention either on something, such as an object, word, or idea, or clearing the mind of all thoughts. Visualization involves the mental creation of a desired state of affairs. Both involve relaxing and becoming quiet within the self. Hundreds of self-help tapes, conferences, and videotapes on these topics are available for further exploration. The important point is to find a method that is doable within the context of one's life-style.

One of the authors used meditation and visualization in family therapy to reduce stress. Since changing family patterns can engender some stress, meditation was used to enhance the family members' well-being as they explored and changed dysfunctional behaviors. Visualization is particularly useful in dealing with triangles, which are automatic, unconscious behavioral patterns that can underlie dysfunctions in families. Triangles include a three-person emotional system in which two people are comfortable and the third is distant. Once the family is aware of how the automatic triangling behaviors contribute to its discomfort, visualization that includes breaking up the triangle is helpful.

Assertiveness training is another stress management strategy of great help to caregivers. The caregiver is often the contact person with large, impersonal bureaucracies or with harried health-care providers who do not give the family enough information. Assertiveness training allows caretakers to feel comfortable in making their needs known, in holding persons responsible for meeting those needs, for offering a referral, or in demanding a reasonable explanation of why a need cannot be met.

Assertiveness training is usually a formal course that gives the learner feedback about his or her assertive behavior and a chance to watch others role-model various aspects of the training. Various tapes and books are available if a course cannot be taken.

✦ ROLE OF THE HEALTH-CARE PROVIDER IN SUPPORT SERVICES

The health-care provider has three basic roles in the support service arena: (1) to develop services, (2) to deliver services, and (3) to advocate for services.

Developer of Support Services

Established health-care institutions and entrepreneurs are developing support services. Such support services can be the basis of a new business venture for the health-care provider. There are many articles, books, and courses on starting a business. Nurse Consultants Association (414 Plaza Drive, Suite 209, Westmont, IL 60559) provides consultation, continuing education, and networking services for nurse entrepreneurs.

Many steps are involved in starting such a business. First, one needs to determine if there is a market for these services. Vogel and Doleysh (1988) take readers through the steps of developing a business plan, establishing a philosophy and goals, selecting offices, finding an image, planning services, and the myriad of details that result in an organization. They also describe marketing and promotional strategies, financial considerations for launching the business, and strategies to guide the growth of the fledgling business. Starting a business can be a very exciting opportunity for the health-care provider.

Deliverer of Support Services

The more usual role for health-care providers is to deliver supportive care. They may deliver care directly, as do many nurses, physical therapists, occupational therapists, and nutritionists. There are legal and ethical dimensions of care to be aware of in in-home, community-based practice. These vary greatly from state to state and will not be discussed here.

Advocate for Support Services

Health-care providers can add their voice to that of families calling for more support for the caregiving they provide. Professionals can contact and inform policymakers and legislators of the contributions families make and of the stress such caregiving may exact on a family. Professionals can advocate for funds for respite care, for tax reductions for family caregivers, and for third-party payment of some of the costs the family now absorbs. Advocacy for families allies professionals with the people who do a great deal of implementing care plans. In the long run, successful advocacy will enhance the health of families.

✦ OBSTACLES TO IMPLEMENTATION OF SUPPORT SERVICES FOR FAMILY CAREGIVERS

In a recent survey of 892 parents of chronically ill children, the General Accounting Office found that home care presented some problems (Poppleton, 1988). Families experienced a gap between hospital services and home care. The primary reasons for the problems were economic and lack of information about, and access to, support services. Most insurance policies cover only medically necessary services, so support services become out-of-pocket expenses for the family. Even if the family is able or willing to pay for such services, they often do not exist. Parents report that it is almost impossible to find day care for a sick child. When an agency finds out that the child has a chronic health problem, they lose interest. Persistence seemed to be the one characteristic successful parents cited as useful in finding and using support services.

Cost Containment

The major obstacle to economic support for family caregivers is the cost-containment efforts that typify the American health-care industry today. The Health Care Financing Administration recently tightened the definitions of "homebound," "intermittent care," and "medical necessity," effectively limiting access to home care services (Poppleton, 1988). Already, some visiting nurses are having difficulty in justifying the time they spend talking with the ill family member and his or her family. Activities such as sitting down with the family to give advice about providing care or to letting a caregiver verbalize frustrations are not reimbursable. Hence, such stress-reducing activities are not occurring. Pileup is a very real outcome for the family caretaker when home visitors are forced to focus only on the medical illness.

Congressional hearings are currently directed toward solving some of the conflict in home health care. Although definite savings can be shown for home health care over institutional services, it is unlikely that respite care and other modalities that could reduce caretaker stresses will be paid for directly by third parties in the near future (Quinn, 1986). Lawmakers are concerned about any changes that would possibly increase the already high cost of American health care.

Arguing from a least restricted environment position, Claude Pepper introduced H.R. 65 in the 100th Congress. (S.455 is the companion bill in the Senate.) This bill would expand Medicare coverage to basic preventive services such as hearing screening and annual physical examinations and cover adult day care and respite services. Exactly how these services would be paid for is not clear. Some reimbursement package will probably be worked out over time, but unless some movement is made to find funding for family caregiver support services, financing these services will be an issue for quite a long time.

Reluctance to Seek Help

The other obstacle to providing support services to caregivers is their reluctance to ask for help and to use the services. The work of Cockerill and Warren (1990) demonstrates that caretakers of multiple sclerosis patients prefer to hire someone to help or to ask family or friends for respite. If this is true of other caretakers, the best interventions may be advocacy programs that provide money to hire a respite worker, either in the form of tax credits or direct payment. Another important strategy is to encourage caregivers to keep in touch with their social network to ensure having family and friends involved in respite care. Church groups, as well as other community groups, can be important in this regard. Most people seem to prefer small-scale help in managing caretaker responsibilities.

Individual Focus

The third obstacle to developing support services for caretakers is the individual orientation of the health-care business. Until we can make the family a legitimate focus of health-care intervention, such approaches always will be a secondary concern.

✦ CONCLUSION

The growth of formal services to support family caregivers is encouraging. However, the fear of increasing health-care costs continues to limit the availability of publicly funded support services. Literature also suggests that family caregivers prefer flexibility in seeking support services.

REFERENCES

Acree, E. L., & Gregory, V. J. (1989). Home health care through an academic nurse–managed center. In National League for Nursing (Ed.), *Nursing centers: Meeting the demand for quality health care* (Pub. No. 21-2311, pp. 135-141). New York: National League for Nursing.

Bader, J. E. (1985). Respite care: Temporary relief for caregivers. *Women and Health, 10*(2), 39-52.

Barger, S. E. (1986). Academic nurse–managed centers: Issues of implementation. *Family and Community Health, 9*(1), 12-22.

Barusch, A. S., & Spaid, W. M. (1989). Gender differences in caregiving: Why do women report greater burden? *The Gerontologist, 29*(5), 667-675.

Baumgarten, M. (1989). The health of persons giving care to the demented elderly: A critical review of the literature. *Journal of Clinical Epidemiology, 42*(12), 1137-1148.

Beckham, E., & Adams, R. (1984). Coping behavior in depression. *Behavioral Research Therapy, 21*, 71-75.

Beckman, L. J. (1981). Effects of social interaction and children's relative inputs on older women's psychological well-being. *Journal of Personality and Social Psychology, 41*, 1075-1086.

Bloom, S., Knorr, E., & Evans, B. J. (1985). Cost of childhood cancer. *Children's Health Care, 14*, 62-71.

Borsuk, N. G. (1989). New Jersey's statewide family caregiver education and support program. *Caring, 8*(12), 14-16.

Borysenko, J. (1987). *Minding the body, mending the mind.* New York: Bantam.

Brody, E. M. (1985). Parent care as a normative family stress. *The Gerontologist, 25*, 19-29.

Cantor, M. (1983). Strain among caregivers: A study of experience in the United States. *The Gerontologist, 23*(6), 597-604.

Cicirelli, V. G. (1990). Family support in relation to health problems of the elderly. In T. H. Brubaker (Ed.), *Family relations in later life* (2nd ed., pp. 212-228). Beverly Hills, CA: Sage.

Cockerill, R., & Warren, S. (1990). Care for caregivers: The needs of family members of MS patients. *Journal of Rehabilitation, 56*(1), 41-44.

Cohen, S., & Warren, R. D. (1985). *Respite care.* Austin, TX: Pro-ed.

Council on Scientific Affairs, American Medical Association. (1990). Home care in the 1990s. *Journal of the American Medical Association, 263*(9), 1241-1244.

Dellasega, C. (1990). Coping with caregiving: Stress management for caregivers of the elderly. *Journal of Psychosocial Nursing, 28*(1), 15-22.

Douglass, M. E., & Douglass, D. N. (1985). *Manage your time, manage your work, manage yourself.* New York: American Management Association.

Gaynor, S. E. (1990). The long haul: The effects of home care on caregivers. *Image, 22*(4), 208-212.

George, L., & Gwyther, L. (1986). Caregiver well-being: A multidimensional examination of family caregivers of demented adults. *The Gerontologist, 26*(3), 253-259.

Gnaedinger, N. (1989). The Alzheimer's household: Who cares for the caregivers? *Community Medical, 141*, 1273-1275.

Group for Advancement of Psychiatry. (1986). *Family affairs: Helping families cope with mental illness.* New York: Brunner/Mazel.

Higgs, Z. R. (1989). Models of academic

nurse–managed centers. In National League for Nursing (Ed.), *Nursing centers: Meeting the demand for quality health care* (Pub. No. 21-2311, pp. 103-109). New York: National League for Nursing.

Kaye, L. W., & Applegate, J. S. (1990). Men as elder caregivers: A response to changing families. *American Journal of Orthopsychiatry, 60*(1), 86-95.

National Institute of Mental Health. (1983). NIMH definition and guiding principles for community support systems (CSSs). Rockville, MD: NJMH.

Orodenker, S. Z. (1990). Family caregiving in a changing society: The effects of employment on caregiver stress. *Family Community Health, 12*(4), 58-70.

Parker, M., & Iverson, L. H. (1988a). *Informal caregiving: Its importance in long-term care.* Interdisciplinary long-term care expansion program: Issue papers. Excelsior, MN: InterStudy Center for Aging and Long-term Care.

Parker, M., & Iverson, L. H. (1988b). *InterStudy's long-term care expansion program: Issue papers.* Excelsior, MN: InterStudy Center for Aging and Long-term Care.

Pearlin, L. I., & Turner, H. A. (1987). Measurement and methodological issues in social support. In S. V. Kasl & C. L. Cooper (Eds.), *Stress in health: Issues in research methodology* (pp. 167-205). New York: John Wiley & Sons.

Pearson, M. A., & Deitrick, E. P. (1989). A volunteer program for in-home respite care. *Caring, 8*(12), 18-20.

Poppleton, L. A. (1988). Home health services: Organizational dilemmas. In *Strategies for long-term care* (pp. 253-262). New York: National League for Nursing.

Quinn, J. (1986). Seeking quality alternatives in the community. *Business and Health, 3*(8), 21-24.

Ram Dass. (1990). *Journey to awakening: A meditator's guidebook.* New York: Bantam.

Robinson, K. M. (1989). Predictors of depression among wife caretakers. *Nursing Research, 38*(6), 359-363.

Scharlach, A. E. (1987). Role strain in mother-daughter relationships in later life. *The Gerontologist, 27,* 627-631.

Siwek, J. (1985). House calls: Current status and rationale. *American Family Physician, 31,* 169-174.

Steinmetz, S. K., & Amsden, D. B. (1983). Dependent elders, family stress, and abuse. In T. H. Brubaker (Ed.), *Family relations in later life* (pp. 173-192). Beverly Hills, CA: Sage.

Vogel, G., & Doleysh, N. (1988). *Entrepreneuring: A nurse's guide to starting a business.* New York: National League for Nursing.

Warren, R., & Cohen, S. (1985). Respite care. *Rehabilitation Literature, 46*(3-4), 66-71.

Warren, S., Cockerill, R., Paterson, M., & Paterson, I. (1986). Planning support services for chronically sick in rural areas. *Canadian Journal of Public Health, 77,* 19-23.

Zarit, J., & Zarit, S. (1983). Families under stress: Interventions for caregivers of senile dementia patients. *Psychotherapy, 19,* 461-471.

Zink, M. R., & Bissonnette, A. M. (1990). A unique multidisciplinary approach for urban geriatric home care. *Nursing Administration Quarterly, 14*(2), 69-73.

Zirul, D. W., Lieberman, A. A., & Rapp, C. A. (1989). Respite care for the chronically mentally ill: Focus for the 1990s. *Community Mental Health Journal, 25*(3), 171-184.

FAMILIES AND
SPECIFIC
ILLNESSES

T HIS part of the book contains four chapters. Each chapter examines in detail the demands of caring for a family member with a specific illness. It is *not* the goal of these chapters to present comprehensive reviews from the literature on the etiology of specific illnesses or to examine the course or methods of treatment of particular diseases. Rather, the illnesses are only a mechanism for illustration, within a particular context, of the impact a family member's illness can have on the entire family system. Each chapter begins with a vignette describing briefly the family situation and the illness they are coping with. Using the components of McCubbin & McCubbin's Resiliency Model of Family Stress, Adjustment, and Adaptation (see Chapter 2), further information in the chapters is organized as follows and addresses the following questions:

✦ The demands of the illness situation—the stressor (A)
  What are the specific demands of the illness on the family?

✦ Resources available to the family—the resources (B/BB/BBB)
  What unique resources are available within the family and its community to cope with the demands of the illness?

✦ Family appraisals of the illness situation—the appraisals (C/CC/CCC)
  What specific appraisals of the illness do families hold, and how do these affect the ability of the family to cope with the demands of the illness?

The last section of each chapter explores family interventions that meet the demands of the illness. The following question will be addressed: What types of interventions seem useful for families confronted with this particular illness?

These four chapters attempt to demonstrate the application and usefulness of the theoretical components of this book to an actual illness situation. We believe this information has universal application for families in other illness situations with similar illness stressor dimensions. These chapters also demonstrate the powerful resource *family interventions* offers the health professional.

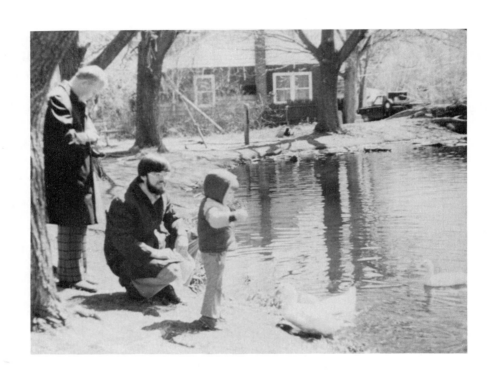

11

Long-term Catastrophic Illness: Spinal Cord Injury

✦

CHAPTER GOALS

✦ To examine the demands a long-term catastrophic illness places on the family and the potential for these demands to cause family strain, stress, and crisis

✦ To illustrate family interventions supportive and useful to families confronted with a long-term catastrophic illness.

OVERVIEW

THIS chapter examines in detail the demands of caring for a family member with a long-term catastrophic illness – spinal cord injury. The dimensions of this illness stressor determining the impact this illness can have on an entire family system are identified and described. The chapter begins with a vignette describing the Graham family situation and the aspects of spinal cord injury with which they are coping. The chapter is organized by the components of the Resiliency Model of Family Stress, Adjustment, and Adaptation (see McCubbin & McCubbin, Chapter 2, Fig. 2-1) and discusses spinal cord injury in relation to: the demands of the illness situation – the stressor (A); resources available to the Grahams – the resources (B/BB/BBB); and the Graham's appraisal of the illness situation – the appraisals (C/CC/CCC). The last section of the chapter offers suggestions for family interventions that meet the demands of this type of illness and concludes with an example of a specific family intervention that demonstrates the need and value of family interventions in a long-term catastrophic illness. We think the information in this chapter can be universally applied to families facing similar long-term catastrophic illness situations.

✦ THE FAMILY SITUATION

Danny Graham is a popular junior in high school. Not the best of students, Danny compensates for his lack of academic prowess by being "one of the guys." On this particular Saturday night he is out with three friends—just cruising, going nowhere in particular. Like many other kids his age, Danny is no stranger to alcohol, although it is hardly a habit. Tonight, the boys have a beer or two. Shortly after midnight, as they are driving home, Tim McGill, the driver, loses control of the car on a corner. The car leaves the road and tumbles down an embankment, landing on its roof. None of the boys are wearing seat belts, and they are all thrown from the car. One boy is killed, two others sustain fractures, and Danny suffers a spinal cord injury.

When Danny's mother, father, and two younger sisters arrive at the hospital they are relieved to learn that he will live, but are shocked to realize that he may never walk again. The accident has left him without the use of his arms and legs; he is paralyzed from his neck down.

This vignette is the beginning of a narrative designed to illustrate how the stressor dimensions of long-term catastrophic illnesses affects families. The Graham family's situation will exemplify common family reactions and needs in this type of illness situation. The box below lists illness stressor dimensions typical of spinal cord injury (see Chapter 4 for general infor-

---

Illness Stressor Dimensions Characteristic of Spinal Cord Injury

Sudden *onset*	Great *severity*
Long-term *duration*	Large *financial* demands
Great social *stigma*	Random *predictability*
Known, man-made *cause*	Limited ability to *control*
Origin from outside the family	High *extent* of family impact

mation on stressor dimensions). Within the context of this long-term illness, the illness stressor dimensions are examined for the demands they put on the family and for their potential to cause family strain, stress, and crisis.

In long-term catastrophic illnesses, family adaptation is often required. Family adaptation can be enhanced by mutually supportive relationships between health-care professionals and families (McCubbin & McCubbin, Chapter 2). Therefore establishing positive, collaborative patient–family–health professional relationships in long-term illnesses can be critical to successful patient outcomes. The nature of this illness provides multiple opportunities for the health professional to empower families dealing with the many challenges this type of illness engenders.

✦ THE ILLNESS – SPINAL CORD INJURY

Severe traumatic injury to the spinal cord can result in total or partial transection of the cord (Schenk, 1991). Total transection causes loss of voluntary function and of all sensations below the level of the lesion. Cervical spine injury, the focus of the Graham family situation, is the most critical of spinal injuries because of its potential to compromise respiratory function and to cause paralysis of all extremities and the trunk (Table 11-1). It is initially treated by realignment and stabilization of the bone fractures. Steroids are given to reduce inflammation. Once the patient's condition is stabilized and swelling subsides, surgery is performed to stabilize the fractures. From this point on the patient and family begin the struggle to achieve maximum rehabilitation, which includes the following:

1. Physical therapy to prevent contractures of muscles and to strengthen muscles still under voluntary control
2. Modifications (with or without equipment) of daily living activities
3. Prevention of pressure sores
4. Maintenance of bowel and bladder function to prevent autonomic dysreflexia (a medical emergency caused by bladder and bowel distention initiating paroxysmal hypertension that can result in a cerebrovascular accident [CVA], blindness, or death)
5. Management of sexual impairments
6. Prevention of urinary and respiratory infections
7. Exploration and development of vocational and independent living potentials.

Table 11-1 *Muscle function and rehabilitation potential after cervical spine injury*

Cervical spinal cord injury	Muscle function present	Rehabilitation potential
C 2-3	*Usually fatal*	
C4	Above the neck	Paralysis of all four extremities; respiratory ventilator needed
C5	Shoulder (partial), elbow (partial)	Needs adaptive devices; may need ventilator
C6	Shoulder, elbow, chest, and partial wrist	Propel wheelchair with knobs on wheels
C7	Shoulder, elbow, wrist, partial hand, partial chest	Transfer to and from wheelchair; propel the wheelchair
C8	Shoulder, arm, weak hands, partial chest	Transfer wheelchair into the car; drive car with adaptations; vocational and recreational goals achievable

Modified from Brunner, L.S., & Suddarth, D.S. (1992). S. Smeltzer & B. Bare (Eds.), *Brunner and Suddarth's textbook of medical-surgical nursing* (7th ed.). Philadelphia: J.B. Lippincott; and Phipps, W., et al. (1991). *Medical-surgical nursing: Concepts and clinical practice* (4th ed.). St. Louis: Mosby-Year Book.

Accompanying these activities is the difficult task of psychosocial adjustment to the disability. These lifelong tasks require continual adjustments and adaptations as the family situation changes and illness complications occur.

Spinal cord injury is a low-incidence, high-cost disability that produces enormous changes in life-style (Geissinger, 1986). Approximately 200,000 persons with spinal cord injury live in the United States (Steinbauer, 1989). This injury most often occurs to males 15 to 29 years old as the result of a motor vehicle accident. The life expectancy of these individuals, with today's medicine, is near normal, and 80% of those having a C6 injury or lower live in the community. As a result, this disability has a long-term impact on families.

In a report describing allocation of health-care benefit dollars to spinal cord–injured patients, the cost of one patient's 80-day hospitalization and rehabilitation was $150,576 (Weingarden, Kuric, Belen, & Graham, 1989). This is only a small part of the financial burden rendered by this kind of disability. After initial care and rehabilitation, the average costs related to spinal cord injury can be $20,000 per year not including income loss (Steinbauer, 1989). Home modifications, equipment, outpatient rehabilitation, nursing care, and follow-up medical care costs account for most of the costs. Insurance coverage for some of these expenses is limited (Weingarden et al., 1989). With such staggering costs, families without strong financial resources can be devastated, and some may be reduced to accepting welfare.

✦ DEMANDS OF THE ILLNESS STRESSOR (A)

Each stressor dimension encompassed in this illness creates varying degrees of demands on the family. This portion of the chapter will explore those demands and their effects on the Graham family. Stressor dimensions that relate to each other or cause similar effects on the family will be discussed together. Family vulnerability (V) and family typology (T) (Fig. 11-1) also will be discussed in relation to the demands they add to the situation. The Graham family has been arbitrarily assigned the family type *bonded family* to study the implications family typology brings to the situation. Bonded families are "low in family flexibility but high in family bonding" (McCubbin & McCubbin, 1989, p. 30). This type of family is part of the resilient family typology (see Fig. 5-3). Their strength resides in their sense of internal unity. They rely on each other for understanding and support and easily make decisions as a family unit. However, their low flexibility makes them resistant to compromise and set in their ways.

Sudden Onset

✦ ✦ ✦ ✦ ✦

The Grahams are terrified when they see Danny in the hospital for the first time. On his head is a metal apparatus (Crutchfield tongs) that is screwed into his skull. He is pale and so still. Fear and anguish are clearly written on their faces as the physician approaches them. The physician reveals to them that Danny may have suffered damage to his cervical spine. Spinal shock has rendered him paralyzed from the neck down at this time. The

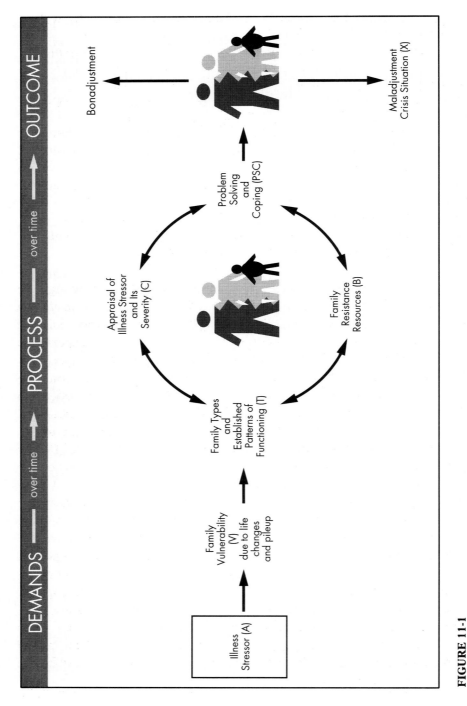

FIGURE 11-1

Adjustment Phase of the Resiliency Model of Family Stress, Adjustment, and Adaptation. This portion of the chapter focuses on the demands of the illness stressor (A).

extent of the damage to the spinal cord and the amount of paralysis that will remain cannot yet be determined. It could be 3 to 6 weeks before an accurate assessment of the injury can be made. The physician explains that the purpose of the cervical traction applied to Danny's head is to immobilize the injury.

The family can barely believe this has happened. They are overwhelmed and in a state of shock. The idea that Danny may never walk again is a loss they find difficult to face and desperately hope they will not have to. They are immobilized, barely knowing what to do next. It is difficult for them to talk to Danny without crying.

As they leave the hospital they are relieved that Danny is alive yet aware of the changes and losses that may be taking place in their lives and Danny's. They are overwhelmed by feelings of helplessness, loss of control, fear, and disorganization. Many tears and hugs are exchanged as the family realizes their potential losses and attempts to support each other.

Danny's accident has suddenly rocketed the Graham family through the Family Cycle of Health and Illness from *Phase 1—Health—*to *Phase 4—Medical Contact* (see Chapter 3, Fig. 3-2). Initially, no time was available to adjust, gather information, plan, or organize for this experience (Cleveland, 1980/1989). The Graham family has no previous experience with an illness stressor of this type to prepare them for this situation. The suddenness and severity of the onset causes strong emotional reactions to reverberate throughout the family. Initially the Graham family is horrified and in disbelief. They ask themselves, "How can this be happening to us? Why did this happen to us? Could we have prevented it? What will Danny be like?" and pray, "Please let him walk again." The result is family chaos and accompanying stress that leads to family crisis.

In a study by Martha Cleveland (1980/1989) of 19 families experiencing spinal cord injury, *all families* described the initial events of this illness/disability as causing an extreme family crisis. Through this crisis a collective coping process begins. Over 50% of the family members reported feeling closer to each other and perceived other family members as having closer relationships. This collective coping process makes mutual support readily available and losses more easily faced. For the Graham family, high in family bonding, this serves to strengthen the sense of internal unity already present. The outcome of this family crisis will depend on family problem solving, coping capabilities, and support received (McCubbin & McCubbin, Chapter 2).

Severity, Stigma, and Extent of Family Impact

✦ ✦ ✦ ✦ ✦

It has been 6 weeks since Danny's accident, and his condition has stabilized. He has been in intensive care most of this time to prevent respiratory failure from spinal shock (a transient flaccid paralysis with loss of reflexes [Schenk, 1991]). The intensive care experience was very frightening and stressful for both Danny and his family. Surgery to repair his fracture was completed, which added further stress to the situation. Spinal cord damage did occur at the C8 level, and his legs are completely paralyzed. However, he does have shoulder and arm movement with weakness of the hands and partial movement of chest muscles.

Danny has been moved from the intensive care unit to a standard hospital unit (much to the relief of his family, a sign of recovery), and more rehabilitation activities are initiated. Realization of the extent of his injuries is beginning to affect Danny. He is moody and often uses abusive language with the staff. It is not easy dealing with him. Mrs. Graham, Sarah, is spending most of her waking hours at the hospital and often needs comforting from the staff as she weeps over Danny's losses. She eats very little and looks drawn and tired. The staff is becoming concerned for her health. Danny's father, Jim, visits after work everyday and is having difficulty dealing with the situation. He is often curt and complaining, as he makes demands on the hospital staff. That he is angry cannot be mistaken. Danny's two younger sisters are being cared for by Jim's parents, who have traveled a great distance to come and help. The grandparents bring the girls into the hospital regularly to see Danny. Although the girls enjoy their grandparents, they miss their accustomed access to their parents. This adds to their anxiety.

The high degree of severity found in this illness strongly contributes to the family crisis present at the onset of the illness. Through the grieving over present and anticipated losses and the drastic, sudden changes in family patterns, every family member is affected by this illness. Mrs. Graham's time at the hospital is greatly disrupting family task organization. Calling on their family resources, she has reallocated tasks to the grandparents. The extended family is now involved. Close friends are affected through their support to the family and assistance to the grandparents in caring for the girls. The severity of this illness makes the need for help clear, fostering high family impact and community involvement.

Severity of this disability makes acceptance difficult. The family confronted with a spinal cord injury can be classified, according to Hill (1958), as being in the most difficult of crisis resolution situations (cited in Cleveland, 1980/1989). This situation includes: (1) "death" of the family member as he normally was; (2) "birth" of the injured family member as a disabled person; and (3) degradation through society's strongly negative view of the disabled person. Society honors roles it needs and accepts and devalues roles, like that of the disabled, that it does not need and wishes to reject (Saylor, 1990b).

Danny's ascribed incapacities are extended to his family (Turnbull & Turnbull, 1985), and the family will carry this stigma for the duration of Danny's life. Therefore this new label—*disabled*—is difficult for the family to accept. Role changes, one of the most difficult kinds of changes (Leventhal, Leventhal, & Van Nguyen 1985), must take place not only within the family but also outside the family; that is, the family must find a new fit with the community. Because of this, accepting this disability and resolving this crisis are not often accomplished early in the illness (Flannery, 1990). This resistance can make it difficult to accept the treatment plan. Even when the disability is accepted, the family acceptance is constantly challenged by new losses realized as advancements through the illness cycle and the milestones of individual and family life occur (Brunner & Suddarth, 1992).

The situation is also difficult for families to resolve because it is a relatively rare occurrence. As a result, no societal guidelines or expectations have been established (Cleveland, 1980/1989). Societal guidelines play a major role in helping families adapt to crisis (McCubbin & McCubbin, Chapter 2). Therefore the absence of guidelines can have some disastrous effects. The family may now go through a series of trial-and-error attempts to adapt to the situation instead of striving in one direction and accomplishing a goal. This trial-and-error process expends family energy, placing additional demands on the family system, which can lead to family crisis (McCubbin & McCubbin, Chapter 2). Also, the process may be detrimental to the family's sense of mastery and control.

Altered social relationships due to the stigma related to the severity of this disability become a reality when Danny eventually returns home. Discomfort can be experienced in family, friends, and other community relationships (Dewis, 1989; Saylor, 1990a). The family may have to tolerate uncomfortable social interactions, pity, and judgmental comments. Avoidance of these situations may cause social isolation, which can hamper development of social support networks so necessary in this type of illness (Saylor, 1990b). A limited social support network can diminish family adaptability (Connelly, 1988). This is something the Graham family, already low in flexibility, cannot afford. Feelings of social isolation are intensified as the freedom to come and go as they please is curtailed by attending to Danny's needs or to the inability to find competent respite care (see Chapter 10). The family strain and stress generated by this isolation and resulting limited social support can increase the potential for family crisis.

Duration, Predictability, and Control

✦ ✦ ✦ ✦ ✦

Danny and his family have been told that, with training, Danny will be able to transfer himself to and from a wheelchair, propel the wheelchair, and drive an automobile with special adaptations (Brunner & Suddarth, 1992). Also, some vocational and recreational goals can be achieved despite his disabilities. Danny and his family seek and explore information on the different rehabilitation programs and facilities available to them. A large, well-known spinal cord facility is a 1-day trip away. A smaller rehabilitation facility with a good reputation is only a 2-hour ride from home. The family chooses the smaller rehabilitation center because of its proximity and the ability to keep the family intact in its normal patterns as much as possible. It is estimated that Danny will be there for at least 3 months.

While Danny is in the rehabilitation center, Sarah goes to see him whenever possible during the week, and the family visits on weekends. The weekend visits are not easy. Each time they see him, it reminds them of their losses. Their grief is mixed with other ambivalent feelings. Jim is beginning to make some of the renovations needed for Danny's return home. A day at the rehabilitation center leaves him only one free weekend day to work on these projects. Because of this, he is afraid that he will have to hire someone to help him finish the work on time. This is an expense he cannot afford. Sarah has resigned from her volunteer work and given up some of the fun things she enjoys doing to fit her visits into her normally busy week. This isolates her from her social support networks and limits activities that have a relaxing influence on her life. Danny's sisters resent the visits to Danny absorbing their free time. They dislike giving up social and school activities on the weekends.

It is 3 months later and Danny has now completed his rehabilitation program. He is ready to return home. The entire family has received information about the extent of Danny's losses and the care involved. Everyone has participated in training sessions, informational exchanges, and support sessions necessary to deal with Danny's physical and emotional care. The remodeling of the house to meet Danny's needs is completed. Anticipation is high.

Danny's presence in the home brings the full impact of Danny's disability with it. The Graham family will be dealing with Danny's disability for the rest of his life, and the burden of care now falls almost completely on Danny and his family. The true impact will be harder to ignore or deny.

The degree of disorganization that occurs when bringing the severely disabled home can be related strongly to the maintenance of accepted roles (Cleveland 1980/1989). Typically the reorganization of a family with a chronically ill child involves addition of tasks to the already existing family structure. Family members stay within their major roles — mother, father, and siblings — and tasks are divided according to those roles. Since the Graham family, low in flexibility, prefers the status quo, they are likely to choose this course. This will decrease family disorganization experienced at Danny's return home. However, family loads are usually not renegotiated in a load-equalizing way. Therefore Sarah takes on the greatest burden of caring for the disabled child. With time, she will feel role strain, which can manifest itself in physical and emotional complaints (Fradkin & Liberti, 1987; Gaynor, 1990) indicating the presence of pileup and possible oncoming exhaustion.

The long-term course of spinal cord injury brings many unexpected setbacks (for example, respiratory infection, kidney infections, bowel impaction, skin breakdown, autonomic dysreflexia) that can occur at any time (Schenk, 1991). Opportunity for pileup exists as these illness complications, family life cycle transitions, and problems of living take place simultaneously or back to back. A sense of helplessness and loss of control may occur (Nordstrom & Lubkin, 1990). This uncertainty can decrease family unity and the sense of mastery (Ferrari, Matthews, & Barabas, 1983/1985) unless the uncertainty is appraised positively as an opportunity for growth (Mishel, 1990). The low flexibility of the Graham family makes a positive appraisal of the situation unlikely. Therefore the uncertainty of the illness generates family strain and stress for the Graham family.

Cause and Origin

When the cause of an illness is known and families are able to develop explanations, families usually cope more effectively (Olson et al., 1989). A sense of control is present. The cause of this illness is known but it originates as a man-made accident — something outside the family and beyond its control. This may counteract feelings of control. Feelings of guilt can develop related to the inability to have controlled or prevented the situation (Flannery, 1990). Anger may arise as the family ponders, "Why me?" or "If only I had. . . ." We see this anger in both Danny and his dad as they take their anger out on the hospital staff.

Pitzele (1985) states that the anger phase of the grieving process can be one of the most difficult phases to resolve (cited in Kahn, 1990). Anger turned inward can cause depression and prevents confrontation of the profound sadness associated with loss of "normal" health and life-style that disability brings. This anger can be maladaptive and manifest behaviors that are annoying and frustrating to others (Savedra & Dibble, 1989; Saylor, 1990a). The demand this poses for the family is to free themselves from the guilt and channel the anger into useful energy (see examples in Chapter 4, Cause of the Stressor). This is especially true for Danny, whose anger can interfere with successful rehabilitation outcomes.

Resource Demands — Financial

◆ ◆ ◆ ◆ ◆

The family's most important tangible resource, money, adequately met family needs before Danny's accident. By working long hours, Jim Graham brings home a salary of about $40,000 a year. He is an electrician and has worked hard to attain that level of success with his own electrical contracting business. The family is proud of his success.

The comprehensiveness of the family's medical insurance is limited. Because Danny's disability was caused by an automobile accident, the maximum benefit the family can receive is $300,000. Once that sum is gone, no further insurance assistance is available. Danny's family is aware that this sum will hardly cover Danny's needs. They may need to sue the driver of the car to increase this resource, yet this may take years to resolve. Danny's 6 weeks of hospitalization and 3 months at the rehabilitation center, a total of 132 days, cost $250,000. This leaves $50,000 for home renovations, equipment, medical costs, and psychological support for the rest of Danny's life. For equipment alone, Danny has many expensive needs.

He needs a special bed, a wheelchair, toileting equipment (for example, urethral catheters) that requires constant replacement, renovations to the toilet area of the home, and car modifications so that he can drive and load his wheelchair. Also, the medical sequelae of his disability may necessitate further hospitalizations. Jim is thankful to members of the extended family who have offered to help as they can with expenses.

The financial demands this illness places on the family can be as catastrophic as the illness. It can create a real source of family anxiety, especially for Danny's father. Reduced family funds can intensify feelings of isolation by limiting entertainment with friends and decreasing the ability to hire respite care for the caregiver or to take vacations (Hennen, Seitz, & Seitz, 1987). The adolescent stage of family development is a stage normally fraught with financial strains (Olson et al., 1989). This illness adds yet another enormous financial strain for the Grahams as they pass through this stage of family development. The overwhelming financial burden of this disability can easily cause pileup and family stress, which can lead to family crisis.

✦ RESOURCES AVAILABLE TO THE FAMILY (B/BB/BBB)

Within the framework of the Resiliency Model of Family Stress, Adjustment, and Adaptation, resources are described as encompassing both tangible and coping capacities of the family and its community (McCubbin & McCubbin, Chapter 2). Three kinds of resources are identified: (1) personal resources of the individual family members, (2) collectively held family resources, and (3) community resources, or social support. To deal with this long-term catastrophic illness and its demands, the Graham family will draw from all three resource areas. This portion of the chapter examines the strengths and weaknesses of resources available to the Graham family (Fig. 11-2).

Personal Resources (B)

Feelings of mastery and self-esteem are essential for the individual to manage demands successfully (McCubbin & McCubbin, Chapter 2). Feelings of control over one's life that support a sense of mastery maintain dignity and encourage participation in life (Dittmar, 1989). With the onset

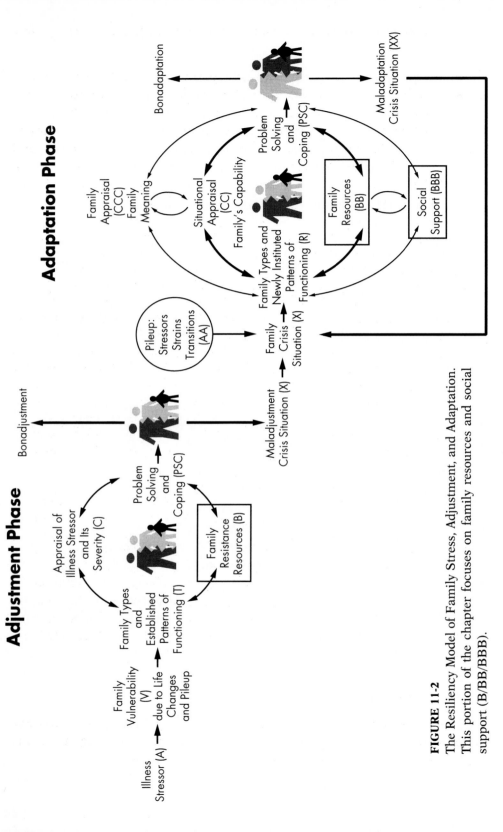

FIGURE 11-2

The Resiliency Model of Family Stress, Adjustment, and Adaptation. This portion of the chapter focuses on family resources and social support (B/BB/BBB).

of illness, the resources of mastery and self-esteem are the most readily affected as illness demands increase. For example, this disability assaults Danny's self-esteem and sense of mastery on many levels — self-identity, sexual function, social and emotional roles, toileting functions, and so forth. Furthermore, Danny is an adolescent whose self-esteem is developing and fragile. This illness crisis superimposes itself on a developmental crisis, intensifying the stress felt by both Danny and his family (Savedra & Dibble, 1989).

✦ ✦ ✦ ✦ ✦

While in the rehabilitation center, Danny is very moody, showing signs of depression that can be found among teenagers (Savedra & Dibble, 1989) and spinal cord patients depending on their personality characteristics before the injury (Steinbauer, 1989). This depression indicates diminished self-esteem that can be destructive to managing demands of the rehabilitation program and producing successful outcomes.

Danny's parents also find their self-esteem and sense of mastery challenged by this disability. Jim's business was doing well, and he had hoped to pass it on to his son. Danny had appeared eager for that to happen as well. Jim feels that dream is destroyed. He is devastated by his son's disability and the financial burdens it creates. Sarah is overwhelmed by the demands Danny's disability creates and grieves for her son. She often sets aside her own needs for Danny's needs. Much of the time she feels tired and helplessly unable to control her life. The sense of mastery that existed for Danny's parents before the accident is missing.

As with other siblings in this type of situation, Danny's sisters, Susan (10 years old) and Jennifer (12 years old), often feel that their needs have been relegated to second place (Walker, 1988; Savedra & Dibble, 1989). Their parents' attention is always diverted to the consuming job of caring and planning for Danny. The girls learn to seek support from each other instead of their parents (Cleveland, 1980/1989). They are resentful and jealous that Danny is not held to the same behavioral standards that they are (Martinson, Gilliss, Colaizzo, Freeman, & Bossert, 1990). All of this threatens their sense of mastery and self-esteem, which is developmentally still evolving.

Family Resources (BB)

Moderate amounts of family cohesion and adaptability have been found to be two of the most important family resources in managing stress and crisis (McCubbin & McCubbin, Chapter 2; Olson et al., 1989). Reiss, Gonzalez, Wolin, Steinglass, and Kramer (1983), in a study of families facing chronic illness, uncovered a positive relationship between family flexibility and openness and patient health outcomes (cited in Steinbauer, 1989). Long-term illnesses that produce family stress and crises require these family attributes for successful outcomes.

The high bonding in the Graham family makes them feel close to each other (McCubbin & McCubbin, 1989). They rely on each other for support and understanding and consider their cohesiveness to be a strength. However, spinal cord injury of a child places chronic strain on marital relationships and communications (Cleveland, 1980/1989). Also, lengthy illnesses with an uncertain course have been shown to produce impaired communications, poor sibling relationships, and less cohesiveness (Damrosch & Perry, 1989; Ferrari et al., 1983/1985; Leventhal et al., 1985). Clearly the cohesiveness and openness of the Graham family will be threatened by Danny's disability.

Surprisingly the threat to the Graham's high amount of bonding or cohesiveness could be helpful in view of the following studies. Reiss et al. (1983) found family coordination, a family trait similar to family bonding, has a negative relationship with patient survival in chronic illness (cited in Steinbauer, 1989). M. A. McCubbin's (1986) study on the success of balanced families (see Fig. 5-2) in dealing with chronic illness appears to indicate that *moderate* amounts of the family trait, cohesion, best serve the Graham's situation (cited in McCubbin & McCubbin, Chapter 2). Therefore the high family bonding in the Graham family could possibly have a negative impact on patient outcomes, but the illness situation that decreases their cohesiveness may counteract that impact.

The initial closeness that develops with this disability often gives way to strong dyadic relationships that can undermine cohesiveness (Cleveland, 1980/1989). This occurs in the Graham family.

✦ ✦ ✦ ✦ ✦

Sarah's overprotectiveness toward Danny causes marital tension. Jim resents Sarah's caregiving role interfering with her role as wife. In turn, Sarah feels anger toward Jim's lack of understanding and assistance. This marital conflict undermines family cohesion. It will be detrimental to the situation if a moderate amount of family cohesion cannot be maintained.

Bonded families such as the Graham family predictably have difficulty adapting because of low flexibility. Bonded families usually resist compromise and rigidly prefer their established patterns (McCubbin & McCubbin, 1989). Shifting responsibilities among family members and including all family members in making decisions is not something often practiced, so this will not come easily to the Grahams. Their way of managing tensions and strains depends on their sense of unity, their strength, and resistance to change, their weakness. This type of stress management may not work with an illness that demands many changes.

Economic stability is a critical resource for family adjustment and adaptation (McCubbin & McCubbin, Chapter 2). Adequate finances also increases family flexibility to find alternative solutions. Danny's disability as discussed earlier, severely threatens the financial stability of the Graham family.

Community Resources (BBB)

✦ ✦ ✦ ✦ ✦

During the initial hospitalization and at the rehabilitation center, the Grahams were given information on the various national and local organizations supportive to families with spinal cord injuries. Rehabilitation services are available nearby, including occupational therapy, physical therapy, psychological support, an organization that supports independent living situations for disabled individuals, and a state vocational center. Danny's care will be managed through the spinal cord clinic at the local hospital and their family physician. The Graham family will need to access most of these services.

The Grahams have many friends that initially offered assistance to the family, but with time this number diminished to a few close friends. Sarah has several friends that occasionally offer assistance and respite from Danny's care, but Danny does not like them caring for him or feeling like he has a babysitter. These friends drop in to see Sarah often. She finds this a great source of support. Jim has friends that helped raise funds to assist in the remodeling of their home. Some of them assisted with the actual construction efforts. Jim was very thankful. Initially, Danny also had many friends coming to see him. Their discomfort with his disability soon decreased these visits to a few close friends. At times, these friends take him on outings with them. Danny's school provided tutoring services for him at first. Eventually he was integrated back into the school system to finish his high school education. This was a difficult time for Danny and his parents, but he enjoyed being back among his peers.

✦ FAMILY APPRAISALS OF THE ILLNESS SITUATION (C/CC/CCC)

The Graham family's appraisal of this illness situation arises from their perception of the existing balance between demands and resources (Fig. 11-3). An appraisal indicating an imbalance could initiate family crisis. At the onset of this illness it is clear that a *threat* exists and losses will be incurred. The societal definition of this disability earmarks it as highly severe with results that isolate the family as "different" from normal (Cleveland, 1980/1989). Because of this, family integrity is threatened. The sudden onset, severity, permanency, and stigma of this disability strongly contribute to their appraisal of the situation as *threatening*. In terms of the Resiliency Model of Family Stress (Fig. 11-3), the Graham family questions its capabilities (B/BB/BBB) to meet the demands of the situation (A). Family crisis (X) develops as they are overwhelmed by the implications of this illness, with its many demands and anticipated losses. A demand-resource imbalance is perceived, and adaptation is required. This produces disorganization and family chaos — family crisis.

Because the initial definition is clear — a "threat" exists — the expectations are also clear. The family is expected to mobilize its resources to meet the challenges of the illness. To their advantage, this collective coping process facilitates production of a shared appraisal making adaptation easier (Olson et al., 1989). Minimal family energy is lost gaining a consensus, and the need for support and assistance is established. Now family energy can be spent gathering information, formulating coping strategies, and adjusting/adapting to the demands.

As time passes, the Graham family attempts to meet the long-term demands of this disability. The appraisal will change depending on the family situation at the time. The lack of flexibility in the Graham family may perpetuate the original appraisal (situation is threatening) and require them to find alternatives to resist change. In many instances, old patterns of behavior do not work.

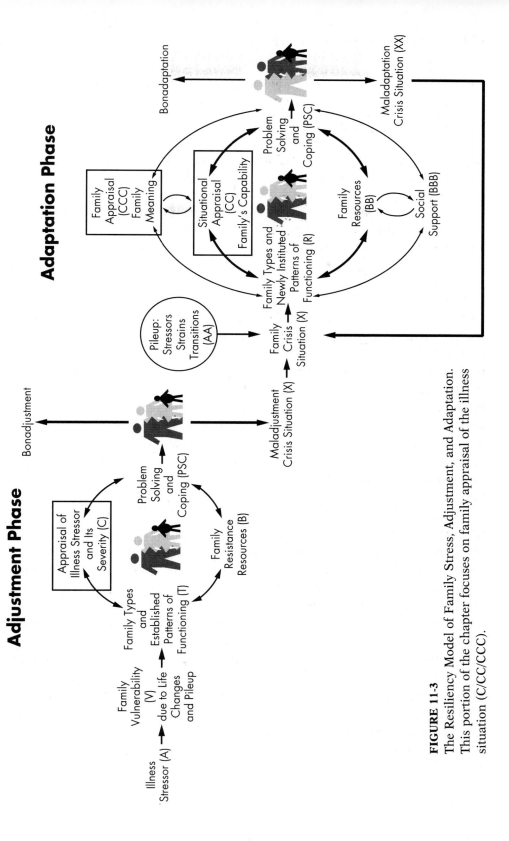

FIGURE 11-3

The Resiliency Model of Family Stress, Adjustment, and Adaptation. This portion of the chapter focuses on family appraisal of the illness situation (C/CC/CCC).

Adjustment Phase

Bonadjustment

Problem Solving and Coping (PSC)

Appraisal of Illness Stressor and Its Severity (C)

Family Types and Established Patterns of Functioning (T)

Family Resistance Resources (B)

Maladjustment Crisis Situation (X)

Family Vulnerability (V) due to Life Changes and Pileup

Illness Stressor (A)

Adaptation Phase

Bonadaptation

Maladaptation Crisis Situation (XX)

Family Appraisal (CCC) Family Meaning

Situational Appraisal (CC) Family's Capability

Problem Solving and Coping (PSC)

Family Types and Newly Instituted Patterns of Functioning (R)

Family Resources (BB)

Social Support (BBB)

Pileup: Stressors Strains Transitions (AA)

Family Crisis Situation (X)

✦ ✦ ✦ ✦ ✦

As new situations arise, the Graham family finds it difficult to attain a balance between resources and demands. This becomes even more evident as finances are exhausted. Attempts to conserve money brings on further social isolation, which limits social support and the flexibility it provides. Sarah is often exhausted from the constant physical drain of caring for Danny. Crises begin to erupt more often. All these things make it difficult for the Grahams to view this disability positively. At times, they feel the whole world is against them and there is no hope.

✦ FAMILY INTERVENTIONS

Opportunities to develop long-standing patient–family–health professional relationships that can assist families through this long-term catastrophic illness are many. The Resiliency Model of Family Stress offers the health professional some insight into directions these relationships can take in offering assistance to families. It is possible to empower families to confront this disability positively by focusing on two components of the model — *resources* (B/BB/BBB) and *appraisal* (C/CC/CCC). This can be done by (1) assisting the family to develop *manageable, positive appraisals* (C/CC/CCC) of the situation, and by (2) maximizing the application and development of *individual, family,* and *community resources* (B/BB/BBB) (see Fig. 11-3).

At the onset of this illness, priorities of care make it unlikely for health professionals to influence family typology (T), vulnerability (V), or the demands of the stressor (A) (see Fig. 11-3). Therefore interventions need to be centered on the appraisal (C/CC/CCC) and resources (B/BB/BBB) components of the model. In both the adjustment and adaptation phases of the model, the appraisal and resource components influence and interact with the family's problem-solving capabilities (PSC). In addition, in the adaptation phase these two components interact with the resiliency component (R) and influence the formation of newly instituted patterns designed by the family to meet demands for adaptation. Thus these two components contribute to the family's level of adjustment/adaptation (McCubbin & McCubbin, Chapter 2). Consequently, interventions concentrating on positively influencing the family's appraisals and resources may contribute to facilitating formation of newly instituted patterns, problem-solving capabilities, and a positive level of family adjustment. This may reduce family strain and stress, preventing crisis or at least reducing its impact. Overall this focus by health-care professionals may increase the opportunity for bonadjustment and bonadaptation and decrease the potential for maladjustment and maladaptation.

Studies show that models supporting self-efficacy and allowing the help-seeker to assume responsibility for solutions correlate positively with health outcomes and enhancement of well-being (Dunst, Trivette, & Deal, 1988). Therefore the health professional's role is to facilitate, encourage, support, and offer information, not to impose ideas and directions.

Convening the family is an excellent vehicle for implementing family interventions that assist in forming manageable family appraisals and maximizing resources (McWhinney, 1989). This family meeting also can provide the opportunity to assess family strengths and weaknesses. To maximize their effectiveness, family meetings need to take place at times of known or expected difficulty in the illness or family situation (for example, during Danny's initial hospitalization and subsequent rehabilitation, upon his return home, at developmental milestones such as Danny's twenty-first birthday, and the like). Decisions to convene the family need to be collaborative, coming from both the family and the health professional. The following section illustrates and discusses family-empowering interventions that address the appraisal and resource components of the Resiliency Model of Family Stress.

Developing Manageable, Positive Appraisals

Assessment of family appraisals can provide a vehicle to understanding family fears and behavioral reactions to illness situations. Understanding the family appraisals offers the health professional clues for facilitating a balance between what the family's perceives as the illness demands and its resources. With knowledge of the appraisal, health professionals can focus interventions on specific (to the particular family) areas of need (for example, information, social support, financial). Interventions will then more likely contribute to a positive appraisal and, in turn, a positive level of family adjustment and adaptation.

Through the use of therapeutic communication skills, interviewing, and observations, the health professional can elicit family appraisals. The duration of this particular disability provides ample time for this kind of intervention and opportunity to use family assessment measuring tools to uncover (1) family strengths and weaknesses, (2) the level of family stress and (3) the presence of family resources to manage stress (see Appendix for family assessment tools). Information sharing, crisis-intervention strategies, counseling skills, or more in-depth psychiatric therapy may be needed to produce a manageable, positive appraisal in an illness such as this that requires a great deal of adaptation.

Generating hope. Prospects for a dismal future can easily be projected with a disability of this kind. Since studies prioritizing family needs during illness list hope very high (Hickey, 1991; Leske, 1986; O'Neill-Norris & Grove, 1986), giving families hope may be important, especially for those confronted with a spinal cord injury. In fact, Zelktzer (1980) studied adolescents with chronic illness and found hope and denial to be two healthy strategies enabling them to manage their lives (cited in Savedra & Dibble, 1989). When hope is operationalized, it is easier to face the future and reality of the situations (Friedman-Campbell & Hart, 1984). Hope offers a sense of control and possible mastery of the situation. Realistic hope can be offered based on family strengths, community resources, and available treatment (Anderson & Holder, 1989). The process of offering hope can mobilize resources and contribute to a positive family appraisal. Offering hope to the Grahams could have a profound effect on their adaptation.

To generate hope, families like the Grahams need information about some possible positive outcomes of this disability. It is possible for Danny to complete his education, be employed, and live independently, but family support is vital to these outcomes (Steinbauer, 1989). Initially, denial and shock may make it difficult for families to "hear" or believe in positive outcomes. Therefore observing for family readiness to receive this information and using creative ways to repeat the information for gradual assimilation need to be considered. Knowledge of these possible outcomes can offer families hope for a more normalized existence.

To reinforce this hope, the family needs knowledge of organizations in the community that can support these efforts. Information from the national and local spinal cord organizations (for example, National Spinal Cord Injury Foundation, National Paraplegic Foundation) and those organizations that deal with disabilities (for example, institutes for independent living and state vocational rehabilitation programs) should be explored for support and possible financial aid. A study of 75 spinal cord patients (DeJong, Branch, & Corcoran, 1984) demonstrated that the more vocational rehabilitation services received the greater the resultant productivity of the individual. A productive Danny is more likely to produce family hope for mastery of this situation.

Redefining normal. The meanings families assign to changes required by illness can determine the family's acceptance of the adaptations made (McCubbin & McCubbin, Chapter 2). An appraisal process that can form positive family meanings for an illness and its demands involves the coping strategy of reframing. Reframing consists of viewing the illness as a challenge to be overcome. In this case, illnesses and their accompanying changes are viewed in a positive, meaningful, acceptable light, making adaptation easier (Olson et al., 1989). Fatalism is another coping mechanism that can have positive impact on appraisal formation in spinal cord injury. This coping mechanism takes into account that certain events are beyond control and therefore can be accepted with minimal discomfort (Olson et al., 1989). Fatalism combined with reframing may overcome feelings of helplessness. Therefore health professionals wishing to enhance family adaptation by facilitating a positive family appraisal need to support and encourage these two coping strategies.

In review articles written by Grolnick (1971) and Bruhn (1977) on the effect of chronic illness on the family, the role expectations of the family appeared to dictate the level of adjustment or adaptation to illness (cited in Steinbauer, 1989). Families may invest in the sick role as a needed family stabilizer or adapt to more normal role expectations. Overinvestment in the sick role with family life revolving around the care of the patient appears to produce poor outcomes for both the patient and the family (Steinbauer, 1989). Better family adaptation to this kind of illness occurs when the expectations produce a more "normal" family situation (Saylor, 1990a). The disabled individual is viewed as an integrated, contributing member of the family, not as a special responsibility. The disability is appraised in a positive light without overreacting or underreacting to genuine physical limitations.

To initiate "normal" expectations, Danny needs to be involved, even if his initial energy levels are low, in family meetings that formulate and choose plans and solutions to deal with his illness. During illness, family patterns of emotional sharing are critical to a sense of belonging and self-esteem (Leventhal et al., 1985). One quadriplegic described being left out of the planning process as being treated like a piece of wood (Aadalen & Stroebel-Kahn, 1981/1989). In Frank and Elliott's study (1989), spinal cord–injured patients who believed they were responsible for their own health demonstrated more adaptive behaviors and less depression than those with an externalized locus of control. These researchers believed that attitudes about controlling health can be learned. Therefore helping models that foster self-efficacy and responsibility for solutions may be best suited for this situation. In fact, if the family can be encouraged to develop a self-efficacy helping model, the family can affect well-being and produce positive outcomes to illness (Dunst et al., 1988). With these facts in mind, promoting a more normal family situation where Danny would be expected to fulfill, within his limitations, his societal and family roles may produce more positive outcomes. Since spinal cord–injured patients are initially ensconced in the sick role, the expectation often is not there for them to take on responsibilities. Over the long term, this clearly is not in their or the family's best interest.

Since society provides few role norms for the disabled (Lubkin, 1990; Saylor, 1990a) and few guidelines for families facing this kind of disability (Cleveland, 1980/1989), information concerning successful family outcomes to these situations may be helpful (McCubbin & McCubbin, Chapter 2). Using studies similar to those described in this chapter to support suggested alternatives that produce successful outcomes may be of particular importance to the Graham family, whose low flexibility makes it difficult to go through multiple trial-and-error efforts to find effective solutions. Offering these possible shortcuts to successful adjustment and adaptation may conserve family energy and the sense of mastery.

For the Graham family this normalization process can have many benefits that need to be suggested when convening the family. The individual and family esteem gained may be central in countering the stigma of this illness (Saylor, 1990a). Increasing Danny's self-esteem and sense of purpose can decrease financial loss from the self-neglect and self-destructive behaviors that can occur with spinal cord patients (Dewis, 1989). The family can be freed from guilt related to the disability, decreasing the opportunity for the disabled person to become an overly powerful member of the family (Cleveland, 1980/1989; Steinbauer, 1989). It may free the mother from the overprotectiveness that causes role strain (Cleveland, 1980/1989). It can decrease social isolation by discouraging retreat from the community into the sick role. If Danny does achieve independence, it will allow the family to go through, to some extent, the normal stages of the family life cycle. As a result, grief may not be felt over loss of certain milestones in Danny's and the family's life. Independent living may assist in decreasing the financial burden, not to mention the physical care burden, placed on the family. The family itself can return to a degree of normalcy.

Dealing with stigma. To achieve a positive family appraisal, it may be necessary to empower the family to confront with confidence those situations that decrease family esteem. For example, Danny's family may find themselves ridiculed or teased, or they may resent being singled out as "different." Instructing the family through role playing and through exploring various methods of handling stigmatized situations can increase its ability to deal with uncomfortable social interactions. In Dewis's study (1989) of adolescents and young adults with spinal cord injuries, these individuals expended great energy and at times were ingenious in attempting to normalize their situation. Efforts by the family to support these behaviors and to do likewise can enhance patient efforts to handle the stigma (Saylor, 1990b). Family strategies to decrease the effects of stigma rely on the family meaning ascribed to the disability. Since the disabled are a culturally devalued population, encouraging the use of cultural and family valued behavior and goals when redefining "normal" can enable these people and their families to live culturally valued lives (Dewis, 1989; Saylor, 1990b). This can contribute to formation of a positive appraisal of the disability that will buffer the effects of stigma.

Health-care professionals are not immune to the stigmas that society establishes and have been shown to engage in nonempathic, discriminating responses to the disabled (Saylor, 1990a). Many opportunities are open to health professionals to relay positive attitudes themselves by maintaining open, respectful, trusting relationships with the family and the disabled. This kind of patient–family–health professional relationship can assist the family in confronting stigma as well as enhance other aspects of care.

Maximizing Family Resources

Maximizing personal, family, and community resources to manage this kind of illness needs to include the following:

1. Maintaining the family system by:
   a. Encouraging open communication lines
   b. Supporting a sense of mastery
   c. Supporting a sense of pride/self-esteem

   2. Assisting family reorganization efforts by:
      a. Fostering moderate amounts of cohesion and adaptability
      b. Encouraging the use of adaptive coping strategies of synergizing, interfacing, and compromising
      c. Facilitating the mourning process
      d. Developing informational, financial, and social support resources

Family system maintenance is vital to the family's survival and ability to use resources. Lack of attention to family needs appears to be a major contributor to family breakdown (McCubbin & McCubbin, 1989). Especially during long-term illness, family needs are often neglected while the family focuses on the patient (Murray, 1988). During this illness, family cohesion, self-esteem, sense of mastery, and open communication lines are constantly challenged and at times undermined. Therefore attention by the health professional to these resources that maintain the family system is vital.

   In an illness of this type, the constant adjustment and adaptation make ongoing family reorganization inevitable. Resources have been shown to influence the family reorganization process by (1) increasing the effectiveness and number of solutions available, (2) impacting the definition of the situation (that is, more resources translates into a positive appraisal and sense of mastery), and (3) softening the impact of pileup (that is, more resources means more ways to resolve problems) (McCubbin & McCubbin, 1989). For example, information gives the family direction in forming plans, and social support makes it all seem possible. Following are suggestions for maximizing resources that maintain the family system and assist family reorganization.

   Facilitating the mourning process. Emotional ventilation is important in the earlier stages of spinal cord injury, as family members need to relive the traumatic event (Richmond & Craig, 1986; Wright & Leahey, 1987). The health professional needs to be comfortable with the strong emotional responses that families can display at this time. Reactions may vary greatly depending on the cultural, ethnic, and social background of the family. Some responses may seem inappropriate or out of control from the health professional's frame of reference but not the family's.

   Families with long-term illnesses or disabilities often experience what has been labeled *chronic sorrow* (Damrosch & Perry, 1989) in response to the constant reminders of shattered expectations and the continual need to alter family life. This sorrow usually is not maladaptive and needs to be acknowledged to allow airing of family concerns. Chronic sorrow needs to be distinguished from the excessive mourning and depression that sometimes occurs during spinal cord injury. Excessive mourning and depression can be destructive to adaptation and reorganization (Steinbauer, 1989) and may need to be treated with psychotherapy. Families undergoing chronic sorrow need to discuss the frustrations and grief they feel over losses. In these discussions, family members will discover that they have many shared concerns and mutual losses. If family cohesiveness is low, this intervention may help increase cohesion.

Encouraging the use of adaptive coping strategies. To support family reorganization, the Graham family needs to be encouraged to use the adaptive coping strategies of synergizing, compromising, and interfacing (McCubbin & McCubbin, Chapter 2). *Synergizing* involves the unification of the family to achieve a common goal. This may be easy for the Graham family, as a bonded family, and extremely helpful in adapting to Danny's return home. With a disability as severe as Danny's, meeting every family member's needs is unlikely. A willingness to accept and support the best possible solution is critical. Therefore *compromise* is necessary for the many family adjustments and adaptations that need to take place. The lack of flexibility in the Graham family may prevent compromise. Therefore encouraging compromise in the family may be a priority. The Graham family also will need to *interface,* or find a new "fit," with their community. Developing a "fit" that preserves the family's self-esteem and sense of worth is essential. This will preserve family pride, which Olsen et al. (1983) found eased the adaptive process for families like the Grahams in the adolescent stage (cited in McCubbin, Needle, & Wilson, 1985). This pride may also assist the family to deal with stigma (Saylor, 1990a).

Need for information. Studies done on family needs during illnesses demonstrate that families prioritize information as their number one need (Leske, 1986; O'Neill-Norris & Grove, 1986). For the Graham family, the need for information and information resources cannot be overrated. It is critical to producing effective family reorganization efforts that maintain a sense of mastery and control. It is important to be sensitive to the amount of information that can be absorbed when anxiety is high; "dosing" information may be necessary. Since these families are vulnerable, information needs to be presented at an understandable level with honesty, openness to questions, and a caring attitude (Leske, 1986; O'Neill-Norris & Grove, 1986).

A central resource person responsible for disseminating information to the family can help provide continuity. Coordinating for continuity between the multiple services—physical therapy, respiratory therapy, occupational therapy, medical staff, nursing staff, psychiatric support staff, and social services—is one of the biggest challenges health professionals face during this kind of illness. Fragmented, disjointed information and care can often be a real source of family stress (Bahnson, 1987). In the hospital, rehabilitation center, and home, the central resource person must be able to follow the family throughout one stage and coordinate transition to the next. Nurses have shown interest and demonstrated expertise in this area and are often found in this role especially in long-term care situations (Freidman-Campbell & Hart, 1984; Gilliss, Rose, Hallburg, & Martinson, 1989).

The family needs information about how to care for a spinal cord injury. Caring for a family member with a spinal cord injury creates great anxiety, especially for the primary caregiver. Learning physical care skills must include several guided practice sessions and opportunity for independent practice with available guidance and evaluation. Convening the family to discuss scheduling these activities into the family's daily routine and sharing the burden may produce a more equal distribution of the tasks. Skills learned in the rehabilitation center may have difficulty transferring to the home situation (Brunner & Suddarth, 1992). This fact should be explained to the family to prevent frustration and a sense of failure.

On Danny's return home it would be helpful to have written instructions or a manual prepared at the rehabilitation center for the family and Danny to refer to if they become hazy about any of the information they received (Aadalen & Stroebel-Kahn, 1981/1989; White, 1989). In the home and community settings (for example, school), support from the visiting nurse, physical therapist, or occupational therapist may be needed to adapt and reinforce physical care skills. Feelings of competence in carrying out these skills in different settings are vital to both Danny and to the family's sense of control and mastery.

Encouraging open communication. Information will be better passed on and used if openness and good communication lines exist within the family. As stated earlier, openness results in a decreased number of serious complications in chronic illness (cited in Steinbauer, 1989). Openness and good communication lines enable more informed decisions to be made and can facilitate consensus on family appraisals (Olson et al., 1989). As a result, more realistic plans are made, and family adaptation is supported. This openness also prevents wasting valuable energy on constructing and maintaining barriers among family members (Richmond & Craig, 1986) and encourages use of every family member as a resource. For example, if Danny's disability was not allowed to be discussed around his sisters, they could become more apprehensive and isolated from the rest of the family. Their usefulness as a resource in Danny's care would be negated. Communication lines with friends also need to remain open to develop the large amount of social support so necessary to producing successful outcomes in an illness of this kind. Health professionals need to encourage open communication lines on family and community levels at family meetings throughout this illness.

Social support. Social support by health professionals can be offered through therapeutic communications, positive reinforcement, and crisis intervention strategies, and by exploring coping mechanisms and organizing problem-solving sessions. Depending on the family, psychiatric skills may be needed to provide adequate support.

Cleveland (1980/1989) suggests that counseling families confronted with a spinal cord injury needs to explore three areas, all of which are reflected in the Graham family's situation. First, Sarah tends to be overprotective of Danny. Counseling efforts need to correct this behavior, which discourages the development of Danny's independence. Sarah may need permission along with concrete suggestions to take "vacations" from caring for Danny and to meet her own needs (Richmond & Craig, 1986). Sarah may experience some guilt as she reduces her protectiveness. Second, equal recognition of Jim's contribution to Danny's adjustment needs to be established. Jim has lost many anticipated dreams for he and his son. Reluctant communication between he and Danny must be exchanged for more open interchange especially in the area of affective relationships and sexual issues. Third, Jim and Sarah's marriage needs to be supported and strengthened, since it is this relationship that sets the family "tone." As Sarah and Jim focus on each other, it allows Danny and his sisters the psychological space to grow and develop emotional and physical independence.

Upon Danny's discharge from the rehabilitation center, sources of community support should be identified for the family and its use encouraged. The spinal cord clinic that Danny will be attending offers social support groups for Danny and the family. Support groups capitalize on the presence of others in similar situations (Richmond & Craig, 1986). These groups allow reality testing that acknowledges feelings and concerns as normal. The cost of participation in these groups is often minimal. Since insurance benefits may be depleted, inexpensive support is a necessity. Developing support from friends and other community resources such as the church needs to be encouraged as well. Religion often can be a real source of strength and meaning in chronic illness (Savedra & Dibble, 1989). Sources of respite care also can be a form of support that sustains family energy. This is difficult to find, and the family may need assistance in exploring options (see Chapter 10).

Financial assistance. The financial burden incurred in spinal cord injuries can be devastating and dash any shred of hope the family may have. Families need information, encouragement, and support to seek financial assistance from all sources.

Some insurers recognize the financial burden of this kind of disability and have taken a closer look at allocation of health benefits in these situations (Weingarden et al., 1989). Case-manager programs have been created in the insurance industry to coordinate distribution of health benefit dollars to maximize their use. In one such program a 30% cut in cost was accomplished by supporting home care or other alternative care programs instead of institutional care (Quinn, 1986). This gained additional time before benefits were exhausted and permitted opportunity to find other financial resources (Weingarden et al., 1989). As our society looks more carefully at its health-care expenditures, our policymakers may come to realize that it may be more economical to support families that are taking on the burden of long-term care at home.

A case-management approach is also developing in the health industry and could contribute to more equitable health and financial outcomes. At present, case management calls for a collaborative registered nurse–physician practice base that manages clinical *and* financial outcomes of patient care (The Center for Nursing Case Management, 1989). It focuses on giving families and patients more opportunity for participation and satisfaction with their health care, as stated by the New England Medical Center (1988) (cited in Center for Nursing Case Management, 1989). In the long-term illness situation this collaborative practice base may need to expand one step further to include the family—a family–RN–MD practice base. Perhaps integrating the case-management approaches in both the insurance and health industries could bring together needed expertise in health and finances to resolve problems. Better dialogue could obtain more realistic solutions.

Specific Intervention — Spinal Cord Injury

The following is an example of the use of crisis intervention skills to facilitate formation of a manageable family appraisal and to maximize family resources in the Graham family situation. The reader is taken back to an earlier point in the family anecdote, when Danny is initially hospitalized for his injury and family crisis is occurring. The few weeks after a crisis are critical in forming new patterns. Through trial and error new patterns emerge, but the family is not yet entrenched or committed to them. Because of this, maladaptive patterns can be more easily altered at this time (Bozett, 1987; Halm, 1990). Also, there is an openness to new ideas and support that will not exist later (McCubbin & McCubbin, 1989). Therefore intervention is critical at this time.

◆ ◆ ◆ ◆ ◆

The diagnosis of a cervical spinal injury has been confirmed and the family is overwhelmed. While Danny is still in the intensive care unit a psychiatric nurse liaison and one of the staff nurses that works with Danny meet with the family. They are part of a collaborative team that will manage Danny and his family's needs throughout his hospital stay. Initially, Danny's physical condition makes it difficult for him to participate in these family meetings. As Danny is more able, he is integrated into this process. He is also receiving individual psychiatric support.

As the first step in crisis intervention, the Grahams are asked to reveal the meaning this illness has for them (Aguilera, 1990). Openness is encouraged. A clear understanding of the situation and the difficulties to be encountered are explored. The family is relieved to know that their feelings, reactions, and needs are normal. The discussion reveals the growing depression and exhaustion Sarah is feeling, and Jim's anger dissipates a degree in the telling. It is discovered that Sarah's parents often looked on the disabled with pity and sometimes disgust. Sarah is having difficulty dealing with those feelings herself.

At subsequent sessions the next steps in crisis intervention take place. The family explores successful coping strategies used in the past for their applicability to this situation, as well as ideas for new strategies (Aguilera, 1990). This situation is difficult for the Graham family, since nothing quite like this has happened to them before, and they find it difficult to know what direction to go. Resistance to change is present, related to their lack of flexibility. The nurses explore alternatives, with the family pointing out the advantages of dealing with Danny as the family member he was, with the disabilities he has. Once the Grahams determine possible strategies, potential consequences of those strategies are considered to determine which will be the most acceptable family choice. These solutions or coping strategies are devised and chosen *by the family*, not the health professional. This produces family investment in the plan, which in turn increases the likelihood of the plan's success (Storer, Frate, Johnson, & Greenberg, 1987).

It is decided that Sarah should spend less time in the hospital to curb her growing exhaustion. Sarah and Jim realize that they have been sharing similar feelings, and this knowledge is comforting. Talking about the situation and uncovering Sarah's feelings about disabilities has brought forth more family support for Sarah to work out these feelings. Danny's sisters are bewildered but find working together reassuring.

Resolution of the present crisis with anticipatory planning for future difficulties is the final step in crisis intervention (Aguilera, 1990). The nurses and a social worker offer the Grahams information on the local rehabilitation centers with the advantages and disadvantages of each. Then they suggest helpful steps for choosing a rehabilitation program. The family draws up a list of priorities related to location, kinds of therapy and vocational programs, available finances, and institutional attitudes and policies (Richmond & Craig, 1986). The Grahams use the list to select their choice. This gives them a sense of control and mastery as they methodically go through this process.

Physicians, nurses, social workers, and physical and occupational therapists are brought into the intervention process as their expertise is needed. A family living close by has been successfully coping with a similar disability and therefore is asked to share thoughts and feelings with the Grahams. This family provides the Grahams with an example of successful coping and a possible source of support.

Successfully bringing the Graham family through this initial crisis is critical to enhancing the family's sense of mastery and starting them on a path that constructively resolves this most difficult of situations. The nurses meet with the family many times to accomplish this before Danny's discharge to the rehabilitation facility.

In this example of family intervention, crisis intervention skills have uncovered the family appraisal, bringing forth potential difficulties the health professional may assist the family in facing. It appears the impact of

Sarah's parents' views on her own attitudes and perhaps the grandparents' reactions to Danny may pose problems for the Graham family. This influence may cause difficulties in establishing Danny as a contributing family member. Sarah's feelings need to be dealt with, since the greatest burden of Danny's care will probably fall on her. The anger that Jim feels may continue to resurface as new adjustments are needed, but its meaning will be understood and alternative responses can be created. Through this process the health professional has gained valuable information to guide further interventions.

This family intervention also began the process of maximizing family resources and encouraging family adaptation. Increased information and social support resources provide greater opportunity to balance demands and resources. A sense of control and mastery was fostered in this way. The initial family crisis that labeled this event as a "threat" could perhaps be altered or at least softened by this early intervention. Coping patterns for future use were established, and the health-care professional was established as a source of information and support. These initial interactions can lay the basis for future health professional–family–patient relationships during this illness.

REFERENCES

Aadalen, S. P., & Stroebel-Kahn, F. (1989). Coping with quadriplegia. In R. H. Moos (Ed.), *Coping with physical illness: 2. New perspectives* (pp. 173-188). New York: Plenum. (Reprinted from *American Journal of Nursing*, 1981, *8*, 141-147)

Aguilera, D. C. (1990). *Crisis intervention: Theory and methodology* (6th ed.). St. Louis: Mosby–Year Book.

Anderson, C. M., & Holder, D. P. (1989). Family systems and behavioral disorders: Schizophrenia, depression, and alcoholism. In C. N. Ramsey (Ed.), *Family systems in medicine* (pp. 487-502). New York: Guilford.

Bahnson, C. B. (1987). The impact of life-threatening illness on the family and the impact of the family on illness: An overview. In M. Leahey & L. M.

Wright (Eds.), *Families and life-threatening illness* (pp. 26-44). Springhouse, PA: Springhouse.

Bozett, F. (1987). Family nursing and life-threatening illness. In M. Leahey & L. M. Wright (Eds.), *Families and life-threatening illness* (pp. 2-25). Springhouse, PA: Springhouse.

Brunner, L. S., & Suddarth, D. S. (1992). *Textbook of medical-surgical nursing* (7th ed.). Philadelphia: J.B. Lippincott.

Center for nursing case management (1989). Boston: Center for Nursing Case Management unpublished handout compiled for the Vermont State Nurses Association's Annual Convention, November 1989.

Cleveland, M. (1989). Family adaptation to traumatic spinal cord injury: Response to crisis. In R. H. Moos (Ed.),

Coping with physical illness: 2. New perspectives (2nd ed., pp. 159-171). New York: Plenum. (Reprinted from *Family Relations*, 1980, *29*(4), 558-565)

Connelly, C. E. (1988). Affiliative relationships: An overview. In P. H. Mitchell, L. Hodges, M. Muuaswes, & C. Walleck (Eds.), *AANN's neuroscience nursing* (pp. 247-267). Norwalk, CT: Appleton & Lange.

Damrosch, S. P., & Perry, L. A. (1989). Self-reported adjustment, chronic sorrow, and coping of parents of children with Down syndrome. *Nursing Research*, 38 (1), 25-30.

DeJong, G., Branch, L. G., & Corcoran, P. J. (1984). Independent living outcomes in spinal cord injury: Multivariate analysis. *Archives of Physical Medicine Rehabilitation*, 65, 66-72.

Dewis, M. E. (1989). Spinal cord–injured adolescents and young adults: The meaning of body changes. *Journal of Advanced Nursing*, *14*, 389-396.

Dittmar, S. (1989). Scope of rehabilitation. In S. Dittmar (Ed.), *Rehabilitation nursing: Process and application* (pp. 2-15). St. Louis: Mosby–Year Book.

Dunst, C. J., Trivette, C. M., & Deal, A. G. (1988). *Enabling and empowering families: Principles and guidelines for practice.* Cambridge, MA: Brookline.

Ferrari, M., Matthews, W. S., & Barabas, G. (1985). The family and the child with epilepsy. In D. H. Olson (Ed.), *Family studies: Review yearbook* (Vol. 3, pp. 63-69). Beverly Hills, CA: Sage. (Reprinted from *Family Process*, 1983, *22*, 53-59)

Flannery, J. (1990). Guilt: A crisis within. *Journal of Neuroscience Nursing*, *22*(2), 92-99.

Fradkin, L., & Liberti, M. (1987). Caregiving. In P. Doress & D. Siegal (Eds.), *Ourselves growing older* (pp. 198-212). New York: Simon & Schuster.

Frank, R. G., & Elliott, T. R. (1989). Spinal cord injury and health locus of control beliefs. *Paraplegia*, *27*, 250-256.

Friedman-Campbell, M., & Hart, C. A. (1984). Theoretical strategies and nursing interventions to promote psychosocial adaptation to spinal cord injuries and disability. *Journal of Neurosurgical Nursing*, *16*(6), 335-342.

Gaynor, S. E. (1990). The long haul: the effects of home care on caregivers. *Image: Journal of Nursing Scholarship*, *22*(4), 208-212.

Geissinger, S. B. (1986). The impact of traumatic injury on the family: A research issue. *Presented to the National Council on Family Relations—Family and Health Section*, Nov 6, 1986.

Gilliss, R., Rose, D. B., Hallburg, J. C., & Martinson, I. M. (1989). The family and chronic illness. In C. Gilliss, B. Highley, B. Roberts, & I. Martinson (Eds.), *Toward a science of family nursing* (pp. 287-299). Menlo Park, CA: Addison-Wesley.

Halm, M. A. (1990). Effects of support groups on anxiety of family members during critical illness. *Heart and Lung*, *19*(1), 62-71.

Hennen, B. K., Seitz, M., & Seitz, B. (1987). The chronically disabled child and the family. In D. B. Shires, B. K. Hennen, & D. I. Rice (Eds.), *A guidebook for practitioners of the art* (2nd ed., pp. 42-50). New York: McGraw-Hill.

Hickey, M. (1990). What are the needs of families of critically ill patients? A review of the literature since 1976. *Heart & Lung*, *19*(1), 401-415.

Kahn, A. M. (1990). Coping with fear and grieving. In I. M. Lubkin (Ed.), *Chronic illness: Impact and interventions* (2nd ed., pp. 65-85). Boston: Jones & Bartlett.

Leske, J. S. (1986). Needs of relatives of critically ill patients: A follow-up. *Heart and Lung, 15*(2), 189-193.

Leventhal, H., Leventhal, E. A., & Van Nguyen, T. (1985). Reactions of families to illness: Theoretical models and perspectives. In D. C. Turk & R. D. Kerns (Eds.), *Health, illness, and families* (pp. 108-145). New York: John Wiley & Sons.

Martinson, I. M., Gilliss, C., Colaizzo, D. C., Freeman, M., & Bossert, E. (1990). Impact of childhood cancer on healthy school-age siblings. *Cancer Nursing, 13*(3), 183-190.

McCubbin, H. I., Needle, R. H., & Wilson, M. (1985). Adolescent health risk behaviors: family stress and adolescent coping as critical factors. *Family Relations, 34*, 51-62.

McCubbin, M. A., & McCubbin, H. I. (1989). Theoretical orientations to family stress and coping. In C. R. Figley (Ed.), *Treating stress in families* (pp. 3-43). New York: Brunner/Mazel.

McWhinney, I. R. (1989). The family in health and disease. In I. R. McWhinney (Ed.), *Textbook of family medicine* (pp. 202-227). New York: Oxford University Press.

Mishel, M. H. (1990). Reconceptualization of the uncertainty in illness theory. *Image: Journal of Nursing Scholarship, 22*(4), 256-262.

Murray, J. L. (1988). Care of the elderly. In Taylor, R. (Ed.), *Fundamentals of family medicine: Principles and practice* (3rd ed., pp. 521-533). New York: Springer-Verlag.

Nordstrom, M., & Lubkin, I. (1990). Impact on client and family. In I. M. Lubkin (Ed.), *Chronic illness: Impact and interventions* (2nd ed., pp. 136-154). Boston: Jones & Bartlett.

Olson, D., McCubbin, H. I., Barnes, H., Larson, A., Max, M., & Wilson, M. (1989). *Families: What makes them work* (2nd ed.). Beverly Hills, CA: Sage.

O'Neill-Norris, L. O., & Grove, S. K. (1986). Investigation of selected psychosocial needs of family members of critically ill adult patients. *Heart and Lung, 15*(2), 194-199.

Quinn, J. (1986). Seeking quality alternatives in the community. *Business and Health, 3*(8), 21-24.

Richmond, T. S., & Craig, M. (1986). Family-centered care for the neurotrauma patient. *Nursing Clinics of North America, 21*(4), 611-651.

Savedra, M. C., & Dibble, S. L. (1989). The family with a chronically ill adolescent. In C. Gilliss, B. Highley, B. Roberts, & I. Martinson (Eds.), *Toward a science of family nursing* (pp. 322-331). Menlo Park, CA: Addison-Wesley.

Saylor, C. (1990a). Stigma. In I. M. Lubkin (Ed.), *Chronic illness: Impact and interventions* (2nd ed., pp. 65-85). Boston: Jones & Bartlett.

Saylor, C. (1990b). The management of stigma: Redefinition and representation. *Holistic Nursing Practice, 5*(1), 45-53.

Schenk, E. (1991). Management of persons with neurological problems. In W. J. Phipps, B. C. Long, N. F. Woods, & V. L. Cassmeyer (Eds.), *Medical-surgical nursing: Concepts and clinical practice* (4th ed., pp. 1817-1896). St. Louis: Mosby–Year Book.

Steinbauer, J. R. (1989). Spinal injury: Impact and implications for family medicine research. In C. N. Ramsey (Ed.), *Family systems in medicine* (pp. 487-502). New York: Guilford.

Storer, J. H., Frate, D. A., Johnson, A., & Greenberg, A. (1987). When the cure seems worse than the disease: Helping families adapt to hypertension treatment. *Family Relations, 36,* 311-315.

Turnbull, H. R., & Turnbull, A. P. (1985). *Parents speak out: Then and now* (2nd ed.). Columbus, OH: Charles E. Merrill.

Walker, C. (1988). Stress and coping in siblings of childhood cancer patients. *Nursing Research, 37*(4), 208-212.

Weingarden, S. I., Kuric, J. P., Belen, J.G., & Graham, P. M. (1989). A new approach to catastrophic injury: Spinal cord injury patients. *Paraplegia, 27*(4), 314-318.

White, B. (1989). The teaching-learning process. In S. Dittmar (Ed.), *Rehabilitation nursing: Process and application* (pp. 63-71). St. Louis: Mosby–Year Book.

Wright, L. M., & Leahey, M. (1987). Families and life-threatening illness: Assumptions, assessment, and intervention. In M. Leahey & L. M. Wright (Eds.), *Families and life-threatening illness* (pp. 45-58). Springhouse, PA: Springhouse.

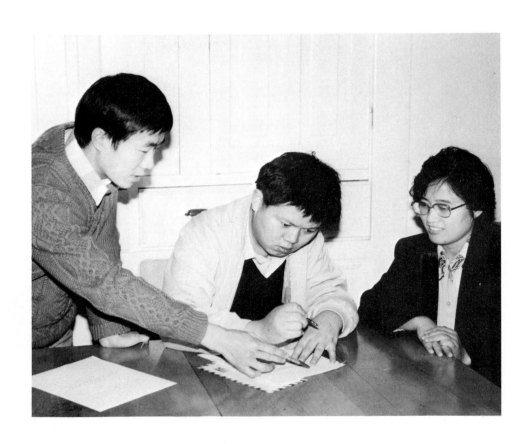

12

Short-term Illness: Cholelithiasis

✦

CHAPTER GOALS

✦ To examine the demands a short-term resolvable illness places on the family and the potential for these demands to cause family strain, stress, and crisis

✦ To describe and illustrate family interventions supportive and useful to families confronted with a short-term resolvable illness

OVERVIEW

THIS chapter examines in detail the demands of caring for a family member with a short-term resolvable illness—cholelithiasis. The dimensions of this illness stressor that determine the impact this illness can have on an entire family system are identified and described. The chapter begins with a vignette describing the Jameses' family situation and the aspects of cholelithiasis with which they are coping. The chapter is organized by the components of the Resiliency Model of Family Stress, Adjustment, and Adaptation (see McCubbin & McCubbin, Chapter 2, Fig. 2-1) and discusses cholelithiasis in relation to: the demands of the illness situation—the stressor (A); resources available to the Jameses—the resources (B/BB/BBB); and the Jameses' appraisal of the illness situation—the appraisals (C/CC/CCC). The last section of the chapter offers suggestions for family interventions that meet the demands of this type of illness and concludes with an example of a specific family intervention that demonstrates the need and value of family interventions in a short-term resolvable illness. We believe the information in this chapter has universal application for families facing similar short-term illness situations.

✦ THE FAMILY SITUATION

✦ ✦ ✦ ✦ ✦

Helen James is a 40-year-old mother of two teenage boys, Patrick, 13, and Miller, 17. Helen and her second husband, Phil, have been married for 5 years. Life seems more difficult to Helen lately. The boys, both in their teens, are more rebellious, especially toward Phil. They continually make it clear that he is not really their father and therefore cannot tell them what to do. Organizing a family schedule to accommodate the boys' many activities seems mind-boggling at times. On top of it all, Helen has had terrible "heartburn" pains that make her uncomfortable after large meals. Her brother had trouble with stomach ulcers and had to have surgery. She is afraid that she also has ulcers. The very idea of surgery frightens her. She shares her fears with her husband and several of her close friends, who all encourage her to see the doctor. At first, she avoids the problem by putting off making the appointment. Then one evening she is so uncomfortable that Phil has to clean up after dinner while she lies down. That night, Helen and Phil discuss the problem, and Helen again shares her fears. These fears and her discomfort make it difficult for Helen to maintain control, and she begins to cry. Now, Phil insists that she see the doctor. The next day Helen makes an appointment, feeling very anxious about the possible outcomes of the visit.

After her initial visit with the doctor and undergoing several diagnostic tests, Helen meets with her physician to discuss her diagnosis. The tests indicate that she has some small cholesterol gallstones that are causing her discomfort. This problem might require surgery if acute inflammation or infection occurs. At this point, she has the option of trying Chenix, a medication that has been successful in dissolving cholesterol gallstones. Treatment also includes a low-cholesterol, weight-reducing diet to forestall recurrence of the stones. With her fear of surgery, Helen is relieved to hear that medication and diet may resolve the problem.

As Helen leaves the office, she has several lingering fears. Is the doctor really sure she does not have the same problem as her brother? Will she need to have surgery despite the medication and diet? These fears preoccupy her, making her irritable with the family for the next few days.

This vignette and its sequels, woven throughout this chapter, are designed to illustrate the stressor demands of and family reactions to a short-term resolvable illness—cholelithiasis. The illness situation, which eventually requires surgery, demands family reorganization during the illness experience but allows the family, if it chooses, to return to its original configurations. Therefore the effects of this case of cholelithiasis on the family are short-lived. Since the onset of this illness situation is gradual, time is available to gather resources and to make decisions. Also, the family will have time to plan for the major stressor in this experience, the surgery. These activities decrease the potential for excessive stress to surround the illness experience. The box below lists the illness stressors dimensions found in this case of cholelithiasis (see Chapter 4 for general information on stressor dimensions).

Family reactions to the stressor dimensions of cholelithiasis are illustrated and examined in this chapter for their potential to cause family strain, stress, and crisis. Interactions with health professionals during this short-term illness can be sporadic and fleeting, yet meaningful, since they occur during the critical events of the illness, which can translate into crisis events for the family. The presence of family crisis provides the practitioner with an opportunity to intervene when the family is most open to assistance (Halm, 1990).

Illness Stressor Dimensions Found in This Case of Cholelithiasis

Gradual *onset*	Areas of expected *predictability*
Short-term *duration*	Little *stigma*
Moderate *severity*	Moderate *financial* demand
Known *cause*	Manageable *control*
Initially low *extent* of family impact, then high at surgery	*Origin* within the family

✦ THE ILLNESS – CHOLELITHIASIS

Cholelithiasis is a condition in which calculi, or stones, form from the solid constituents of the bile salts in the gallbladder or bile duct. These gallstones vary in composition, size, shape, and consistency and can interfere with the normal drainage of the biliary system into the duodenum. About 75% of gallstones in the United States are formed from cholesterol (Cassmeyer, 1991). If a gallstone obstructs the cystic duct, the gallbladder becomes distended causing biliary colic. Biliary colic is a nonacute transient condition consisting of right upper quadrant pain, dyspepsia, fatty food intolerance, and flatulence. These symptoms disappear as the stone dislodges. When unrelenting obstruction occurs, cholecystitis, an inflammation of the gallbladder, can ensue and lead to infection. In these acute cases, cholecystectomy, surgical removal of the gallbladder, is the current treatment of choice. This surgery is performed either at the time of the attack or 4 to 8 weeks later, after antimicrobial therapy has reduced the inflammation and fluid deficits from the acute attack are corrected.

As many as 20 million Americans are affected with cholelithiasis, and an estimated 1 million new cases are diagnosed each year (Way & Sleigenger, 1989). Three times as many women as men are affected by gallbladder disease (Cassmeyer, 1991). These women are usually 40 years of age or older, multiparous, and obese. Dietary changes (low fat, low cholesterol, and weight reduction), analgesics, anticholinergics, and antacids help relieve symptoms but does not stop the disease process. Chenodeoxycholic acid (CDCA, Chenix) and urodeoxycholic acid (UDCA) are bile acids in the form of oral medication that are used to dissolve small radiolucent cholesterol stones. These medications are effective about 50% to 60% of the time in dissolving this kind of stone (Greenberger & Isselbacher, 1991). If acute symptoms of cholecystitis continue, this pharmacological treatment is considered a poor substitute for surgery.

Gallstones ranks fifth among reasons for hospitalization, and cholecystectomy is the third most common type of surgery performed (Way & Sleigenger, 1989). Endoscopic laser surgery is now being used for gallbladder removal (Jackson, Martin, Evans, & Rudio, 1990). This method of surgery considerably decreases discomfort, recovery time, and complications when compared with previous surgical methods. For example, recovery time is 7 to 10 days as opposed to 4 to 6 weeks. Extracorporeal shock wave lithotripsy and direct dissolution therapy with methyl tertiary butyl ether via percutaneous biliary catheters are treatments currently used on some patients (Greenberger & Isselbacher, 1991). These methods appear to have promise. In our vignette involving the James family, the surgical method of treatment has been chosen to demonstrate the demands it places on the family.

✦ DEMANDS OF THE ILLNESS STRESSOR (A)

This portion of the chapter describes and illustrates the demands this short-term illness stressor (A) places on the James family (Fig. 12-1). Since an illness's stressor dimensions can influence the demands of an illness on the family (see Chapter 4), we examine the stressor dimensions of this short-term illness for the impact their demands impose on the James family. Those stressor dimensions that are related to or cause similar family responses will be discussed together. The discussion will illustrate that the degree to which illness demands affect family life is directly related to the need for change.

Where applicable, family vulnerability (V) and family typology (T), both components of the Resiliency Model, are discussed in relation to the demands they add to the situation. The James family has been arbitrarily assigned the family type *secure family*. These families are low in family coherence and high in family hardiness (McCubbin & McCubbin, 1989). This type of family is part of the regenerative family typology (see Fig. 5-3). The strength of secure families is their sense of purpose and control and their ability to plan ahead. They are active and willing to try new things. However, family members lack supportiveness, caring, and loyalty when faced with hardships.

Onset

As seen in the vignette at the beginning of this chapter, the onset of this case of cholelithiasis is gradual and undramatic. Initially the gradual onset allows Helen and the family to ignore the problem until it becomes clear that something *is* wrong (Hirsch, 1988). Once this appraisal is made, they have time to gather information and plan for the medical contact, which can be integrated into the family's schedule. Since the James family has time to

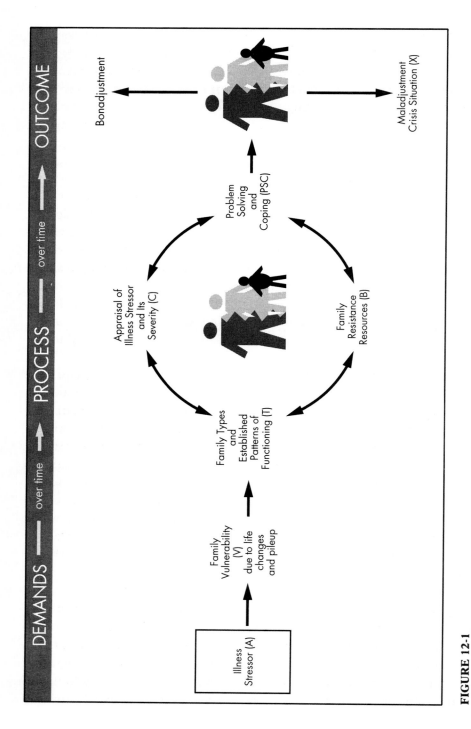

FIGURE 12-1

Adjustment Phase of the Resiliency Model of Family Stress, Adjustment, and Adaptation. This portion of the chapter focuses on the demands of the illness stressor (A).

gather information and plan, a family crisis is less likely to result at the onset of this illness (Halm, 1990). Their appraisal reflects this in feelings and attitudes demonstrating that the situation is under control. This illness dimension—gradual onset—enables the family to maintain its sense of mastery so vital to its functioning.

However, other family factors at the onset of this situation may increase the possibility for family stress and crisis. The James family is in the adolescent phase of the family life cycle, a phase fraught with conflict, pressures, and the need for constant family adjustments (Olson et al., 1989). This increases the family's vulnerability to stress, making it possible for even an illness with a gradual onset to cause a family crisis. Certainly, Helen's energy to manage the illness situation is decreased. Also, her fear of possible surgery could increase the potential for crisis. Both of these situational factors have probably contributed to her initial attempts to ignore her problem and tend to other family problems.

Severity, Origin, and Extent of Family Impact

Since the illness originates within a family member and not outside the family, the family is expected to assume responsibility in managing it (Leventhal, Leventhal, & Van Nguyen, 1985). However, the gradual onset indicates to the family a lack of severity with an apparent low urgency for family involvement and support. As this illness begins, only Phil is involved, as he supports Helen and encourages medical contact to evaluate the problem. The boys are relatively unaffected. Demands of the illness situation appear low. The control and the maintenance of family organizational patterns are present. The demand for change or even adjustment is not apparent and therefore does not cause undue family strain or stress. This low severity with resultant low demand has the inherent value of making it easier for the family to maintain its sense of mastery (see Chapter 4).

The situation, however, does have some disadvantages. The lack of an appraisal, indicating that family involvement is needed, makes mobilization of family support more difficult. The difficulties this poses become apparent when Helen attempts the dietary changes required by her physician's treatment plan. Helen is expected to adhere to a weight-reducing, low-cholesterol diet. Changes in family eating patterns may be needed, requiring greater family involvement. Life-style changes such as this can be easily undermined by family members unaware of the need and the significance of their support (Anderson & Holder, 1989). In the James family, resistance to the dietary changes may be high because the need for change and family support is not evident, especially to the teenage boys. The family will resist change by attempting to keep its established, comfortable patterns. In fact, that is what happens.

✦ ✦ ✦ ✦ ✦

The two teenage boys, Patrick and Miller, strenuously object to the changes in their food and its preparation. They liked things just the way they were. Helen is frustrated by the extra work this will cause if she prepares her own food separately. This lack of support increases the chance that Helen will not follow the diet.

However, changes occur in Helen's illness that alter this situation.

✦ ✦ ✦ ✦ ✦

Despite the fact that Helen is taking her medication and is trying to adhere to her diet regimen, she continues to have some intermittent biliary colic. Today's attack is much more severe than the others. The pain is more intense and is not subsiding. She is nauseated and has vomited several times. She also has chills and feels feverish. Finally, Helen calls a friend and asks for a ride to the doctor. After examining her in his office, the doctor sends Helen immediately to the hospital for further tests and treatment. As she is being admitted, Phil arrives with the boys.

The next few hours are filled with anxiety for both Helen and her family. Helen is put through a number of tests, while Phil and the boys wait nervously for news of the outcome. Finally, the physician tells them that Helen has acute cholecystitis, an inflammation, and in this case an infection, of the gallbladder due to an obstruction caused by gallstones. She will need to remain in the hospital for antibiotic therapy, analgesics, intravenous fluids, and nasogastric suction. Her condition should improve within the next 24 hours. At that time they will perform further tests. The physician explains that in Helen's case this condition is most successfully treated by surgically removing the gallbladder, known as a cholecystectomy. This can be performed any time from 4 to 8 weeks after Helen returns home. This will give Helen time to regain her strength and her family time to plan for the experience.

Family support now may be easier to mobilize. The severity of the situation is evidenced by Helen's hospital admission and need for surgery.

In this case the demands are clear and the need for temporary change a possibility. Helen's surgery may require family reorganization and temporary changes that will involve the whole family. The severity of the illness appears to have significance in determining the visibility of illness demands. If family consensus determines that resources are inadequate to meet demands of the situation, the potential for family crisis will be high (McCubbin & McCubbin, Chapter 2).

As the severity of an illness increases, the extent and invasiveness of its impact on the family escalates. Helen's hospitalization requires reassigning her tasks to other members of the family or friends (Halm, 1990). Temporarily, Phil will need to take over some aspects of the role of mother, and Helen's role as housekeeper may need to be reallocated. Since the boys might be an unwilling resource, a temporary maid service is an option, or cleaning can be ignored for awhile — one of the advantages of the short-term illness. Fortunately, both Patrick and Miller are old enough to care for themselves. However, they require transportation to their activities. Friends or relatives may be asked to carry this out. The family also may need to relinquish some community responsibilities. Helen was to chair a church meeting at this time. As a result, a friend must be sought to take over the responsibility. Along with these demands, the family will need to support and encourage Helen as she faces surgery and recovery.

Pileup can easily occur for Phil as he tries to support Helen and manage the home. Time spent at the hospital makes it difficult to carry out home activities. Conflicts with Patrick and Miller occur as Phil takes over monitoring their activities. Phil also is concerned about Helen's medical bills. Will he be able to meet these expenses if his insurance does not? Furthermore, he worries about taking time off from work to help Helen when she returns home.

Just as the severity of an illness influences the level of family involvement, the family situation with its demands also determines the extent of family involvement in a family member's illness. For example, the James boys are old enough to provide help; therefore they will feel some pressure to meet demands. However, adolescents are not always so willing to assist.

✦ ✦ ✦ ✦ ✦

Miller is center for the school basketball team. Winning the state championship is a priority for him, and his team has the potential. Practices give him little time available to help at home, and he often uses his sports activities as an excuse to get out of tasks. In turn, Patrick gets asked to pick up the slack, and the tasks have increased with Helen's absence. He feels like he is doing everything, and it is "not fair!"

As the family faces these behaviors and other crises at the time of the illness, its vulnerability to stress increases. This may determine the extent of family involvement and the energy the family members have to deal with the illness (Loveys, 1990). Pileup of family demands combined with illness demands increase the potential for family crisis (McCubbin & McCubbin, Chapter 2).

Family typology also can determine the extent of family involvement and the development of family crisis. The James family is a *secure family* type; these families are less tolerant of difficulties and hardships and typically offer less support to each other during difficult times (McCubbin & McCubbin, 1989). This illness produces difficulties and hardships, and we already see the predictable behaviors of a *secure family* from the teenage boys. They are intolerant of the dietary changes and the need to absorb Helen's household tasks. Furthermore, this type of family deals with problems by getting upset — another factor that could potentially precipitate family crisis.

Duration

Because this case of cholelithiasis is short term, its demands and burdens are short-lived. Therefore the James family perceives the demands as more bearable and manageable. For example, Patrick and Miller know they will not have to help with Helen's household tasks forever. Phil knows that other responsibilities can be postponed to a later date when normalcy returns. Consequently, opportunity for pileup can be decreased. These factors decrease family stress levels and reduce the potential for crisis.

The short-term nature of this illness determines that no *permanent* changes need to be made. Therefore the easier to implement adjustment behaviors may be sufficient to manage the illness. After her surgery and recovery, Helen will be able to resume her place in the family system. In the end, the James family will be able to return to their established patterns. Studies have shown that after surgery families return to normal social function within 3 to 4 months (cited in Leventhal et al., 1985). Since the family will return to configurations that are familiar and comfortable, the resistance to readjusting back to "normal" can be fairly low. The family can choose to keep only those changes they value or are willing to make work.

Predictability

Although Helen's biliary colic and her acute episode of cholecystitis were not predictable, a major component of the treatment plan, the surgery, is a planned experience with a predictable course. Predictable stressors do not cause family crisis (Montgomery, 1982). Therefore, if the predictability of the situation is used to advantage, the situation can be more comfortable for the family. To do this, the family must receive appropriate information concerning the surgical event (Halm, 1990).

Essentially the James family must become information gatherers to understand the demands of the surgical experience; they must find out what to expect. How long will Helen be hospitalized? When will the surgery start and end? What will be happening to Helen? How dangerous is this for her? How uncomfortable will she be? For how long? What can the family do to help her? How long will her recovery be? Once they have all the information they need, the Jameses can use their problem-solving skills to plan family life around the event. For example, Patrick and Miller must decide if they should make alternative plans to participate in their activities or if they should omit them temporarily. Phil must decide whether to take time off from work when Helen comes home from the hospital. Once they have gathered their information, determined the availability of their resources, and developed a plan, they will be prepared for the surgery. The information gathering is not finished, however. Throughout the experience the family will continue to gather more information, evaluate effectiveness of resources, and adjust plans to meet both Helen's needs and those of the family. These activities will decrease the likelihood of family crisis.

Families with poor problem-solving skills and few adaptive coping strategies and resources may find adjustment and adaptation to the surgical experience difficult. However, the James family, as a *secure family* type, has a sense of purpose and can plan ahead (McCubbin & McCubbin, 1989). This family type believes it can influence things that happen to them. The health-care practitioner can perhaps use this family characteristic to overcome the lack of support among family members typically seen with these families during hardships by developing support through the planning process.

Cause, Control, and Stigma

Once medical diagnosis establishes its presence, cholelithiasis is a well-understood disease that can be concretely defined and explained. Cures are available, and the disease is controllable. Because of these factors, minimal social stigma surrounds the disease. With negligible stigma, the illness can be discussed openly, thus maintaining communication lines for support. In this situation, cause, control, and stigma of the illness produce few demands and therefore bring little potential for family stress or crisis. Their impact is positive in allowing the family to maintain its sense of control.

Resource Demands — Financial

The James family has health insurance through Phil's employer. The insurance plan is modest, however, and the Jameses will have some out-of-pocket expenses that will place a burden on family finances. Phil's salary is $30,000 and accounts for the majority of the family's income. Helen's part-time job brings in another $10,000 but offers no insurance benefits. The initial doctor visits Helen makes for this illness must be paid for at the time of service; the insurance company reimburses them later. Only 80% of the cost is covered by insurance. The fee for Helen's diagnostic tests is completely covered, as is her medication. Phil is paying off several loans at this time, and Helen's expenses strain the situation. Sometimes several months pass before he receives reimbursement checks from the insurance company, and he wonders if he will have enough cash available to cover the void left by payments for the medical visits.

The deductible portion for the hospital insurance coverage must be paid upon hospital admission. This $800 bill worries Phil and Helen, since they will need to withdraw money from their modest savings account to pay this. This deductible will have to be paid twice if Helen's second hospital admission occurs later than 60 days after her first. When they discover this, they quickly call to schedule the surgery, hoping the hospital can accommodate them within the 60-day limit. The rest of the hospital and doctor bills for the surgery will be covered. This is a relief to Helen and Phil.

Upon discharge, their insurance covers only those nursing services that the doctor deems necessary. It is hoped and expected that Helen will not need any at-home services. The family with the help of friends will deal with Helen's limited physical strength and the tasks she cannot yet fulfill.

✦ RESOURCES AVAILABLE TO THE FAMILY (B/BB/BBB)

This part of the chapter focuses on the resource components (B/BB/BBB) of the Resiliency Model (Fig. 12-2). Resources are the tools families use to adjust and adapt to changes in their lives. These tools include tangible resources and coping capabilities; they are family strengths used to buffer the impact of demands. In this way, resources assist in decreasing stress and preventing crisis. According to McCubbin and McCubbin (see Chapter 2), the three kinds of family resources are (1) personal resources of individual family members; (2) collectively held internal family resources; and (3) community or social support resources. The James family will draw from all three resources to manage this illness situation.

Personal Resources (B)

Feelings of self-esteem and mastery have been cited in the stress literature as being the two most critical personal resources for effective management of demands (McCubbin & McCubbin, Chapter 2). The following vignette examines the levels of self-esteem and mastery found in the James family members.

✦ ✦ ✦ ✦ ✦

As the James family enters this illness, it appears Helen has a decreased sense of mastery. The boys' many activities are sending her in many directions, and her sense of balance with this confusion, her other home responsibilities, and her part-time job is precarious. She is also upset by her boys' defiant attitude toward their stepfather. Phil is upset by this too. However, things are going well for him. Phil just received a raise for managing a project well. He feels good about himself and his mastery of life up to this point. Although the divorce process was difficult, he knows divorce made his life better. He certainly is much happier with Helen

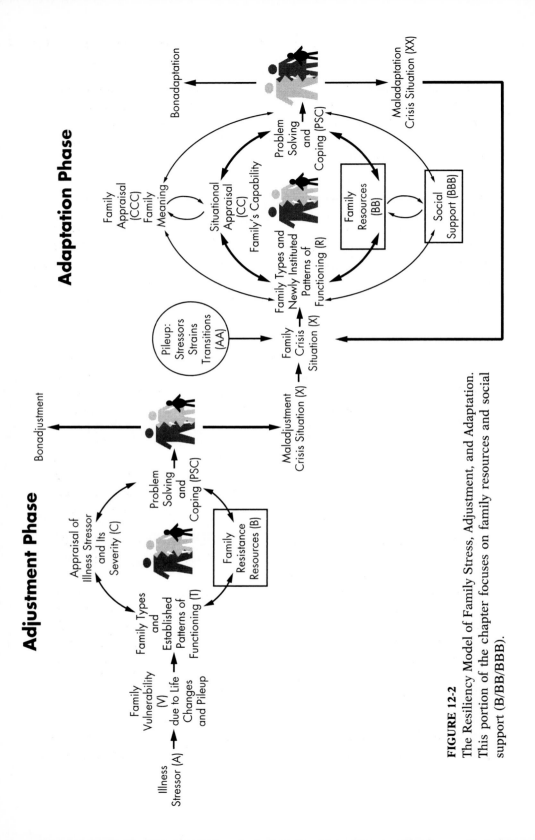

FIGURE 12-2

The Resiliency Model of Family Stress, Adjustment, and Adaptation. This portion of the chapter focuses on family resources and social support (B/BB/BBB).

despite the conflict with the boys. Both Patrick and Miller as teenagers are at a developmental point where the personal resources of self-esteem and mastery are a fragile, vacillating commodity. As a result, these personal resources may or may not be available for Patrick and Miller to use during the different phases of this illness.

Family Resources (BB)

Moderate amounts of cohesion and adaptability are important resources for families managing crisis (McCubbin & McCubbin, Chapter 2; Olson et al., 1989). The James family is neither rigid nor chaotic and therefore can be considered moderately adaptive (Olson et al., 1989). However, as a secure family type, cohesion is low.

◆ ◆ ◆ ◆ ◆

Helen and Phil share the parenting responsibilities of the boys, although it is difficult for Phil as a stepfather. When it was decided that increased family income would help, the family was able to adapt successfully to Helen's acquisition of a part-time job. Phil took over some of the grocery shopping and made himself more available to drive the boys to activities on the days Helen worked. The boys began to make their own lunches for school and helped prepare supper on Helen's work days. These efforts demonstrate the family's ability to successfully apply the adaptive coping strategy of synergy (pulling together for a shared life-style). This successful adaptation has allowed them to increase their tangible resources and demonstrates their sense of control over life events. It appears the family has the sense of worth vital to maintaining the family system. This would be expected, since the James family, as a *secure family* type, is high in family hardiness (McCubbin & McCubbin, 1989).

Low coherence (similar to cohesion), also a characteristic of secure families (McCubbin & McCubbin, 1989), appears present in the James family. Each individual in the family has boundaries and is differentiated. However, relations between the boys and their stepfather are strained. The boys cope with their problems by getting upset and showing disrespect for Phil. This often hinders communication lines and lowers cohesion, which makes it difficult to maintain the family system.

In general, the James family is low in family cohesion and high in adaptability. This has implications for family interventions that are discussed later in this chapter. The family's most valuable tangible resource, money, was discussed earlier. Its importance as a family resource in illness situations should not be forgotten.

Community Resources (BBB)

The James family is respected and liked in the community and has many community resources and sources of social support to draw on.

✦ ✦ ✦ ✦ ✦

Phil is considered successful in his job and has several close friends whom he plays tennis with regularly. The family is active in their church, a real source of support for them. Helen is an involved and respected member of the church women's organization and has many good friends there. This organization has an Outreach program that helps families through difficult times. Helen's part-time job has been a positive experience. Her boss and other individuals in the office have praised her calm, organized manner. The boys are doing well in school. Miller is on the first string of the basketball team and respected for his athletic ability. Patrick is interested in computers and participates in the school computer club, which he enjoys a great deal.

Medically, the family has access to the health-care system through their family physician. Phil, Helen, and the boys see him for physical checkups and other medical needs. Phil's insurance from work helps with the expense incurred here.

✦ FAMILY APPRAISALS OF THE ILLNESS SITUATION (C/CC/CCC)

The family's subjective appraisal of the illness situation greatly determines whether an illness will cause family crisis (McCubbin & McCubbin, Chapter 2). The appraisal is formed from family perceptions of the demands (A) of the situation and their resource capabilities (B/BB/BBB) (Fig. 12-3). The family's perceived balance between these two factors, *demands* and *resources*, determines its movement away or toward crisis. This family appraisal changes throughout the illness cycle. In this short-term illness, the health professional needs to be aware of the family's appraisal at key times,

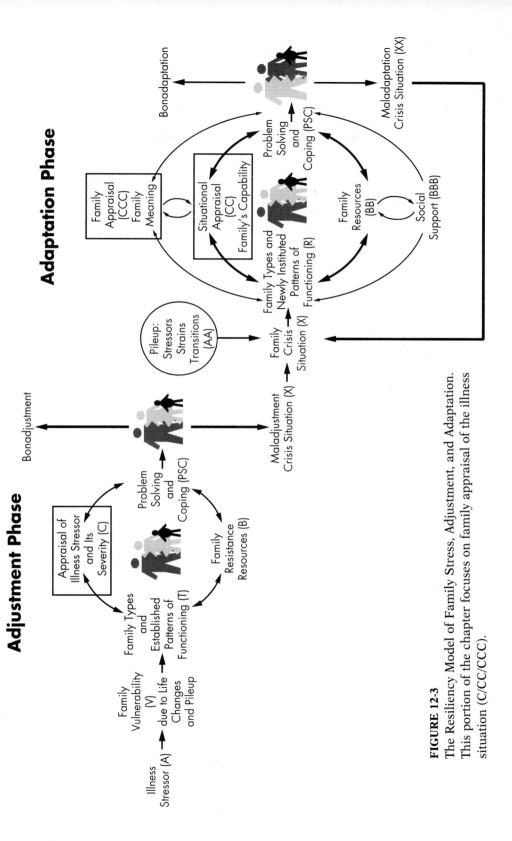

Adaptation Phase

Bonadaptation

Maladaptation Crisis Situation (XX)

Family Appraisal (CCC) Family Meaning

Situational Appraisal (CC) Family's Capability

Problem Solving and Coping (PSC)

Family Resources (BB)

Social Support (BBB)

Family Types and Newly Instituted Patterns of Functioning (R)

Pileup: Stressors Strains Transitions (AA)

Family Crisis Situation (X)

Adjustment Phase

Bonadjustment

Maladjustment Crisis Situation (X)

Appraisal of Illness Stressor and Its Severity (C)

Problem Solving and Coping (PSC)

Family Resistance Resources (B)

Family Types and Established Patterns of Functioning (T)

Family Vulnerability (V) due to Life Changes and Pileup

Illness Stressor (A)

FIGURE 12-3

The Resiliency Model of Family Stress, Adjustment, and Adaptation. This portion of the chapter focuses on family appraisal of the illness situation (C/CC/CCC).

including initial medical contact, first hospitalization, preoperative state, recovery to the home, and reentry into health.

Initial Medical Contact

With the increased intensity of Helen's signs and symptoms, the family has provisionally assigned Helen to the sick role; it has appraised the situation as beyond its ability to solve and therefore as one requiring medical contact. The family has time to plan and integrate this medical contact into its schedule. Phil's insurance will cover most of the expenses. Because of these favorable conditions, a feeling of control exists. The situation is manageable.

However, Helen comes to the doctor's office with many fears. She has applied her knowledge from other similar illness situations (for example, her brother's ulcers) in an attempt to understand her problem. Since the signs and symptoms of stomach ulcers are similar, she equates her brother's illness with hers, which increases her fears. Her brother was very ill and needed surgery that followed with several complications. She concludes that surgery is something to avoid. With this meaning applied to the situation, Helen's fears impact the family, especially Phil. The thought that Helen might ever need surgery frightens Phil also. Two years ago, Phil had a friend who died during abdominal surgery, thus explaining his uneasy feelings about any kind of surgery.

The James family brings these perceptions to the medical consultation. They wonder if the doctor will confirm their worst fears. This visit is an anxious one for Helen and her family. When the doctor diagnoses Helen's problem as cholelithiasis, the family is relieved to know the illness appears manageable. With medicine and dietary changes, the problem may be solved. Little change is demanded, so no real threat is seen. Demands are perceived as balanced by resources. These feelings of control trickle down to the boys, who barely feel any impact. Because of this, the need for the boys to mobilize support for the dietary changes is not evident, and as Helen discovers, their resistance to change is high.

Helen's Hospitalization

The safe, in control feelings vanish as Helen is admitted to the hospital on an emergency basis. This need for hospitalization now defines the situation as serious and threatening and therefore stressful (Bozett, 1987). Society reinforces this perception with its own stigmatization of hospitals (Kemp, Pillitteri, & Brown, 1989).

✦ ✦ ✦ ✦ ✦

As Phil and the boys drive to the hospital, they are afraid. How ill will Helen be? What is the problem? Will she be OK? Her appearance does not reassure them. She is uncomfortable and has a fever. She has a nasogastric tube inserted into her nose and intravenous fluid flowing into her arm. Some of their fears are confirmed, and their concern deepens. Helen is *really* sick. The need to mobilize support and gather information about the problem is evident.

The doctor reassures them by explaining that the problem is manageable and that Helen's health will return with treatment. Even though the cure is frightening—surgery—the problem can be resolved. The family knows they will have the opportunity to plan and prepare for the experience, something the James family, as a *secure family*, does well.

The fact that this illness is short-term with a known cause that is curable (controllable) has greatly influenced the family's perceptions. These stressor dimensions make the situation appear manageable. Yet, the thought of surgery is overwhelming for Helen and Phil. Will Helen have the many complications her brother had with his surgery? Will Helen die, as Phil's friend did? Helen has been afraid of this possibility and now it has become a reality. Helen seeks and yearns for support from her family and friends.

The boys do not understand much about the surgery, but they are aware of the seriousness of the situation. When they tell their friends and teachers about their mother, everyone stops and sympathizes, showing concern. This behavior only emphasizes to them the seriousness of the situation. Not wishing to upset Helen and unwilling to talk with Phil, they share their concerns with each other. The boys conclude that the situation is serious. Yet, they have so many other important things on their minds with activities at school. Why does this have to be happening now!

As a *secure family*, offering support to each other is not a strength of the James family (McCubbin & McCubbin, 1989). With Helen and Phil's fearful thoughts about the surgery and the ambivalent feelings of the boys, the potential for family crisis is high. More than minimal family support will be needed to meet the demands of this situation. A demand-resource imbalance may be present.

Surgery

✦ ✦ ✦ ✦ ✦

The night before surgery, Phil and the boys are truly frightened for Helen. This interferes with their ability to offer support to Helen, who is equally frightened. The boys have worked out some of their differences with Phil in planning for the experience. To do all that needs to be done and meet some of their own needs, the boys have decided it was in their best interest to cooperate. Life on the home front is a little chaotic but manageable. However, Helen feels isolated and longs for more comfort from her family, but it is not forthcoming. She wonders why this is happening to her and if she'll make it through the surgery.

On the day of surgery, Phil and the boys stay with Helen until she goes to the operating room. The next few hours are anxious ones as they wait. Finally, the surgery is over, and they are told that she is doing well. What a relief! However, when they get to see her she looks terrible, reminding them of her previous hospitalization. She is obviously uncomfortable. They wonder if she really is alright. It is hard for them to feel confident that everything is going well. They seek further information for reassurance. It is not easy to find out about Helen's progress. The nurses and doctors are all busy and rushed. It is even hard to know where to look for this information. An element of unrest and a decreased sense of mastery invade the family system. Their ability to meet demands is precarious. A demand-resource imbalance continues to be present. They are also concerned about her return home.

Recovery

✦ ✦ ✦ ✦ ✦

The James family is relieved that the worst is over and look forward to a gradual return to normal. As they anticipate Helen's return home, they know the extra work they are doing now will soon be over. The boys are helpful to a point, and Phil plans to spend a few days home with Helen. Many of Helen's friends from church have offered assistance and support, and they have activated the Outreach program to assist the James family. This support lends to the manageability of the situation. As a result, a sense of mastery grows.

Some of the medical bills are starting to arrive, but most are covered by insurance. Although Phil thinks money is tight, he will be able to cover the costs. The illness demands are diminishing, and resources are adequate. The family feels successful.

Reentry into Health

✦ ✦ ✦ ✦ ✦

It has been 3 weeks since Helen arrived home from the hospital. She has had no complications, and her energy has returned. The whole family is happy that the ordeal is over and they can get on with their lives. As the seriousness of the situation fades, the experience is looked on as positive. A closeness that did not exist before is present. Do they want to keep this closeness? This will be decided as the family returns to normal.

✦ ✦ ✦ ✦ ✦

As reflected in this fictitious story, the perceptions that existed throughout this illness experience are closely linked to the demands of the illness stressor dimensions, the family situation, previous experiences, available information, and resource capabilities. The health-care professional has many opportunities to help form these perceptions. This assistance can have a strong influence on the family's ability to form positive, manageable appraisals of the illness situation.

✦   FAMILY INTERVENTIONS

Application of the Resiliency Model to the Jameses' family situation provides health-care professionals with valuable guidelines for action. In the short-term illness situations, health professionals may have little opportunity to influence changes in the family situation, especially if contacts are brief and minimal. However, to meet the family's needs for information and the illness situation's demands for family reorganization and resources, the health professional can assist by giving attention to the family's *appraisals* (C/CC/CCC) of the situation and to the presence of *resources* (B/BB/BBB). These two components of the Resiliency Model influence and contribute to the family's problem-solving capacities (PSC) and therefore may govern the level of family adjustment/adaptation that occurs (Fig. 12-3) (McCubbin & McCubbin, Chapter 2). Input by health professionals into these two areas can assist in empowering families to better deal with illness stressors and to perhaps prevent or soften family crisis. Therefore, when dealing with or trying to prevent family crisis during illness, the health professional may wish to focus on the following:

1. Assisting the family in developing manageable, positive *appraisals* (C/CC/CCC) of the situation

2. Maximizing the application and development of *individual, family,* and *community resources* (B/BB/BBB).

The purpose of this focus is to increase the opportunity for family bonadjustment and bonadaptation to the illness stressor and decrease the potential for maladjustment and maladaptation.

Developing Manageable, Positive Appraisals

By applying the skills of observing, interviewing, and therapeutic communications, the health professional can assess the family and the family's appraisal of illness situations. Family assessment tools can be used to evaluate family strengths and weaknesses, but these may be impractical for the brief contacts made during short-term illnesses. Health professionals need to understand the meaning the family has assigned to the illness. Understanding the family appraisal is necessary to planning appropriate interventions (Wright & Leahey, 1987). Knowledge of the family's appraisal can provide a point from which promotion or reinforcement of a positive, manageable family appraisal can begin. The family's appraisal can reveal implications for maximizing existing resources and coping behaviors and for developing new resources and capabilities. Interventions based on assessments of the *family's* appraisal, *not* the health professional's appraisal, will be more likely to fit family needs.

In the Jameses' family situation, it will be important to find out early in the illness that Helen equates her illness with that of her brother. This will bring forth her fears of surgery and establish the meaning she has applied to her symptoms. Helen's appraisal of her symptoms can affect the whole family. Without understanding *her* interpretation, the health professional cannot focus on correcting or reinforcing the family outlook or allaying fears. If this interaction does not occur, a patient may leave the initial medical contacts with unnecessary fears. These fears can then be brought back to the family, as they were in Helen's case, and become a potential contributor to family crisis. Using family interventions, we will explore how gathering information on the family's appraisal can be valuable during Helen's first visits to the doctor and how knowledge of the appraisal can bring awareness of potential problems.

◆ ◆ ◆ ◆ ◆

When Helen first visits her family physician about her problem, he inquires into Helen's perceptions of the signs and symptoms and their possible causes. By doing so, he uncovers some real fears. She thinks she might have peptic ulcers and need surgery like her brother. After tests are done, Helen returns to learn her diagnosis. Phil has come along at the doctor's request. The doctor wishes Phil to have access to the information too and to be able to ask any questions he might have. With both Helen and Phil there, the doctor hopes to have stronger input into the family appraisal and create better support for Helen. Phil and Helen will start out with equal information and the doctor will have the chance to uncover Phil's concerns, which he finds are grave, too, especially regarding surgery.

   Because he is aware of Helen's and Phil's fears, the doctor makes it clear that Helen does not have a stomach ulcer like her brother, although the symptoms are similar. He explains that, unfortunately, like her brother's situation, her problem will require surgery if the medication and diet are ineffective. However, surgery for her problem is much less complicated than the surgery her brother received. He explains that she should not compare the two types of surgery. Hopefully, she will not have to have surgery in any case. He is realistic and shows respect for Helen's original summation of the situation. He now knows that if Helen did eventually need surgery, many preconceived fears would be governing family behavior and extra support may be needed to assist the family through the surgical experience.

Studies have shown that families consider information their number one need during illness (Hickey, 1990; Leske, 1986; O'Neill-Norris & Grove, 1986). Health-care professionals can tend to see short-term illnesses as relatively minor when compared with other major health problems and therefore gloss over or omit information. Yet, the family's need for information in short-term illnesses is no less than that in more serious or chronic illness situations.

   As Helen's family progresses through the illness cycle, information is needed to understand the illness and its demands more fully. In this illness, information is an essential resource needed at diagnosis and before Helen's surgery. This information can empower Helen's family to form manageable appraisals and effective plans that meet both illness and family demands (Dunst, Trivette, & Deal, 1988). Information can offer the family a sense of control (Halm, 1990). In turn, this sense of control can itself positively impact the family's appraisals. Presenting information to the family in a group when possible can be effective in transmitting accurate information throughout the family system, getting many questions answered, and stilling many fears (Anderson & Holder, 1989). This kind of family meeting may lead to a more realistic and manageable family appraisal.

Maximizing Family Resources

Maximizing family resources to deal with this short-term illness needs to include the following components:

1. Maintaining the family system by:
   a. Encouraging open communication lines
   b. Supporting a sense of mastery
   c. Supporting a sense of pride and self-esteem
2. Assisting family reorganization efforts by:
   a. Fostering moderate amounts of cohesion and adaptability
   b. Encouraging use of the adaptive coping strategies of synergizing, interfacing, and compromising
   c. Developing informational, financial, and social support resources

Let us look at a family intervention that maximizes family resources in the Jameses' family situation.

✦ ✦ ✦ ✦ ✦

The family doctor knows that the gradual onset and the initial low severity of Helen's illness does not establish a clear need for the family to rally around the dietary changes he proposes. Also, he is aware that the James family's typology (assessed earlier during health checkups) increases the potential for resistance to the diet changes. For these reasons he invites the James family to attend a series of classes. He and one of his office nurses have designed a series of classes to offer information, support, and problem-solving time to families needing dietary changes. The nurse teaches the classes, bringing in experts as needed. As many family members will attend as is appropriate and feasible. Two other families from the doctor's practice will be attending this series of classes.

The family must pay for these classes, since insurance does not cover this kind of intervention. Fortunately the James family has the resources to pay for these classes and is willing to do so.

To foster adaptation, the purpose of these classes is threefold. First, the classes offer the family information concerning the need for diet changes in relation to their family member's future health. A low-cholesterol, weight-reducing diet also can have implications for everyone's health, and this can be used to make the sessions meaningful for the whole family. The information will make Helen's problem more evident to the family. As a result, support for the changes may be more forthcoming.

Second, these classes can be a source of support to the family as they undergo these changes. Formal support from the health professional can be established, as well as informal support among family members and the other families in the class. In light of the fact that families find informal support more helpful and acceptable (Dunst et al., 1988), fostering informal support among the different families in the class may become an important part of the intervention. With the proper encouragement, the interactions among these families can foster support akin to that in self-help groups. If the family continues to deny Helen the support she needs, support established in the classes from outside her family may be important to her.

Third, these classes offer specific time for family problem solving and planning for these changes. The health professional can facilitate family efforts to arrive at a solution they "own" by reviewing typical family meals and having the family modify them. These activities can foster the adaptive behaviors of compromising and synergizing by getting the family to rally around the problem. Studies have shown that allowing families to "own" and plan for medical treatments produces better compliance (Storer, Frate, Johnson, & Greenberg, 1987). Since compliance with the needed diet changes is at risk in the James family situation, family "ownership" of the problem will be important to foster.

The family problem-solving activities also can be used to foster the Jameses' family strength of family hardiness (a sense of control and meaningfulness, ability to plan, commitment to learning, and exploring new experiences [McCubbin & McCubbin, 1989]), and to build up family coherence (caring, pride, shared values in the management of tensions and strain [McCubbin & McCubbin, 1989]), which is a family weakness. The sharing of thoughts and ideas also may increase communication lines. Sharing with the children, a communication link sometimes neglected (Martinson, Gilliss, Colaizzo, Freeman, & Bossert, 1990), may be of particular importance in the Jameses' family situation, since it is the boys that have the greatest objections to the changes. Open communication lines also may reveal Helen's frustrations with the family's resistance to change and her own needs to change. In the end the family's solutions would demonstrate to the instructor the family's level of understanding. Congratulating them on their success would support the family's sense of mastery and pride, both of which are important resources for adaptation (McCubbin, Needle, & Wilson, 1985).

Doherty and Baird (1983) propose that the need for life-style changes, such as dietary changes, is a significant time for health professionals to convene the family (cited in Anderson & Holder, 1989). For health professionals and families, the value convening the family can hold in promoting a life-style change is demonstrated in this vignette. Health professionals can reap the benefit of better compliance with medical regimens. Families have the potential to maximize family information, self-esteem, problem solving, communication lines and social support resources, as well as the ability to produce a manageable family appraisal. These factors can assist in facilitating a more positive level of family adaptation.

This vignette also demonstrates the usefulness of examining illness stressor dimensions (for example, gradual onset, low severity) and family typology to determine the focus of interventions. Both the gradual onset and low severity of this illness situation contributed to the unclear family appraisal. The family's unclear appraisal along with the family typology caused resistance to change. The dietary classes that convened the family to confront and discuss problems or a similar intervention could be used to correct the situation. Convening the family would be an especially important intervention to apply to families with low cohesion or adaptability. Overall the vignette illustrates how attention by health-care professionals to the family's resources (B/BB/BBB) and the family's appraisals (C/CC/CCC), two components of the Resiliency Model, can be an enabling force in reducing resistance to change, producing family acceptance and involvement in the treatment plan, and decreasing the potential for family crisis.

Specific Interventions — Cholecystectomy

Family interventions also can be very effective in preparing for the surgical experience (Halm, 1990). In fact, Schmidt (1983/1985) proposes and supports with research that convening the family during the surgical experience is an effective intervention health professionals need to use. Because of the Jameses' fears of surgery, the risks of forming a family appraisal that labels the experience "overwhelming" are high. These fears increase the potential for family crisis. The family will need a great deal of reassurance to form a positive, manageable appraisal. Furthermore the situational needs for family reorganization, information, and support require resources from all three resource areas — personal, family, and community. To assist the family in accomplishing these tasks, attention to the family's appraisal and to maximizing resources continues to be a priority for the health professional. The following is an example of a family intervention that can accomplish this purpose during the surgical phase of this illness.

✦ ✦ ✦ ✦ ✦

Before Helen returns home from her initial hospitalization to prepare for her surgery, the doctor who will perform her surgery meets with the family. He brings with him Rebecca, a case manager nurse who assists in preparing and managing families undergoing surgical experiences. She works closely with the surgeon. With permission from the family the nurse has communicated with Helen's family physician and is aware of the James family's perceptions and attitudes surrounding the surgery.

During this initial family meeting, the nurse and surgeon explain what the surgical experience will be like and encourage family communication of fears. Both the doctor and the nurse are aware that family members find information helpful in preparing them for the unknown (Aguilera, 1990; Lovejoy, 1986) and that predictable situations have less potential to produce family crisis (Montgomery, 1982).

Rebecca organizes subsequent meetings to assess the family appraisal, plans, and coping resources. Meetings may take place in the home if that appears to facilitate the situation. She asks the family to make a list of its needs and consider how they plan to meet them. A meeting may be arranged with other families also preparing for surgery. This offers the opportunity for families to validate feelings and concerns, observe role models, and develop mutual support (Gilbey, 1989; Halm, 1990). The number of meetings depends on the difficulties Rebecca sees brewing in the family's preparations. She also takes the family on a hospital tour. Rebecca will continue to meet with the family throughout the experience to provide information and support and to coordinate services.

The current trend in nursing toward a case-management approach lends itself well to this kind of situation. This approach calls for a registered nurse–physician collaborative practice base responsible for overseeing the clinical and financial outcomes of the patient's care (Center for Nursing

Case Management, 1989). New England Medical Center (1988) describes this approach as focusing on giving patients and their families "more participation, security, and satisfaction with the health-care delivery system" (cited in Center for Nursing Case Management, 1989, p. 2). The approach is not just hospital based but calls for integration and follow-through with community care as well. In this case the nurse (case manager) can then provide a stabilizing influence as she offers consistency before, during, and after the surgical experience. The present success of the case-management approach in hospital settings lends hope for future elaboration and implementation of this kind of intervention with its strong family focus.

Feelings of helplessness and lack of control often persist with hospitalization especially for surgery (Bozett, 1987; Hickey, 1990). This can *negatively* impact a sense of mastery and control, which, in turn, *negatively* impacts the family appraisal. Acting as an information resource, the health-care professional can *positively* impact the family's feelings of mastery and control, thus *positively* impacting the family's appraisal. McCubbin and McCubbin (Chapter 2) and Olson et al. (1989) describe the ability of the cognitive appraisal to neutralize a stressful situation. With the fears that Helen and Phil hold surrounding surgery, they need knowledge of the decreased risks and complications that laser surgery brings to Helen's situation (Jackson et al., 1990). Only four small puncture wounds are necessary to perform the surgery. Helen will be admitted to the hospital on the day of surgery and can go home the next day. Normal activities can be resumed within the next few days after discharge. It can be explained that the surgery Helen's brother and Phil's friend underwent was more serious with greater potential for complications and therefore is not comparable to Helen's situation. This information may assist in neutralizing their fears.

However, information and social support from the health professional alone may be inadequate to counteract overwhelming family fears (Dunst et al., 1988). Therefore encouraging the family to seek emotional support from friends and to tap religious resources that reduce fears are important (Olson et al., 1989). Secure families are not supportive of each other during hardships (McCubbin & McCubbin, 1989). This factor also may increase Helen's need for informal support systems outside of the home.

When convening the James family, many adaptive coping strategies can be supported to assist reorganizational efforts. During planning discussions, supporting synergy and compromise are particularly significant, since some antagonism exists between Phil and the boys. To do this, open communication lines need to be encouraged. During the surgical experience the family needs to interface, that is, form a new, temporary "fit" with the community. Along with seeking social support from friends, community responsibilities may need to be temporarily relinquished. Both Helen and Phil have to request time off from their jobs. Helen needs to find others to carry out her church responsibilities. Financial resources may need to be sought. As in the previously discussed intervention concerning life-style changes, using these family planning activities to develop intrafamilial lines of support may be very effective.

Some families may need great assistance to plan for this experience effectively, whereas others who already have well-developed strategies and resources may need very little. Since the Jameses' strength is family hardiness, they may need only minimal encouragement to plan for the experience. Their low family coherence, however, compels the health professional to prioritize the facilitation of support between family members and extrafamilial sources. With this assistance, the James family may be empowered to maintain or increase family functioning that buffers stress. The fact that planning time is available before Helen's surgery and that the situation is predictable gives the health professional the opportunity to convene the family and carry out interventions of this kind.

✦ CONCLUSION

This short-term illness involving the James family has been used as a vehicle to demonstrate the demands of this kind of illness on the family and family interventions effective in meeting those demands. Although less intense when compared with other more serious or chronic illness situations, short-term illnesses can benefit from family interventions. Health practitioners interacting with families will have a better understanding of their patients' needs and behaviors. The rewards of these interventions are evident in the developed strategies and resources that can be orchestrated by the family and the potentially less strenuous course taken during illness. The health professional can enhance the health of the whole family, which translates into successful patient outcomes.

Pivotal questions regarding family interventions come to the foreground in this illness situation. First, who will carry out these interventions? Nurses and physicians, either singly or collaboratively, can intervene by convening the family in the hospital, the office, or the home setting. Nurses and physicians need to explore the use of family interventions in all health-care settings and decide who will take responsibility for the family. Second, how will these services be paid for? At present, third-party payment is aimed at high-tech services and lends little support to low-tech services of this type. Research and studies are beginning to demonstrate the value of these low-tech services (Anderson & Holder, 1989; Anderson, Reiss, & Hogarty, 1986; Schmidt, 1983/1985; Storer et al., 1987). However, further research is needed to establish an equal value. Presently a family approach, case management, is being successfully used to ensure positive patient outcomes *and* to decrease health costs. This may give impetus to looking at the value of other family-oriented interventions in containing health-care costs. Since our society is currently taking a hard look at the cost of health care, this may be an opportune time to advocate for family interventions.

REFERENCES

Aguilera, D. C. (1990). *Crisis intervention: Theory and methodology* (6th ed.). St. Louis: Mosby–Year Book.

Anderson, C. M., & Holder, D. P. (1989). Family systems and behavioral disorders: Schizophrenia, depression, and alcoholism. In C. N. Ramsey (Ed.), *Family systems in medicine* (pp. 487-502). New York: Guilford.

Anderson, C. M., Reiss, D. J., & Hogarty, G. E. (1986). *Schizophrenia and the family*. New York: Guilford.

Bozett, F. (1987). Family nursing and life-threatening illness. In M. Leahey & L. M. Wright (Eds.), *Families and life-threatening illness* (pp. 2-25). Springhouse, PA: Springhouse.

Cassmeyer, V. L. (1991). Management of persons with problems of the gallbladder and exocrine pancreas. In W. J. Phipps, B. C. Long, N. F. Woods, & V. L. Cassmeyer (Eds.), *Medical-surgical nursing: Concepts and clinical practice* (4th ed., pp. 1363-1384). St. Louis: Mosby–Year Book.

Center for nursing case management (1989). Boston: Center for Nursing Case Management unpublished handout compiled for the Vermont State Nurses Association's Annual Convention, November 1989.

Dunst, C. J., Trivette, C. M., & Deal, A. G. (1988). *Enabling and empowering families: Principles and guidelines for practice*. Cambridge, MA: Brookline.

Gilbey, V. J. (1989). Will the health professional meet the challenge? *Canadian Journal of Public Health, 80,* 373-374.

Greenberger, N. J., & Isselbacher, K. J. (1991). Diseases of the gallbladder and bile ducts. In J. D. Wilson, E. Braunwald, K. J. Isselbacher, R. Petersdorf, J. B. Martin, A. S. Fanci, & R. K. Root (Eds.), *Harrison's principles of internal medicine* (12th ed., pp. 1358-1368). New York: McGraw-Hill.

Halm, M. A. (1990). Effects of support groups on anxiety of family members

during critical illness. *Heart and Lung,*
19(1), 62-71.

Hickey, M. (1990). What are the needs of
families of critically ill patients? A
review of the literature since 1976.
Heart and Lung, 19(1), 401-415.

Hirsch, L. L. (1988). Problem differentiation. In R. B. Taylor (Ed.), *Family
medicine* (3rd ed., pp. 58-65). New
York: Springer-Verlag.

Jackson, D. C., Martin, T., Evans, M. M.,
& Rudio, P. A. (1990). Endoscopic
laser cholecystectomy: New approach
to gallbladder removal. *North Carolina
Medical Journal, 51*(7), 324-325.

Kemp, B., Pillitteri, A., & Brown, P.
(1989). *Fundamentals of nursing: a
framework for practice.* New York:
Springer-Verlag.

Leske, J. (1986). Needs of relatives of
critically ill patients: A follow-up.
Heart and Lung, 15(2), 189-193.

Leventhal, H., Leventhal, E. A., & Van
Nguyen, T. (1985). Reactions of families to illness: Theoretical models and
perspectives. In D. C. Turk & R. D.
Kerns (Eds.), *Health, illness, and families* (pp. 108-145). New York: John
Wiley & Sons.

Lovejoy, N. (1986). Family response to
cancer hospitalization. *Oncology
Nursing Forum, 13*(2), 33-37.

Loveys, B. (1990). Transitions in chronic
illness: The at-risk role. *Holistic Nursing Practice, 4*(3), 56-64.

Martinson, I. M., Gilliss, C., Colaizzo, D.
C., Freeman, M., & Bossert, E. (1990).
Impact of childhood cancer on healthy
school-age siblings. *Cancer Nursing,
13*(3), 183-190.

McCubbin, H. I., Needle, R. H., & Wilson, M. (1985). Adolescent health-risk
behaviors: Family stress and adolescent coping as critical factors. *Family
Relations, 34*, 51-62.

McCubbin, M. A., & McCubbin, H. I.
(1989). Theoretical orientations to
family stress and coping. In C. R.
Figley, (Ed.), *Treating stress in families*
(pp. 3-43). New York: Brunner/Mazel.

Montgomery, J. (1982). *Family crisis as
process: Persistence and change.* Washington, D.C.: University Press of America.

Olson, D., McCubbin, H. I., Barnes, H.,
Larsen, A., Muxen, M., & Wilson, M.
(1989). *Families: What makes them
work* (2nd ed.). Newbury Park, CA:
Saga.

O'Neill-Norris, L., & Grove, S. (1986).
Investigation of selected psychosocial
needs of family members of critically
ill adult patients. *Heart and Lung,
15*(2), 194-199.

Schmidt, D. (1985). When is it helpful to
convene the family? In D. Olson, (Ed.),
Family studies review yearbook (Vol. 3,
pp. 38-43). Beverly Hills, CA: Sage.
(Reprinted from *Journal of Family
Practice,* 1983, *16*(5), 967-973)

Storer, J. H., Frate, D.A., Johnson, A., &
Greenburg, A. (1987). When the cure
seems worse than the disease: helping
families adapt to hypertension treatment. *Family Relations, 36*, 311-315.

Way, L. W., & Sleigenger, M. H. (1989).
Acute and chronic cholecystitis. In M.
H. Sleigenger & J. S. Fordtran (Eds.),
Gastrointestinal disease (4th ed., pp.
1691-1714). Philadelphia: W. B. Saun-
ders.

Wright, L. M., & Leahey, M. (1987).
Families and life-threatening illness:
Assumptions, assessment, and inter-
vention. In M. Leahey & L. M. Wright
(Eds.), *Families and life-threatening
illness* (pp. 45-48). Springhouse, PA:
Springhouse.

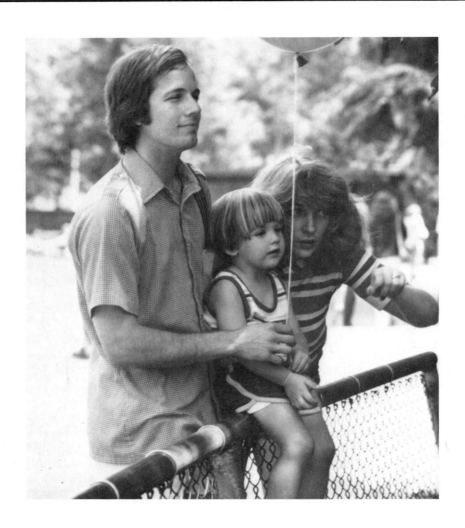

CHAPTER

13

Life-threatening Illness: Cancer

✦

CHAPTER GOALS

✦ To illustrate the impact that cancer, as a life-threatening illness, has on the entire family

✦ To exemplify the range of coping mechanisms observed among families confronted by a life-threatening illness

✦ To propose possible family-oriented interventions that might be used in a life-threatening illness situation

OVERVIEW

THIS chapter examines in detail the demands of caring for a family member with a life-threatening illness—cancer. The discussion about the demands of cancer illustrates the variety of illness stressor dimensions found in a life-threatening illness that are important in determining the impact this illness can have on an entire family system. The chapter begins with a vignette describing the Matthews' family situation and the aspects of cancer with which they are coping. The chapter is organized by the components of the McCubbin's Resiliency Model of Family Stress, Adjustment, and Adaptation (see Chapter 2) and discusses cancer in relation: to the demands of the illness situation—the stressor (A); resources available to the Matthews—the resources (B/BB/BBB); and the Matthews' appraisals of the illness situation—the appraisals (C/CC/CCC). The last section of the chapter offers suggestions for family interventions that meet the demands of a life-threatening illness and concludes with an example of a specific family intervention demonstrating the need and value of family interventions during cancer.

✦ THE FAMILY SITUATION

✦ ✦ ✦ ✦ ✦

Bill and Rita Matthews are in their late twenties, have professional careers, a new house in the "right" neighborhood, and a 4-year-old daughter named Wendy. Both are enthusiastic health-fitness buffs — Bill leaning toward jogging, whereas Rita prefers swimming. Their lives seem rich, full, and blessed with prosperity.

One morning, as Rita is getting dressed, Bill notices that the mole in the small of her back seems larger. During the next year, on and off, Rita keeps track of the discoloration, which seems to be growing and becoming more irregular. Finally, worried about what it could be, Rita makes an appointment with her physician. Things move quickly from that point: a biopsy is taken, a specialist is consulted, and then the announcement that she has a malignant melanoma — a lethal form of skin cancer. Bill and Rita are devastated. Although Rita begins immediate treatment at a respected cancer center, both she and Bill fear that Rita is going to die.

The Matthews' situation is designed to illustrate the impact that stressor dimensions of a life-threatening illness such as cancer can place on families. Their family situation exemplifies common family reactions and needs in a life-threatening illness situation. The box on p. 347 lists illness stressor dimensions found in this case of cancer. (See also Chapter 4 for information on stressor dimensions.)

Life-threatening illnesses such as cancer require ongoing family adjustment and adaptation. The amount of family adjustment and adaptation is directly related to the degree of cancer invasion. Family coping can certainly be enhanced by timely and supportive relationships with health-care professionals (McCubbin & McCubbin, Chapter 2). The life-threatening nature of cancer brings the family and the health-care professional together for numerous opportunities to intervene during the various phases of the illness from prevention to death or recovery.

Illness Stressor Dimensions Characteristic of *the Matthews' Case of Cancer*	
Gradual *onset*	*Origin* from inside the family
Moderate *duration*	Great *severity*
Uncertain *predictability*	Large *resource demands*
Great *social stigma*	Limited ability to *control*
Unknown *causes*	High *extent* of family impact

✦ THE ILLNESS — CANCER

According to the American Cancer Society, cancer is the second leading cause of death in the United States, outnumbered only by cardiovascular disorders (American Cancer Society, 1989). It claims nearly 500,000 lives per year and another 1,010,000 people are diagnosed with it. It affects one of every four people, resulting in a national death rate of 171 people per 100,000. Cancer occurs in approximately three out of four families over the years. Thus, within the United States and throughout the world, cancer has a tremendous economic and sociologic impact. It influences families and their members in every realm of their lives.

Cancer is an economic burden for both families and society. Cancer cost the United States an estimated $71.5 billion in 1985 (American Cancer Society, 1989). As technology advances and medical costs increase, the cost of cancer care becomes even greater in comparison to the costs of other diseases; 9% of health-care costs relates to oncology. Costs may be direct or indirect. Direct costs involve prevention, diagnosis, and intervention, and include payments for chronic and acute care facilities, nursing and medical services, research, and professional education. Indirect costs include loss of national productivity due to absences of people with cancer or their family members from the work force. Programs that focus on prevention are currently the most promising weapons against rising costs of cancer care (American Cancer Society, 1989).

For too many people, the diagnosis of cancer still means death. As recently as 20 years ago most people thought cancer was incurable. But research and technology, together with advances in diagnosis and treatment, have helped cure cancer in many people. In fact, about 5 million

Americans with a history of cancer are alive today. Research indicates that some survivors with an internal locus of control and a high level of self-esteem have an increased perception of well-being in spite of their previous diagnosis of cancer (Dirksen, 1989). Family communication can be a source of strength for some cancer victims. Family issues once dormant may now be opened for discussion and problem solving. Moreover, families who view themselves as people at risk for hereditary cancer can incorporate preventive care plans in their life-styles and remain optimistic for the future (Dirksen, 1989; Longman & Graham, 1986).

Based on cancer research, the understanding of and intervention for cancer is ever-changing. It is even difficult for health professionals to keep abreast of the current theories regarding the nature of cancer, its different types and sites, its prevalence, etiology, pathogenesis, and diagnosis. The multiple possibilities and debates leave families with numerous misunderstandings about cancer, possible victims for quackery solutions, and with the fear of disfigurement, alteration in abilities, and eventual death. Let us examine what might occur in family situation like the Matthews' where the diagnosis of cancer is experienced.

◆ DEMANDS OF THE ILLNESS STRESSOR (A)

This portion of the chapter describes and illustrates the demands this life-threatening illness stressor (A) places on the Matthews family (Fig. 13-1). Each illness stressor dimension encountered with cancer forms demands on the Matthews in various ways. The Matthews are a *fragile family* type with low family bonding and low family flexibility (see Fig. 5-3). This type of family is hesitant to depend on the family for support and understanding. Family members prefer to confide in persons outside the family and encourage members to go their own way. This family resists compromise and is inexperienced in reassigning responsibilities among family members (McCubbin & McCubbin, 1989). The impact of this family typology (T) on the illness situation is indicated.

Onset

The speed of onset varies with cancer. The spreading of melanoma throughout the layers of the skin can last several months or years. The

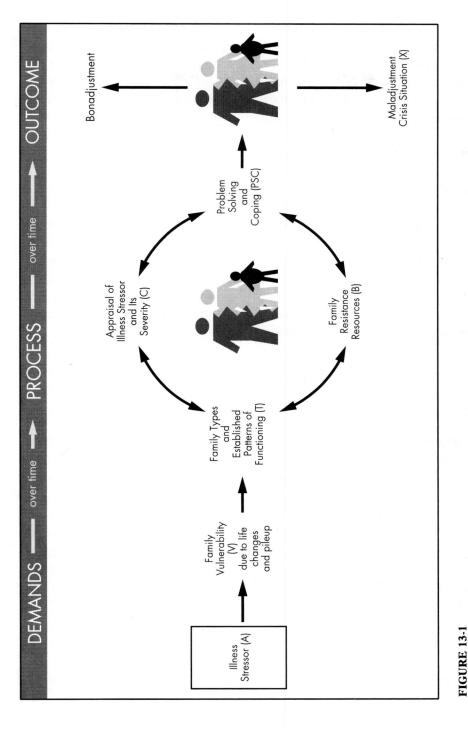

FIGURE 13-1

Adjustment Phase of the Resiliency Model of Family Stress, Adjustment, and Adaptation. This portion of the chapter focuses on the demands of the illness stressor (A).

malignant cells invade the skin and underlying tissue. First, the cells spread laterally across the skin. Then, the tumor grows inward and becomes invasive, spreading into the lymphatic system and bloodstream. In this way the tumor acquires the ability to metastasize. Melanoma becomes noticeable due to its irregular pigmentation of red, white, and blue, with variations from red-purple, to blue-black, to gray-white. The lesion's surface becomes uneven and the borders irregular and notched. Satellite lesions may surface. At later stages, bleeding and ulceration develop.

As in Rita's case, the diagnosis of melanoma is confirmed with the biopsy of the changed or suspicious skin lesion. The patient has no other warning signs. Rita noted the change in her mole over a year's time. For other families the lesion may go unnoticed. Thus the onset of this illness may *seem* sudden. Additionally, confirmation of the diagnosis is shocking for the family and for the unaware victim. A mole is considered to be benign and common. Moles are certainly not cosmetically pleasing, but they are not thought to be killers. Once the implications of this illness are learned by the family, they are startled and shocked (Starr, 1985). Each member reacts differently, but at this point accurate information about the illness helps the family appraise the nature of the demand and plan for dealing with the illness.

Severity and Stigma

Malignant melanoma is the most common fatal skin disorder. It has a great potential to produce widespread metastases. It is one of the most deadly of all cancers, yet it is potentially curable through early detection and treatment. Unfortunately, it is increasing at a rate exceeding all other cancers, except lung cancer. In the United States, malignant melanoma affects about 27,000 people annually. It has a 20% mortality in spite of the fact that it is curable through surgery if recognized early. Malignant melanoma has great potential to have a devastating effect on the family especially if the family loses its member (American Cancer Society, 1989; Fraser, 1982; Lawler & Schreiber, 1989; Schleper, 1984). Even if the illness does not result in death, the search for a cure, the fear that may disrupt interfamily communication, and the disorganization due to surgical intervention and subsequent treatments will stress the family.

As Sontag (1977) notes, cancer is so highly stigmatized that it is treated as a mystery. It is so acutely feared that some people act as if it is contagious (Levanthal, Levanthal, & Van Nguyen, 1985). A surprisingly large number of people with cancer find themselves shunned by relatives and friends and the object of decontamination practices by members of their household, as if cancer were an infectious disease.

Sontag (1977) further discusses the fact that no one thinks of concealing the truth from a cardiac patient; nothing is shameful about a heart attack. Cardiac disease implies a weakness that is mechanical and not disgraceful. Cancer patients are lied to, not only because the disease is thought to be a death sentence, but also because it is considered obscene, ill-omened, and repugnant to the senses. The metaphors attached to cancer imply living processes of a horrid kind.

Extent of the Illness's Impact on the Family

Adjustment phase

✦ ✦ ✦ ✦ ✦

In spite of the positive attitudes expressed by the staff at the cancer center about advances made in cancer treatment, the Matthews fear that Rita's condition will not be cured. After the initial surgical excision of the tumor, the family agrees informally that the next 6 months will be a "wait-and-see" situation. The family feels overwhelmed by the shock and fear regarding Rita's health status.

Previous to this illness, Bill and Rita prided themselves on their individual independence and ability to maintain separate careers. Bill is a successful civil engineer, and Rita owns a graphic design company. Roles and tasks in the family were well defined before this illness situation. Bill and Rita's need for independence contributes to the low bonding found in their fragile family typology; they are hesitant to depend on each other.

At the time of the initial surgical excision of her tumor, Rita tells Bill and the staff that she does not want to know the results of the biopsy. In addition, she does not want family and friends to learn about her prognosis. She feels distracted and cannot concentrate on listening to others. Family members and friends find her distant, tearful, and anxious. She refuses to talk about her condition with anyone. She passively goes along with treatment, asking no questions.

Results of the level of invasion and resection of Rita's lymph nodes indicate that her melanoma has advanced beyond the primary site. Bill is at a loss as to what to do. The family's worst fears are now confirmed. Bill continues to worry about Rita. His anxiety pervades all aspects of his life. He decides to be cheerful when he talks with Rita and speak with her as if nothing has happened. Bill, typical of individuals in fragile families, shares his plan with the staff at the cancer center but not with his family. This behavior is maladaptive and could send the family into crisis.

Metastatic involvement of lymph nodes or other organs requires chemotherapy and immunotherapy. Radiation therapy is currently used only for palliation of bone and brain metastases. Since Rita has metastases to the lymph nodes and other organs, chemotherapy is used. The treatment and recovery will have a severe impact on her family because she is likely to have side effects, either acute or delayed from the chemotherapy. This will make her illness more obvious to family members, increase time away from childcare and work, and lengthen her recovery time. Moreover, due to the advancement of the illness, recovery is uncertain and unpredictable.

The extent of the impact of malignant melanoma on the family can be significant, especially if a cure is unlikely. The impact will be financial, physical, psychological, social, and spiritual. These demands will reverberate throughout the family unit and affect all of its members.

Adaptation phase

◆ ◆ ◆ ◆ ◆

A year passes and Rita's condition deteriorates to the end stages of cancer. She is bedridden and cared for by the tertiary unit at the cancer center. The staff has worked with the Matthews throughout this time. Although the Matthews initially denied the diagnosis and avoided discussing the true nature of Rita's illness, they have come to accept the reality of Rita's impending death. The family has been consumed with grief. Bill dealt with the situation by trying to be cheerful in front of Rita, then reverted to beers with his friends after work. Rita's mother moved into the household to help with Wendy, meal preparation and household chores. The staff held grief work groups with the Matthews to help them communicate with each other. Rita had great difficulty in giving up the control in her life but finally was able to discuss her feelings and illness with her family. Make Today Count, a self-help, mutual support group also was a useful resource. Family members felt much anger and resentment toward Rita's illness, and they continue to express this. They have agreed to spend as much quality time with Rita as possible until her death. Over time it is expected that the

Matthews will be able to give meaning and legitimacy to new family patterns without Rita and come to accept the situation.

Duration, Predictability, and Control

The duration, predictability, and ability to control the illness depends on the degree of invasion and the metastases of the tumor. The survival rate in all forms of melanoma depends on the penetration of malignant cells into deeper skin layers. Penetration depth is measured in millimeters or by reference to anatomical landmarks in the skin. The thicker the tumor or the deeper the invasion into the skin, the greater the likelihood that metastatic growth has occurred. Obviously, early detection and biopsy of suspicious skin lesions is the ideal method of intervention.

✦ ✦ ✦ ✦ ✦

Rita received the treatment of choice, which is a wide local surgical excision with a 3- to 5-cm border. A full-thickness excision biopsy that preceded the treatment helped to determine the level of invasion. Grafting may be necessary, depending on the width of the tumor's border. With a more deeply invasive lesion, regional lymph nodes are resected to measure the progress of the disease.

At this point, the duration and predictability of this illness are uncertain. This uncertainty contributes to a sense of lost control within the family. Fear of the unknown is ever present.

If the melanoma is primary and has not spread, patient treatment is brief and has a limited effect on the family (Greany & Goldsmith, 1985). Treatment for a noninvasive primary melanoma could be limited to the initial surgical excision. Patients have some disfigurement and then must undergo dermatological assessment follow-up and implement future preventive behaviors. Postoperative wound care is another aspect of self-care. Medical supervision and dermatological assessment are necessary every 3 to 6 months, both of which are covered by most health insurance programs. The family is advised of preventive guidelines to implement in the future. Patients with melanoma also must perform a monthly self-assessment of the scalp, trunk, and intertriginous and genital areas to identify pigmented lesions. Medical follow-up is necessary for any changes in pigmented areas. Blood relatives such as parents, siblings, and children should also seek dermatological assessment. All persons are advised to limit sun exposure and are encouraged to use the various photoprotection measures available.

Cause and Origin

The cause of melanoma remains unclear. Experts have identified some risk factors, both personal and environmental, clearly related to its occurrence. Melanoma occurs most often among adults 30 to 60 years of age and affects men and women equally. It most commonly affects individuals with fair skin and light-colored eyes and hair. Although uncommon, it affects people with dark skin, on lightly pigmented areas. The most common sites are the head, neck, and lower extremities, but it also can occur on the perineum or scalp. A positive family history of displastic nevi or malignant melanoma is one risk factor. The presence of increased hormonal activity, such as estrogen or progesterone during adolescence and pregnancy, are also risk factors. A history of considerable sun exposure either by direct sunlight or by tanning beds is an additional significant risk factor (Stewart, 1990). Melanoma occurs more frequently in populations living latitudinally close to the equator. Those living in the Sunbelt in the United States also show a marked increase in incidence. The Matthews were familiar with the word *melanoma* from television health reports, but no one in their family had ever been diagnosed with cancer.

Resource Demands
Financial demands. Generally speaking, cancer recovery is expensive. Interventions are technical and lengthy. Moreover, Rita may need substantial care at home after release from the health-care facility. The financial consequences of Rita's illness are a major concern to her and Bill. A lengthy stay in, or frequent outpatient visits to, a health-care facility takes time from work and managing the household. Rita may experience decreased energy and find it necessary to return to work with a reduced schedule, find a different line of work, or discontinue working altogether. Moreover, cancer frequently has the same kind of social stigma once assigned to tuberculosis. Many people find that they are denied their former jobs or assigned to isolated areas once their cancer becomes common knowledge.

Physical demands

✦ ✦ ✦ ✦ ✦

When Rita undergoes chemotherapy, side effects pervade all her body systems. She is tired and weak, often feeling bodily changes that affect her self-concept. Nausea, vomiting, anorexia, taste distortion, urinary output changes, diarrhea, and constipation are common occurrences. She feels pain due to dermatitis in general, as well as infusion site problems, liver enlargement, hair loss, and darkening of skin pigmentation and nails. Her self-concept is further upset by decreased sexual interest and amenorrhea, even though she knows these aspects of life return to normal after chemotherapy. Her ability to care for herself is diminished as she experiences anemia, tingling in her extremities, cerebellar disturbances, cardiac toxicity, photosensitivity, and ototoxicity. The onset of these side effects is acute and delayed, mild and then severe. These physical changes make Rita more dependent on her family. Her discomfort is obvious and very unsettling for the family. The presence of Rita's mother in the household helps decrease the impact of Rita's increasing dependency, which would be much harder for Bill to manage alone.

Emotional demands

✦ ✦ ✦ ✦ ✦

Coping with cancer is as much an emotional battle as a physical one for the family. Rita's most common fears are of pain, abandonment, dependency, disfigurement, and death. Families are vital in helping afflicted members cope with these fears. Rita feels a loss of control over her life and situation. She has decreased self-respect, changes in her self-image, and an inability to work or maintain the household. She has a kaleidoscope of feelings ranging from anger, denial, sadness, resignation, fear, and acceptance (Friedman, 1980). As expected from members of a fragile family type, it is difficult for Rita to share these feelings with Bill and Wendy.

The Matthews family experiences these emotions also. When Rita receives the diagnosis of cancer, her crisis becomes the family's crisis. Communication and routine are impaired. Helplessness, grief, frustration, anger, false cheer, and guilt can become permanent companions (Friedman, 1980). Individuals within the family must face their unique feelings while trying to be sensitive to the feelings of the person with cancer.

✦ ✦ ✦ ✦ ✦

Stress is present during all phases of the illness. It peaks during the prediagnosis phase. It peaks again during recurrence of advanced disease. The patient and family wonder what procedure could be left to treat the cancer, which has returned despite previous treatment. They often question the treatment and whether it will be worth it. They know treatments, no matter how sound, may fail. Fear of pain and addiction to pain medications are common. Families may want information on death that cannot be given definitively.

Even in the most open of families, some unique features of anxiety may merit attention. Families confront double anxiety: what they hear from the patient and what they feel within themselves. They may hesitate to share worries they may have about cancer or role demands with the patient. This may increase their sense of aloneness. The anxiety may be increased by other family members who ask others for information about the patient. Receiving information at secondhand also may potentiate family anxiety if they are unsure about its accuracy or if they have unanswerable questions. Being right there to hear news of the patient's condition firsthand is always more desirable.

Demands for role changes may exacerbate family anxiety. The patient is often relieved of his or her usual roles due to the illness. The remaining family members must assume the patient's responsibilities often while continuing to work and carrying on their usual routine. Wendy may experience a decrease in attention in relation to her developmental needs as her family copes with the illness.

Discharge from the acute care setting may require 24-hour caretaking responsibility by the family. Responsibilities may include physical care and emotional support, especially as the terminal stages of the illness approach. Stress increases if extended family and community resources are minimal. Stress is also heightened if family members are not clear about indicators of problems and when they should call a physician.

Social demands. Socially, cancer can be an isolating and overwhelming illness for families. Studies indicate that family members are more interested in having the focus of care on the patient, thus putting the needs of their loved one before themselves (Lewandowski & Jones, 1988). Many role changes take place for family members as their time is consumed in adjusting to these new demands and needs. These changes are more difficult for the Matthews because they are a fragile family with low flexibility.

✦ ✦ ✦ ✦ ✦

Bill finds it exhausting to come home from work, prepare dinner, oversee Wendy's care, change bedding and dressings, and still try to provide companionship and emotional support for Wendy and Rita. Bill, who was sharing the load, now becomes the sole breadwinner and primary homemaker. Rita, one of the heads of the household, is now its most dependent member. Time previously spent on involvement in community, recreation, and general socializing is now consumed by seeking medical attention, caregiving tasks, maintaining the household, and resting. Because of their isolation, Bill and Rita are beginning to feel that everyone else is managing nicely while they are floundering.

These changes can cause great upheaval in family interaction. The usual patterns are gone. Bill might look to Wendy for emotional support at a time when she needs a supportive father. Wendy reverts to infantile behavior. She begins to wet her bed and have nightmares, indicating her distress. Friends do not know how to help and so withdraw. The sheer weight of responsibility and fear of cancer can become overwhelming.

Spiritual demands. A family member diagnosed with cancer can be one of the most spiritually disabling events for a family. Since attitudes about cancer are often negative and include fears of death, families feel little hope for recovery. This negative attitude has a significant impact on coping abilities. If the patient and family believe there is no future together, they are more likely to lose hope and abandon life, which can distance them from the patient (Scanlon, 1989). Hickey (1986) finds that hope not only enables the healthy to continue living, but also provides the patient with a reason to live and feel needed. Hope is an essential element in the lives of cancer patients and their families.

The challenge for Rita and her family is to maintain hope. The family's task is to involve Rita in work and activity and to keep her immersed in living and fighting. As much attention needs to be given to helping her maintain the quality of her life as to prolonging it. She needs to continue to live to the fullest to understand her illness and its suffering and fit it into her life. Emphasis is best placed on what the patient has and less on what she has lost.

✦ RESOURCES AVAILABLE TO THE FAMILY (B/BB/BBB)

This portion of the chapter examines the strengths and weaknesses of resources available to the Matthews family (Fig. 13-2). Within the framework of the Resiliency Model, resources encompass both tangible and coping capacities of the family and its community (McCubbin & McCubbin, Chapter 2). Resources include the personal resources of the individual family members, collectively held family resources, and community resources including social support. The Matthews family use all three resource areas to manage the demands of this life-threatening illness. These resources serve as family strengths in decreasing stress and preventing crisis during the illness situation.

Personal Resources (B)

It is easier to come to grips with the reality of any crisis if families replace ignorance with information. There is much to learn about cancer, its treatment, possibility for recovery, and methods of rehabilitation. Well versed in the facts, individual family members are less likely to fall prey to old wives' tales, to quacks touting worthless cures, or to depressing stories of what happened to Aunt Gracie when she got cancer (American Cancer Society, 1989). Often the more families know, the less they will fear.

When cancer develops, many families need to learn to ask for and accept help for the first time. Many medical questions arise. There might be confusion or disagreement over the prognosis: What did the physician mean when he said "guarded prognosis?" What do the various terms mean? For example, *skin biopsy*, *metastases*, and *chemotherapy* are common medical terms that lay people may or may not know in a specific context. As individuals, Bill and Rita have good personal resources. They are educated and intelligent. As a 4-year-old, Wendy has limited ability to comprehend the situation, but if explanations are designed to be developmentally appropriate, she can gain an understanding. The Matthews have the ability to learn much about the illness stressor, if they can emotionally handle the situation. During the period of active treatment, pressing decisions need to be made about the treatment itself and about the future.

Family Resources (BB)

Financial resources. Financial burdens can be crushing. For the most part, the family's medical expenses are covered by a comprehensive

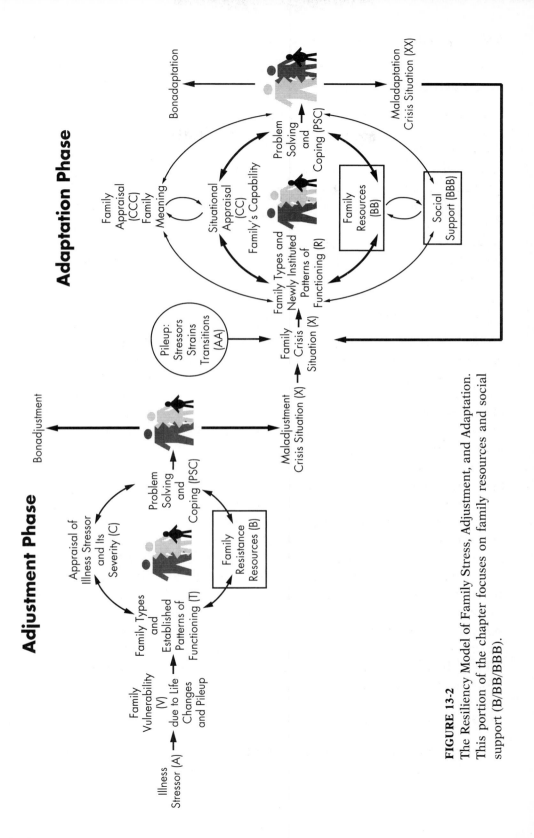

FIGURE 13-2
The Resiliency Model of Family Stress, Adjustment, and Adaptation. This portion of the chapter focuses on family resources and social support (B/BB/BBB).

insurance health-care plan. This will take care of the central expenses related to the needed treatment. However, costs are incurred beyond medical expenses. Transportation to and from treatment can be a major frustrating expense. Also, as Rita's illness progresses, other needs arise, such as a hospital bed, a night nurse, and a person to look after Wendy. These additional expenses become a source of anxiety when they are coupled with the loss of Rita's income.

The stress of handling such responsibilities can be enormous. A new kind of communication and acceptance becomes necessary, such as asking for and accepting outside help, which may be an entirely new role for Rita and Bill. They were raised to believe that "keeping a stiff upper lip" or "going it alone" indicated strength. Now, they have to overcome their discomfort with not being in total control of their lives and seeking resources outside the family.

Family coping resources. Families that cope best are naturally optimistic, confront facts, accept and seek support, and deal with problems as they appear (Donovan & Girton, 1984). Such a family assists the patient with cancer through the phases of adjustment and adaptation that begin at diagnosis and proceed throughout treatment to recovery or death. Overall, this characteristically anxiety-filled time for patient and family can be lessened if the family's problem-solving skills and support systems are adequate. Because Bill and Rita are a *fragile family* type, they struggle with role changes and Rita's increasing dependency. Adequate support among Rita, Bill, and Wendy is lacking.

Cancer patients are generally more anxious than patients with other diseases (Donovan & Girton, 1984). This is explained in part by our society's perception of cancer as always being incurable and inevitably ending in a lingering, painful death. How families feel about cancer as a general concept affects coping when a family member receives definitive diagnosis of cancer. In particular, families that are highly organized, in control, and have the need to predict find the cancer situation highly anxiety-laden. In the final analysis, most families in crisis tend to rely on coping devices that served them well in the past.

The Matthews family chose to ignore the symptoms at first. Other families may be noncompliant with recommendations or treatment because of anxiety over a potential or real cancer diagnosis. It is important to realize that denial creates a distortion of reality. The patient and family can at times benefit from denial but it can hinder coping at other times (Donovan &

Girton, 1984). The prediagnostic period is often marked by acute anxiety when cancer is considered as a possible cause of the suspicious symptom. If the symptom is nonspecific and no cause can be found, patients may leave the consulting physician in a state of stressful uncertainty. The anxiety around the time of diagnosis is intensified by the waiting period between diagnostic tests and hearing the final medical reports. Once anxiety is expressed over the possibility of cancer, worry predominates. Anxious negative thoughts of the outcome are often coupled with hope during the prediagnostic phase.

Many times coping during the prediagnostic stage represents a gradual adaptation, with many people not realizing the intensity of the anxiety until the episode is over. Thus health-care professionals meet the patient and family at a time when anxiety is significantly heightened. Since families often do not absorb all that is taught them, they are at risk for additional anxiety associated with confusion over the treatment that could overwhelm them. Moreover, the emotional stress associated with a diagnosis of cancer is more intense in patients with little family support and diminished emotional coping mechanisms.

The Matthews family feels the most intense anxiety during the treatment phase. The operative period was a time when anxiety peaked for both Rita and the family. Anxiety grew before the chemotherapy treatment. Chemotherapy leads to emesis, invasive procedures, and the helplessness associated with the patient role. Anxiety plays a role in the nausea, vomiting, and physical toxicity of multiple treatments. Concerns about fertility, sexual performance, and sexual desirability surfaced for Rita when chemotherapy ceased. New worries over future tumor growth and the distance to the health-care facility that she depends on began to bother Rita.

Hospitalizations also increased anxiety for Rita. Sensory changes such as having strange roommates, interacting with many health-care professionals, being confined to a bed, undergoing painful procedures, and being isolated were sources of stress. A lack of reassurance that anxiety is a normal reaction to this kind of stress is another factor that increased anxiety. The greatest stressor for Rita was having a roommate with cancer die during her stay. The reality that her life would be limited was overwhelming for Rita.

One effort that seems to help patients cope, and also is a good indication of whether one is coping, is returning to employment. Patients who resume work show fewer signs of low self-esteem, poor morale, anxiety, and depression and seem to feel less threatened by cancer than do their nonworking counterparts. This involves the individual in work and keeps him or her maintaining the quality of life as while trying to prolong it. Rita was able to continue working at least part-time for several months. Then it became apparent she could not continue to work as hard as was necessary to maintain her business. She became depressed when she finally had to sell the business she created. Fortunately the business was bought by a colleague who respected Rita's competence and consulted her on a regular basis.

Stoic acceptance of the inevitable and preparation to accept death implies surrendering one's will. When little hope exist for survival, preparation for death is indicative of a healthy acceptance of reality. The same is true of acceptance of the limitations resulting from the disease. Neither comes easily for the family; both involve time and struggle.

Community Resources (BBB)

The health-care team may be a good first source of answers to medical questions. Physicians and nurses can answer questions about the cancer, its treatment, any side effects from it or any limitations treatment may place on Rita's activities. Other members of the health-care team such as physical therapists, nutritionists, radiation technologists, social workers, and psychologists can explain the reason for a specific aspect of therapy.

Families can be overwhelmed by emotion during times when it is important to have information. It is helpful if more than one member or as many members as possible attend these discussions so that the information can be heard firsthand. Writing questions down makes them easier to remember at the next treatment appointment. Some families not only take notes but also tape-record sessions.

Local libraries, local divisions of voluntary agencies such as the American Cancer Society or the Leukemia Society of America, and major cancer research and treatment institutions are sources of information about cancer and its treatment, equipment for caregiving at home, and financial assistance. On a national level, the National Cancer Institute (NCI), which is part of the National Institutes of Health, operates an information office for the public. Its information specialists can answer many general questions about cancer and its diagnosis and treatment. In addition, the NCI coordinates a network of information offices among the nation's top cancer research and treatment centers. Cancer Information Service (CIS) counselors can provide the names of facilities that are most appropriate in terms of both location and specialization. They also have written materials and information about local self-help and service organizations for cancer patients and their families.

Numerous self-help groups from local chapters of national organizations or from the grass roots offer informal social support assistance. Some are designed for patients only, whereas others include family members. They exist to help patients work through feelings and frustrations, provide skills training and helpful tips, and emotional support. Examples of these groups are Make Today Count, United Ostomy Association, International Association of Laryngectomies, Reach to Recovery, I Can Surmount, and I Can Cope. The location and the family's previous experience with support are factors in indicating if use of a support group can be encouraged and, if so, which one.

More formal emotional assistance from trained counselors, psychologists, and psychiatrists is an additional resource that some families find supportive. These emotional support services are often incorporated into cancer treatment. Individual and group counseling are available for patients and families to explore feelings in depth and to look for the best ways to face problems. Some services incorporate music, poetry, role-playing, visual imagery, relaxation, and action-oriented techniques. Family counseling can help families absorb the shock and manage the stresses of cancer.

✦ FAMILY APPRAISALS OF THE ILLNESS SITUATION (C/CC/CCC)

The Matthews' appraisals of cancer arise from their perception of the existing balance between demands of the illness and resources for the illness situation (Fig. 13-3). During Rita's initial encounter with cancer, the duration of her illness has the potential to be short-term, and the family quickly adjusts to the situation. They take a "wait-and-see" approach and consider the first battle with cancer won, although the final outcome is worrisome and uncertain. The Matthews realize a *threat* to the integrity of the family exists with progression of the cancer beyond the primary site and its accompanying long-term treatment. The eventual increasing invasion of the cancer with its uncertain outcome as well as emotional, physical, financial, social, and spiritual demands, confirm the threatening appraisal.

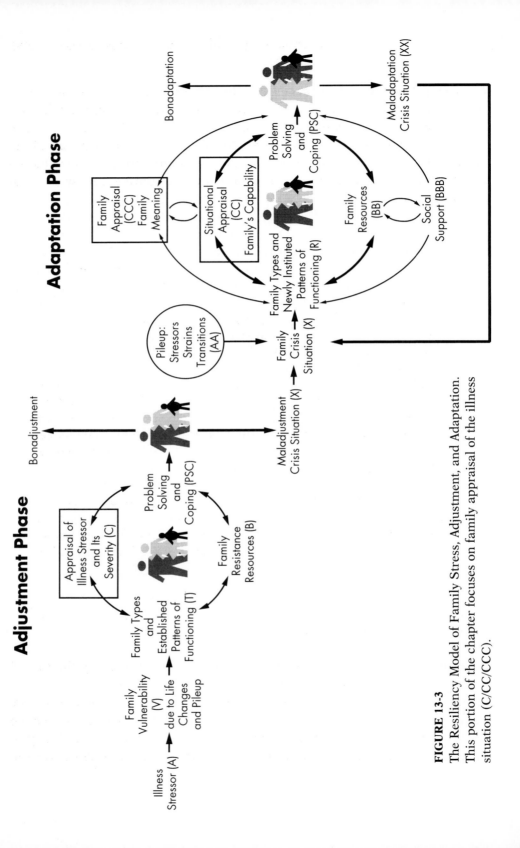

FIGURE 13-3

The Resiliency Model of Family Stress, Adjustment, and Adaptation. This portion of the chapter focuses on family appraisal of the illness situation (C/CC/CCC).

Their worst fears may be realized — the loss of a significant family member. In view of the Resiliency Model, the Matthews question their capabilities (B/BB/BBB) to meet the demands of the situation (A) (Fig. 13-3). The potential for family crisis (X) develops from the strains and stresses of the Matthews' attempts to face the progressive invasion of cancer. As the family perceives the imbalance of demands and resources, they are aware that adaptation is required.

✦ ✦ ✦ ✦ ✦

Initially, Bill and Rita react with dismay to the diagnosis. Bill feels some guilt because one of his first reactions is "thank God, it isn't me." Rita cannot believe that her independent approach to life that has brought her commercial success does not protect her from disease. In spite of the emotional upheaval, their initial appraisal of the situation is that Bill has extensive health insurance and treatment can be attempted. Unfortunately, as time passes and the cancer progresses, Rita and Bill's pessimism and fear about a lack of cure are fulfilled.

The Matthews are emotionally overwhelmed by the illness situation because of their negative appraisal. Rita reacts by isolating herself from others, denying the illness, and does not wish to discuss the circumstances. Bill, as he tries to be cheerful in Rita's presence, initially supports her retreat from reality. The news of the diagnosis is "kept hidden" from other family members, friends, and business associates. As a *fragile family* type, the Matthews' coping devices that served them well in the past will not enable them to cope with this crisis. The low flexibility and low bonding in the Matthews family may assist in perpetuating the threatening appraisal. As the situation progresses, the Matthews find it more difficult to balance resources and demands. This imbalance requires a search for alternatives to deal with the illness.

✦ FAMILY INTERVENTIONS

Application of the Resiliency Model to this life-threatening illness and its impact on the Matthews family provides health-care professionals with important guidelines for intervention. During this life-threatening illness, health-care professionals have numerous opportunities to influence changes in the family situation. Key anxiety-laden times that are likely to occur during the prediagnosis phase, all phases of treatment, during recurrence of advanced disease, at impending death, and death itself carry with them opportunities for family interventions. The Matthews' primary needs are for information about the cancer's demands to plan family reorganization and gather resources and for support in managing the situation. The health-care professional can assist by attending to the family *appraisals* (C/CC/CCC) and to the availability of *resources* (B/BB/BBB). The family appraisal and the resources components of the Resiliency Model influence and contribute to the family's problem-solving capacities (PSC) and therefore govern the level of family adjustment and adaptation (McCubbin & McCubbin, Chapter 2; Fig. 13-3). During this illness situation, the health-care professional's primary focus is to assist the family in developing *manageable* and *positive appraisals* and to maximize the application and development of *individual, family,* and *community resources*. The overall goal of this focus is to increase the opportunity for family bonadjustment and bonadaptation and to decrease the potential for maladjustment and maladaptation.

Developing Manageable, Positive Appraisals

A family's ability to cope with a member with cancer is based on that family's previous coping styles, crisis experiences, perceptions of the illness, and present appraisal of the situation. The health-care professional can prevent maladjustments/maladaptations in those families facing the reality of cancer by helping families develop manageable appraisals of the cancer situation. Many maladaptive family appraisals can easily be corrected in the healthy functioning family. This discussion focuses on those maladaptive appraisals healthy functioning families use to deal with cancer rather than those reflective of preexisting unhealthy functioning of the family system.

In general, certain unfavorable life situations, experiences, and emotional problems appear to predispose the oncology patient to difficulty in coping with cancer. Those with the most trouble suppress, avoid, and deny the truth. As described earlier, Rita had difficulty accepting the diagnosis of cancer. In-control people such as Bill and Rita or domineering individuals in the family may also have difficulty tolerating the loss of control over their lives or the dependency on others. Families with these types of individuals experience a great deal of anger, hostility, and, at times, manipulative behavior. The health-care professional can provide families with constructive avenues for expressing their anger and hostility and encourage problem solving that constructs realistic appraisals.

Previously existing emotional problems are aggravated by cancer. Pessimists show more vulnerability as patients than do those with a more positive outlook. Simonton, Mathews-Simonton, & Creighton (1978) found that these negative attitudes also affect remission rates. Pessimists also have more marital difficulties, experience more depression, feel worthless and destructive, regret their past, and feel a lack of resources that strengthen their lives. Responses common to such people are suppression of emotion, acting-out behaviors, withdrawal, and a feeling of victimization. Thus emotionally unstable families become more so when confronted with cancer. Therefore it is important that health-care professionals work directly with the family's attitude about cancer. Positive imagery and relaxation exercises help.

The period right after a diagnosis of cancer is often a time of anger, fear, and inner confusion. Time to sort out conflicting emotions is needed before a family can express them. Sometimes family members lash out in anger, wishing to find a target for anger and frustration. Family members, including the patient, can become longstanding targets of anger and be blamed for the illness situation (Bluglass, 1986). The health-care professional can prepare families for these emotional reactions and encourage their expression in a supportive, nonaccusatory environment.

A final example of maladaptation is the family that becomes overwhelmed by the threatening appraisal. These families often cannot function as a unit, and disintegrates. Each family member is left to cope on his or her own. Some members retreat and avoid responsibilities. In the extreme situation, although rare, escape can come through suicide. Others, such as Bill, use less destructive tension-reduction strategies such as smoking, drug abuse, and overeating. In these situations the health professional needs to encourage or facilitate alternative appraisals that redefine the situation as a challenge to be faced, thus giving meaning to the situation.

Assessment of the appraisal. The health-care professional is in the crucial position of facilitating the Matthews' adaptation to the diagnosis of cancer. To do this, he or she needs to be cognizant of the demands, existing and needed resources, appraisals of the illness and situation, common maladaptations, and coping characteristics of families facing this illness situation. The health professional attempts to ease the family's adjustment/

adaptation during the ordeal and realizes that each family copes with cancer in its own way depending on its appraisals, strengths, and past experiences. The most useful interventions that health-care professionals can implement fall under the broad categories of assessment, education, and support (Dufault, et al. 1985).

Because each family differs somewhat in its needs while dealing with cancer, health-care professionals need to assess each family carefully. So as to not make assumptions about their appraisal of the situation, health professionals should ask questions about the family's feelings, behavioral symptoms, present coping strategies, and current stressors. Intervention can be based in part on what is worrying the family most at the time. The family receives help in voicing what, when, and how information is being relayed to them. Assessing family typologies can help a health-care professional predict potential problems for the family and plan preventive measures (see Chapter 7 for assessment parameters).

Maximizing Family Resources

Education. Because anxiety is heightened by a family's lack of information or misunderstanding of cancer, education is a major intervention. Today's trend toward sharing information on the cancer diagnosis with the patient and family is well established among health-care professionals. Yet, the family and patient need time and space to adjust to the knowledge of the diagnosis. It is best to give only the necessary information at first. Specific questions are answered, but the family is not bombarded with nonessential facts. Information is repeated as needed and offered in written form. The educational level of the family needs to be considered when giving information. The professional needs to request verbal feedback to assess the family's understanding. Encouraging use of a pocket calendar to record appointment times, diagnostic tests, test preparations, and questions is a helpful suggestion. Others who have experienced similar treatment regimens may help to reinforce information and offer support.

Education is an ongoing process between the health-care professional and family. The patient and family are helped to attain and maintain control when given information about the treatment's purpose, adverse reactions and how to minimize them, as well as the signs and symptoms to report to the health-care provider. Test results, studies, and future interventions are explained.

✦ ✦ ✦ ✦ ✦

The Matthews are fortunate to have an oncologist who is very good at explaining the medical aspects of the illness and a nursing staff that is active with various cancer self-help groups. Bill and Rita are always able to get accurate, timely information. The support from these persons overcomes some of the fear of dependency that characterizes a fragile family such as the Matthews.

Open family communication lines. Some family members can deny the reality of cancer to the extent that they not only refuse to discuss it but also try to hide it from the patient. This makes it almost impossible to support the rest of the family if the diagnosis is hidden from the person with cancer; he or she inevitably learns the truth. The consequences can be deep anger, hurt, or bitterness. The patient might believe that no one is being honest about the diagnosis because the cancer is terminal. Conversely, the person with cancer also can try to protect family and friends from learning the truth. Then each ends up suffering alone, with thoughts and feelings locked within.

Patient, family, and friends usually learn the diagnosis sooner or later. Most people find it easier if everybody can share their feelings instead of hiding them. This frees people to offer each other support. Patients usually agree that hiding the diagnosis from them denies them the right to make important choices about their lives and treatment. Families say patients who try to keep the diagnosis a secret rob loved ones of the chance to express that love and to offer help and support. Family members and intimate friends also bear great emotional burdens and should be able to share them openly with each other and the patient.

False cheer is similar to hiding the truth. In trying to uplift the person with cancer, families may actually cut off his or her attempts to express feelings. When sensing despondency, some people rush in with false reassurances that everything will be all right. Everything is not all right in reality. The person with cancer is left feeling closed off, deserted, and left to face an uncertain world alone. Health-care professionals can encourage families to enjoy the positive and quality moments and to approach the difficulties.

Frequently, family members do not know how to help or what to say to the patient. They avoid interaction, and so do not visit the patient. Family members, by preparing themselves for the possibility of death, can isolate the patient unintentionally. Role play sessions and discussion of what to say can help families approach the situation. The health-care professional is crucial in helping families keep the lines of communication open and honest.

◆ ◆ ◆ ◆ ◆

Rita's prolonged denial of her diagnosis challenged the health-care providers. Directly challenging denial often intensifies it and was not considered an appropriate intervention by the health-care team. To open communication lines, the team worked with Bill to increase his comfort with discussing the illness with Rita. His stated goal of being cheerful in Rita's presence was not supported by the nursing staff. They explained to him the importance of everyone being realistic about the disease. With support, Bill could say the word *cancer* with Rita. His matter-of-fact attitude influenced Rita, who slowly began to participate in her care by asking questions about chemotherapy. The successful decline in denial was demonstrated when Rita bought a wig, anticipating hair loss from the chemotherapy.

Support. Abundant emotional support from others can be facilitated by the health-care professional. The patient and family may be preoccupied with thoughts and questions about life and death. It is important to help the family share thoughts and feelings. Problems can then be defined and solutions discussed. The attention of caring people in the environment helps to relieve possible feelings of despair and isolation.

The health-care professional can refer the family to groups in the community. Participating in a group exposes the family to others coping with similar situations and to recognize that solutions exist for problems that seem overwhelming at the moment. Moreover, the family can realize that feelings and fears are acceptable and appropriate. Group participation encourages the family to care for its own needs through available resources. Prompt relief of the patient's pain through the use of drugs, as well as respect for privacy and dignity, can be enhanced by participating in a group.

Overall, the family appreciates honesty tempered by kindness, sincere optimism, and facilitation of open communication from the health-care professional. Staff can provide the freedom to grieve, a gentle exposure to reality, including viewing disfigurements, while in a protective environment. It is essential to encourage the family to take part in the decision-making process to retain some feeling of control and to maintain a mutually satisfying relationship with the health-care provider.

Sometimes, fragile families, such as the Matthews, when confronted by a crisis (cancer) find strengths they did not know they had. In such situations, a fragile family may change. This did not happen with the Matthews. The health-care professionals needed to offer them information and support continuously as the family had few resources to manage living with cancer and Rita's ultimate death.

Specific Intervention—Cancer

The following is an example of the Matthews' situation and interventions that the health-care professional might employ to facilitate the formation of a manageable family appraisal and to maximize family resources. The announcement of the recurrence of malignant melanoma is a critical time for family intervention since the Matthews are experiencing strong emotions. As they realize that previous ways of coping will not work with this crisis, maladaptive family behaviors may be more easily prevented at this time (Halm, 1990). The family as it struggles to manage the illness stressors is more open to new ideas and support (McCubbin & McCubbin, 1989).

✦ ✦ ✦ ✦ ✦

Bill learns from the oncologist that Rita has been informed about the most recent tests that indicate the cancer has advanced beyond the primary site. When he tries to talk with Rita she becomes tearful, curls up in the fetal position on the couch, and refuses to discuss it. Bill is bewildered and confused as to what is best to do now. The family's worst fears are indeed confirmed. Bill recalls that the staff at the cancer center advised him to be open, honest, and to avoid false cheerfulness during discussions with Rita. He is feeling depressed himself about this latest news and is afraid he will cry in front of Rita if and when she decides to discuss the recurrence. He is missing more days from work and spending more time drinking beers with the boys at their favorite tavern until late in the evening. A housekeeper has been hired and stays with Rita during the day, helps her with Wendy, runs errands, and does grocery shopping for the family. Rita's mother prepares dinner for the family and remains with them for the evenings. She confronts Bill about his late evening hours and remonstrates him about neglecting his family responsibilities. She tells him that Wendy has been complaining about his absences and is having increasing difficulty going to sleep at bedtime. Bill feels increasingly anxious about his family situation and guilty about his own actions.

A family meeting is scheduled at the cancer center to discuss the next step in treatment needed to deal with the recurrence. During discussions with Rita and Bill, the staff notes obvious distress. The staff encourages them to discuss their present state of affairs and feelings with them. Bill and Rita find it easier to discuss their concerns with the help of the staff rather than with just each other. The staff postpones further discussions about treatment and attend to the Matthews' crisis. They conclude the family has an unmanageable appraisal of the illness situation, which in turn is preventing them from using available resources. They need education about the next treatment approaches available and support during the treatment process. The family's communication patterns are not open enough to elicit the needed role changes and mutual support. The staff decides to assist the family first with gaining a manageable appraisal of the illness situation.

Rita and Bill are engaged in a 5-week program to improve their negative attitude toward cancer. They are asked to go through visual imagery and relaxation exercises two times a day. Rita visualizes the cancer being eliminated by radiation treatment. She walks a mile per day. Twice a week the entire family including the grandmother is encouraged to meet to discuss with one of the staff present the meaning this illness has for them. They also explore the impact this situation has on their lives and how they might manage it. The Matthews find this assistance from the staff very reassuring. Their confusion, bewilderment, and avoidance is gradually replaced with hope that this illness situation, although difficult, can be managed. Rita now can visualize her life proceeding in spite of the cancer. She still cries often and begins to ask "why me." The staff is available to listen to her concerns.

The staff soon realizes that Wendy has never been told about Rita's illness. Wendy is a precocious 4 year old and is very aware that her parents and grandmother are very upset. She has been confiding to her grandmother that she knows something is wrong with her mother and believes it is her fault. She knows she has been a "bad girl" and is afraid her mother and father have been avoiding her because of this. She misses the nightly bedtime stories her father used to tell her. Now it seems that he does not get home in time. During a family meeting the staff encourages the Matthews to discuss Rita's illness with Wendy. Rita does not want to be the one to tell Wendy but agrees that someone should tell her. Bill does not wish to tell her either because he fears he will become too emotional and frighten her even more. The staff suggests enlisting the grandmother's help. Wendy is close to her grandmother and has confided in her about previous concerns. The grandmother is agreeable to this suggestion. During additional family meetings the staff teaches the grandmother how much and how to tell Wendy, using her age and level of maturity as a guide. The grandmother uses a doll to demonstrate the problem and the treatment. The goal is to let Wendy express her feelings and ask questions about the cancer. Bill and Rita also explore with the staff ways to respond to Wendy's feelings and questions.

Gradually, the staff helps the Matthews open their lines of communication with each other. Foundations of mutual understanding and trust are established through sharing concerns about the cancer's recurrence. The family is helped with what they can say to and do for each other. Attention on Rita is refocused on what she has to offer rather than on what she has lost.

This chapter has illustrated the application and usefulness of the theoretical components of McCubbin and McCubbin's Resiliency Model of Family Stress, Adjustment, and Adaptation. It demonstrated the powerful impact a family's typology, resources, and appraisal of cancer has on coping ability. The health-care professional provides valuable assistance to the family facing crisis through the family interventions of assessment, education, and support. The information in this chapter has significance for families and health-care professionals dealing with other life-threatening illnesses with similar stressor dimensions.

REFERENCES

American Cancer Society (1989). *Cancer facts and figures*. New York: American Cancer Society.

Bluglass, K. (1986). Caring for the family. In B. A. Stoll (Ed.), *Coping with cancer stress* (pp. 149-154). Boston: Martinus Nijhoff.

Dirksen, S. R. (1989). Perceived well-being in malignant melanoma survivors. *Oncology Nursing Forum, 16*(3), 353-358.

Donovan, M. I., & Girton, S. E. (1984). *Cancer care nursing* (2nd ed.). Norwalk, CT: Appleton-Century-Crofts.

DuFault, K., Sr., Firsich, S. C., Gardner, A., Jones, M., Mosley J. R., & Stone, S. (1985). Ineffective family coping. In J. C. McNally, J. C. Stair, & E. T. Somerville (Eds.), *Guidelines for cancer nursing practice* (pp. 66-72). Orlando, FL: Grune & Stratton.

Fraser, M. (1982). The role of the nurse in the prevention and early detection of malignant melanoma. *Cancer Nursing, 5*(5), 351-360.

Friedman, B. D. (1980). Coping with cancer: A guide for health care professionals. *Cancer Nursing, 3*(2), 105-110.

Greany, D., & Goldsmith, H. S. (1985). Cutaneous melanoma: diagnosis and surgical intervention. *AORN, 42*(1), 43-49.

Halm, M. A. (1990). Effects of support groups on anxiety of family members during critical illness. *Heart and Lung, 19*(1), 62-71.

Hickey, S. S. (1986). Enabling hope. *Cancer Nursing, 9*(3), 133-137.

Lawler, P. E., & Schreiber, S. (1989). Cutaneous malignant melanoma: Nursing's role in prevention and early detection. *Oncology Nursing Forum, 16*(3), 345-352.

Levanthal, H., Levanthal, E. A., & Van

Nguyen, T. (1985). Reactions of families to illness: Theoretical models and perspectives. In D. C. Turk & R. D. Kerns (Eds.), *Health, illness, and families* (pp. 108-145). New York: John Wiley and Sons.

Lewandowski, W., & Jones, S. L. (1988). The family with cancer: Nursing interventions throughout the course of living with cancer. *Cancer Nursing, 11*(6), 313-321.

Longman, A. J., & Graham, K. Y. (1986). Living with melanoma: Content analysis of interviews. *Oncology Nursing Forum, 13*(4), 58-64.

McCubbin, M. A., & McCubbin, H. I.

(1989). Theoretical orientations to family stress and coping. In C. F. Figley (Ed.), *Treating stress in families* (pp. 3-43). New York: Brunner/Mazel.

Scanlon, C. (1989). Creating a vision of hope: The challenge of palliative care. *Oncology Nursing Forum, 16*(4), 491-496.

Schleper, J. (1984). Cancer prevention and detection: Skin cancer. *Cancer Nursing, 7*(1), 67-84.

Simonton, O., Mathews-Simonton, S., & Creighton, J. (1978). *Getting well again: A step-by-step, self-help guide to overcome cancer for patients and families.* (pp. 1-125). Los Angeles: Tarcher.

Sontag, S. (1977). *Illness as metaphor.* New York: Vintage.

Starr, J. C. (1985). Knowledge deficit related to prevention and early detection of malignant melanoma. In J. C. McNally, J. C. Stair, & E. T. Somerville (Eds.), *Guidelines for cancer nursing practice* (pp. 23-27). Orlando, FL: Grune & Stratton.

Stewart, D. S. (1990). Indoor tanning: The nurse's role in preventing skin damage. In C. R. Ash & J. F. Jenkins (Eds.), *Enhancing the role of cancer nursing* (pp. 79-94). New York: Raven.

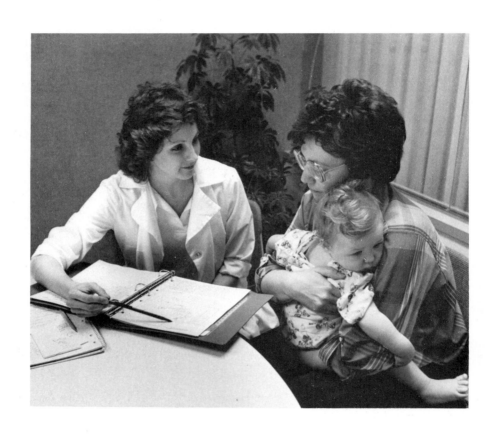

Acute, Recurrent, and Resolvable Mental Illness: Depression

✦

CHAPTER GOALS

✦ To illustrate the impact that depression, as an acute, recurrent mental illness, can have on a family system

✦ To analyze the demands of supporting and caring for a depressed family member

✦ To exemplify the range of coping mechanisms observed among families confronted with mental illness

✦ To propose possible family-oriented interventions that might be used with mental illness

OVERVIEW

THIS chapter examines in detail the demands of caring for a family member with an acute mental illness—depression. The discussion about the demands of depression illustrates the variety of illness stressor dimensions found in mental illness that are important in determining the impact this illness can have on an entire family system. The chapter begins with a vignette describing the Mendelsons' family situation and the aspects of depression with which they are coping. The chapter is organized by the components of the Resiliency Model (see Chapter 2) and discusses depression in relation to the demands of the illness situation—the stressor (A); resources available to the Mendelsons—the resources (B/BB/BBB); and the Mendelsons' appraisals of the illness situation—the appraisals (C/CC/CCC). The last section of the chapter offers suggestions for family interventions that meet the demands of a mental illness and concludes with an example of the need and value of family interventions during depression.

✦ THE FAMILY SITUATION

✦ ✦ ✦ ✦ ✦

Jeremiah Mendelson is a successful 59-year-old businessman. For the past 30 years he has built BPS Business Associates into one of the most respected and profitable accounting firms in the region. Started in the extra bedroom in the family home, the firm now occupies its own building in a new office complex and employs 17 people.

However, Jeremiah is unhappy. To him it seems that everything in his life is falling apart, including himself. It began 2 years ago when his mother died; it never seemed right to have placed her in that nursing home. Then last year when their youngest son, Jeff, went off to college, the big new house on Brentwood Drive seemed so empty. Most days Jeremiah feels old and useless. The work that had once been so important to him now seems mundane and insignificant. In fact, some days he cannot muster the energy to go to work; he does not call in sick, and no one there mentions his absence. Margaret, his wife of 35 years, is worried about him. However, she has never "meddled" in his business affairs.

Jeremiah finds himself waking up at 3:00 or 4:00 AM and lying awake for the next 4 hours thinking about things he has done wrong in the past. He is aware of his poor appetite and that he has lost about 10 pounds over the past 2 months. Jeremiah becomes more nervous and is easily upset. Margaret suggests he go for a physical checkup. His family physician recognizes that he is suffering from a depressive syndrome and refers him to a psychiatrist for treatment.

Jeremiah describes himself to the psychiatrist as feeling extremely anxious, worthless, and sad. He feels great remorse over some business decisions he had to make in firing some staff and over allowing his mother to be admitted to the nursing home. He thinks his family would be better off without him and has considered shooting himself. He fears he would even fail at that and so has not taken action. The psychiatrist decides to admit Jeremiah to an inpatient treatment unit. He is treated with tricyclic

> ### *Illness Stressor Dimensions Characteristic of the Mendelsons' Case of Depression*
>
> ---
>
> Gradual *onset*
> Short *duration* with possible recurrence
> Uncertain *predictability*
> Great *social stigma*
> Unknown *causes*
> *Origin* from both inside and outside the family
> Moderate *severity*
> Medium to large *resource demands*
> Manageable *control*
> High *extent* of family impact

antidepressant medication. He improves markedly within 3 weeks and returns home to resume his business.

The preceding vignette is the beginning of a narrative designed to illustrate the impact that stressor dimensions found in acute, recurrent mental illnesses can place on families. The Mendelsons' situation exemplifies common family reactions and needs in mental illness. The box above lists illness stressor dimensions characteristic of the Mendelsons' case of depression (see also Chapter 4).

Acute, recurrent mental illnesses such as depression require continuing family adjustment and adaptation. Due to the negative stigma and recurrent nature of depression, the family unlikely will ever return to its previous configurations. The effects of depression are ongoing and recur with each new episode of the illness. Family adjustment and adaptation can certainly be enhanced by mutually supportive relationships with health-care professionals (McCubbin & McCubbin, Chapter 2). The recurrent nature of depression begs for health-care professional intervention around the coordination of family and community support systems.

✦ THE ILLNESS: DEPRESSION

Recent government studies show that approximately 29 million adults, one in five, suffer from some form of mental or emotional illness in any

6-m onth period. (U. S. Department of Health and Human Services, 1986). An additional 50 million suffer the anxiety of relating to a family member with this disability. In fact, more hospital beds are occupied by the mentally ill than by the total number of patients with cancer and lung and heart diseases.

Some $30 billion is spent each year on behalf of patients afflicted with mental illness. Yet, third-party payers often offer only minimum coverage for psychiatric illness. There are many different types of mental illness, just as there are many different medical diseases. Mental illnesses differ greatly in severity, symptoms, outcome, and effect on the patient and family. Basically, four common types of severe mental illness exist: affective disorders, schizophrenia, anxiety disorders, and dementias. Unfortunately, causes, cures, and treatments are still being sought and need much more research. A stigma is attached to those suffering from these mental illnesses.

At any given time, four people out of 100 are suffering from a relatively severe depressive syndrome, an affective disorder. Yet, psychotic depression is relatively uncommon, accounting for less than 10% of all depressions. Only about 25% of depressed people seek attention from a mental health provider. Depression is high among patients hospitalized for physical illnesses. This depression is associated with different conditions such as the amount of pain and the severity of the physical illness (Derogatis & Wise, 1989). Gastrointestinal, neurological, and respiratory diseases frequently bring on depression. Unfortunately, depression can be masked by such symptoms as headaches, gastrointestinal complaints, weakness, fatigue, dizziness, and other physical symptoms that cannot otherwise be explained. (Cassem, 1987). Therefore these depressions are largely unrecognized and untreated by health-care professionals (Derogatis & Wise, 1989).

Families have confronted mental illness for years. Mental illness has been a dreadful experience for those patients suffering from it and has a varying impact on the family. Families who do the direct caregiving or maintain the patient close to home have a heavier burden (Morgan, 1989). The meaning the illness has for the family influences the emotional burden. Mental health professionals have added to the family's anguish by bringing forth one family trait after another as the cause of mental illness. Families' abilities to cope with mental illness depend in a large part on the adequacy of community support available to them. A study by Morgan (1989) reports that relatives of the mentally ill often have a difficult, at times traumatic, experience when seeking emergency care for a family member who is deteriorating mentally and who may be unwilling to seek assistance.

✦ DEMANDS OF THE ILLNESS STRESSOR (A)

This portion of the chapter describes and illustrates the demands a mental illness stressor (A) places on the Mendelson family (Fig. 14-1). Each stressor dimension encompassed in depression forms demands on the Mendelsons in varying degrees. The Mendelsons are a *resilient family* type with high family bonding and high family flexibility. This family's major strengths lie in their ability to change and their sense of internal unity (McCubbin & McCubbin, 1989). The impact of this family typology (T) on the illness situation is indicated.

Onset, Origin, and Cause

In comparison to illnesses due to physical injury or infection, the onset of depression is slow and insidious. What triggers it is not fully understood. For some depressions, such as Jeremiah's, there are obvious precipitants while for others there are no precipitants. Current psychiatric thought contends that a range of causative factors such as genetic vulnerability, family processes, developmental events, and physiological and psychosocial stressors may be responsible for depression. In Jeremiah's situation such factors would be the death of his mother, stress from his business, and possible biochemical changes of aging.

Severity

Depression is the most common psychiatric disorder. Early Egyptian medical texts described the syndrome at least 3000 years ago. It is part of the human condition that is familiar to all and yet mysterious to many. Its impact on the community is difficult to determine. Child care, marital relations, and general productivity are all affected (Munoz, 1987). Depression may range from mild and moderate states to severe states with psychotic features. Approximately 10 to 14 million Americans currently have some form of a major affective disorder. The World Health Organization states that the annual worldwide rate of depression is 3% to 5%, or 100 million people (Charney & Weisman, 1988). It is estimated that 15% to 30% of adults have depressive episodes, most often of moderate severity, at some point in their lives, with the onset peaking in their forties and fifties. This is Jeremiah's situation.

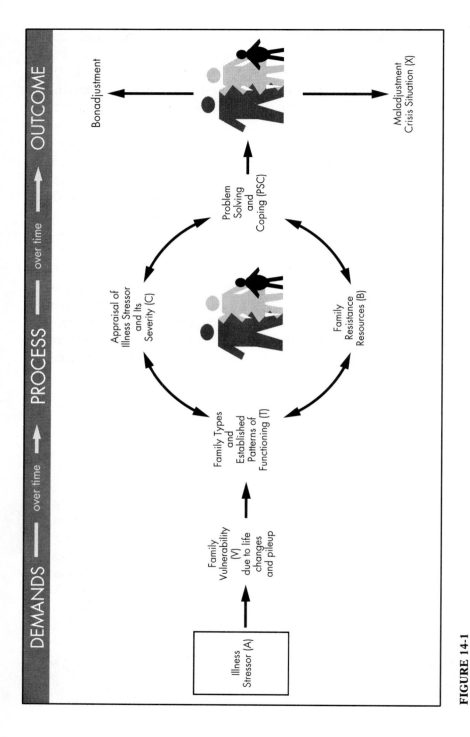

FIGURE 14-1

Adjustment Phase of the Resiliency Model of Family Stress, Adjustment, and Adaptation. This portion of the chapter focuses on the demands of the illness stressor (A).

Suicide, the potential risk in Jeremiah's case, is the most serious complication. Although more women than men attempt suicide, men are more successful and have the highest suicide rate (Lindenthal, 1988). Suicide is the tenth leading cause of death in the United States. Of all psychiatric visits to the emergency room 15% were by individuals with suicide ideation or attempts (Boyer & Guthrie, 1985). About 15% of all hospitalized patients suffering from depression die by suicide eventually. As it is common practice to hospitalize the more severely depressed individuals, suicide is more common in hospital psychiatric units than in the community (Fish & Snyder, 1985). Approximately 60% of all suicides reported by Barradaugh and Palin were attributable to depression, but other studies report lower rates of 30% to 45% (Montgomery, 1990).

Social and personal complications also are common, as in Jeremiah's situation. Decreased energy, poor concentration, and lack of interest cause poor performance at work. Apathy and decreased sexual interest lead to marital tension. Unlike Jeremiah, some patients may attempt to treat depressive symptoms themselves with sedatives, alcohol, or stimulants, thus starting problems with drug and alcohol abuse. All these complications serve to increase the degree to which the demands of the illness reverberate throughout the entire family system.

Stigma and the Extent of the Illness's Impact on the Family

Adjustment phase

✦ ✦ ✦ ✦ ✦

The Mendelsons are pleased with the outcome of Jeremiah's psychiatric treatment. They view his depression as a resolvable condition. From this perspective, whatever adjustments were needed to cope with the illness would be only temporary, since Jeremiah now appears to be back to normal. Health insurance covered 80% of the hospitalization costs. Jeremiah's time away from his business was not much different from his yearly 3-week vacation. Business matters were handled by his office staff.

The home regimen went unchanged except for Jeremiah's absence. Margaret carried on household chores and meal preparations as usual. Jeremiah's condition did cause her to worry for awhile. It was unpleasant to see him so listless and down on himself. Margaret never knew he felt so guilty about his past decisions. It was frightening to consider the possibility of his death or the loss of his business if he had committed suicide or the continuance of his depression. The Mendelsons are financially stable and well invested for retirement, but they would miss their current life-style should Jeremiah be unable to work. Also, their responsibility to continue supporting Jeff throughout college would be difficult if not impossible. Margaret hopes Jeremiah's condition was only temporary, caused by their youngest child leaving home and the realization of approaching old age.

Margaret and Jeremiah's two oldest children, Marie, age 30, and Pat, age 34, are married with their own homes and families to manage. They live in nearby states. Marie and Pat demonstrate the strong bonds of unity found in resilient family types by keeping in frequent telephone contact and visiting the house on Brentwood Drive for major holidays. They have been worried about their dad's condition. Family members easily talk concerns through and readily offer mutual support for each other. Marie and Pat took turns staying with their mother while Jeremiah was hospitalized. The family views outside help from the psychiatrist as being the best solution, since the medication seems to have ensured Jeremiah's recovery. In general, the flexibility of the resilient family type serves them well, as the family has no difficulty deciding what to do as a family unit.

When Jeremiah returns to his business and full-time work hours, tensions for the family begin building again. Jeremiah has some mild side effects from the medication such as dryness of mouth and hand tremors. He feels like he is in "a fog" and finds that his thinking processes are slower. He wonders if people at work notice these changes because he overhears them commenting about his trip to the "looney bin." Neighbors and friends have made similar remarks about his psychiatric treatment. Jeremiah tells Margaret that he is thinking about discontinuing his medication. Margaret becomes very upset about this and asks that he take the medications with her watching from now on. Both fear a recurrence of his depression.

Adaptation phase

✦ ✦ ✦ ✦ ✦

The Mendelsons make every effort to cope with Jeremiah's depression while maintaining the family's routines and basic patterns of functioning established long before his first illness. Six months pass. Jeremiah continues to be troubled about the medication's side effects. Suicidal thoughts return, and he tells Margaret about them. The family decides to change psychiatrists and seeks help at a nationally known psychiatric center. Jeremiah's medication is adjusted, and different combinations of medications are tried.

The family is invited to participate in a group designed to support families with mental illness. The Mendelsons are able to discuss and confront their concerns about the depression recurring and what to do with people's attitudes and comments about psychiatric care. Jeremiah enters into individual treatment to help him process his concerns about his mother and present feelings of guilt. The Mendelsons accept that Jeremiah may need treatment on an ongoing basis. This acceptance and the family's active participation in treatment help reduce tension.

Duration, Predictability, and Control

Jeremiah's situation illustrates many common features of depression. Depression is psychologically very painful, and its pain is not easily forgotten. The fear of suffering another depression tends to haunt people, even when they have responded well to medication in the past and know they would likely do so again. The outlook for patients suffering from depression is very good. The treatment of choice is a combination of drug therapy and family therapy (American Psychiatric Association, 1989). The overall success rate of drugs for the treatment of depression is 60% to 80%. Electroconvulsive therapy can help those who do not respond well to medication. Some control over the illness is therefore possible. Even untreated, a depressive episode seldom lasts more than 9 months. On the other hand, depression tends to recur. The patient is typically well for many months or years, but approximately 30% to 50% are likely to have a recurrence. So the concern about recurrence is justified (Kaplan & Sadock, 1981; Taylor, 1990). Treatment can reduce symptoms but not guarantee a cure. Its onset is relatively unpredictable, and its intensity and severity can greatly vary.

Resource Demands

Family care of a depressed person offers many benefits to the mentally ill member but also makes special demands on the household. This partial or episodic disability in an adult member can strain family resources. As in Jeremiah's situation, the family experiences the stress of caregiving, emotional burden, and residential problems. Certain general family characteristics help people cope with mental illness. The Mendelson family may need to develop these characteristics.

Caregiving. When a family assumes a caregiving or supervisory function, it takes on roles that involve additional stress. Medication supervision often raises concerns about "policing" a loved one. Liaison activities with health and social services take time and effort, since they often demand negotiation of services within complex and poorly coordinated systems. Although some health professionals now believe that attempts to treat the mentally ill individual independently of the family are futile, many mental health systems are designed to communicate with clients as individuals and not their relatives. This kind of communication can be frustrating. Families may feel rebuffed if they act on behalf of their members and neglectful if they leave them to fend for themselves. If the acute illness recurs, it may raise intense feelings in the family, including fears of betraying the ill family member by calling for outside help. They may have doubts about what might have been done to prevent recurrence and disappointment about the relapse.

Emotional burden. Goldman (1982) notes that emotional problems burden families of the mentally ill as heavily as economic concerns. Families report distress about behaviors they consider embarrassing or inappropriate. They have problems with the stigma of mental illness (Geiser, Hich, & King, 1988). One additional and unfortunate problem for families is the guilt surrounding mental illness, which not only adds to the emotional burden but also distances families from sources of support and assistance. This sense of guilt is in part attributed to the psychodynamic theories that consider family interaction to be a factor contributing to mental illness. Indeed, family interaction influences the course of the illness.

Mental illness, especially if recurrent, can put great strain on marriages. The mentally ill spouse may be unable to contribute to the relationship and may require the partner to become a care provider (Group for Advancement of Psychiatry, 1986). Tessler, Bernstein, Rosen, and Goldman (1982) found that only 12% of a sample of persons with mental illness receiving community support services were currently married. For single adult clients, family dependence means dependence on families of origin, generally parents. As mentally ill persons near middle age, parents may be elderly and ill-equipped to manage a home for them. Older clients may have no living relatives.

Residential burdens. Aging or illness of other members of a household may influence a family's ability to maintain the member at home. Practical concerns are also important. Nuclear families often live in homes that are too small to accommodate an additional adult. It may even be difficult for concerned relatives to make room for an extra person. Mobile families may become scattered geographically, so there may be no relatives in the client's community who are able to share a stable home.

Needed family characteristics. Some general characteristics help families cope with a mentally disabled or ill member. These characteristics include the ability to go through some life-style changes that may alter physical, emotional, intellectual, social, and spiritual areas. Nutrition and physical fitness are important areas of a family's life-style. Proper nutrition and physical fitness can help to sustain the assault of stress.

Spiritual development can reduce the family's stress. Spirituality involves finding a meaning in life. Meaning provides a perspective from which to view the struggle of life. Such insight can help a family to integrate the confusing and disorienting impact of their stresses. A family with the ability to develop a positive meaning of the illness situation can appreciate the larger picture and be more compassionate and understanding.

Attitudinal shifts toward the appreciation of individual worth are important for coping with depression in a family member. Family members' potential for personal, organizational, and legislative influence increases as their appreciation of their own worth increases. They learn to reach to others for support to cope with daily stresses, solve problems, and advocate for specific reforms. As families become more helpful to themselves and others, they feel more hopeful. They learn to take charge of their lives through increased information, skills, and support.

✦ ✦ ✦ ✦ ✦

In considering the demands on Jeremiah Mendelson's family, all members have the potential to face all the previously discussed problems. Jeremiah's absence and unusual behavior at work will influence his employees' and colleagues' opinions about him. His business may be affected. It will be difficult for people to understand why a man who has everything should be depressed. They may perceive it as a fault in his character and abilities. He and his wife will need help in discussing the problem and then consider ways to include their son and daughters. The fear of recurrence will be an uncertainty that both Jeremiah and his wife find troubling.

◆ RESOURCES AVAILABLE TO THE FAMILY (B/BB/BBB)

This portion of the chapter examines the strengths and weaknesses of resources available to the Mendelson family. Within the framework of the Resiliency Model, resources are described as encompassing both tangible and coping resources of the family and its community (Fig. 14-2; see McCubbin & McCubbin, Chapter 2). These resources are (1) personal resources of the individual family members, (2) collectively held family resources, and (3) community resources including social support. The Mendelson family will use all three resources to deal with the demands of this mental illness. These resources serve as family strengths in decreasing stress and preventing crisis during the illness situation.

Personal and Family Resources (B/BB)

◆ ◆ ◆ ◆ ◆

As individuals, both Jeremiah and Margaret have good personal resources. They are intelligent and educated, as are their children. They have coped with previous crises in their lives. They have personal leisure activities that give them pleasure and a sense of well-being. Their children, although grown and living away from home, are a source of pride and support.

As a resilient family type, the Mendelsons have many strengths that assist in managing this mental illness. Their sense of internal unity forms the needed supports and their flexibility makes adaptation easier. Resilient families are emotionally close and enjoy being with one another (McCubbin & McCubbin, 1989). They approach problems with a sense of curiosity and optimism that they will be alright, no matter what the outcome of the problem. Shifting roles and responsibilities within the family are easily accomplished for these families. They are able to give and receive support from one another.

The financial aspects of this situation are adequate. Jeremiah has a good income, and his business subscribes to a health insurance plan that covers mental illness services. Only 80% of his hospital expenses were covered, however. The financial burden in this case is minimal but not necessarily typical. Many health insurance plans have poor coverage for mental illness services. Therefore the majority of costs must be paid directly by the family, or the family goes without the services. Families with low incomes would find it difficult to pay for these services.

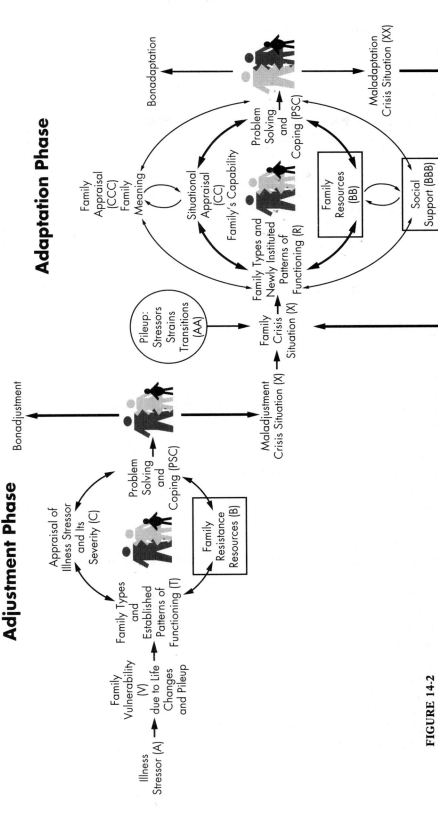

Adjustment Phase

Adaptation Phase

FIGURE 14-2

The Resiliency Model of Family Stress, Adjustment, and Adaptation. This portion of the chapter focuses on family resources and social support (B/BB/BBB).

Community Resources (BBB)

✦ ✦ ✦ ✦ ✦

The Mendelsons live in a large city with many available resources. Their physician is a family practitioner who has cared for the whole family since the children were young. Many psychiatrists practice in the area, some specializing in family therapy. This gives the Mendelsons choices in treatment of the illness. Nearby is a large medical center with a psychiatric unit that encourages family participation. Several mental health centers are in the area as well. The local chapter of the National Alliance for the Mentally Ill is very active and sponsors mutual support groups for families with mentally ill members. The fee for participating in these mutual support groups is minimal.

The Mendelsons are active in their church, and the clergyman has made himself available to them. They have many friends in the church that have been helpful. However, several friends are not comfortable with mental illness and are clearly avoiding the Mendelsons.

✦ FAMILY APPRAISALS OF THE ILLNESS SITUATION (C/CC/CCC)

The family's appraisal of depression arises from its perception of the existing balance between demands and resources for the illness situation (Fig. 14-3). During Jeremiah's initial encounter with depression, the duration of his illness is short-term, and the family quickly adjusts to the situation. Depression is viewed as a perplexing yet resolvable entity. It is with the depression's recurrence and attached societal stigma that the Mendelsons realize its *threat* to the integrity of the family. The recurrent duration, great social stigma, lack of unpredictability, and strain on emotional family resources strongly contribute to the development of this threatening appraisal. The greatest threat to the Mendelsons is meeting the long-term demands of the treatment, the social stigma, and the fear of recurrence of depression. In view of the Resiliency Model (Fig. 14-3), the Mendelson family may question its capabilities (B/BB/BBB) to meet the demands of the situation (A). The potential for family crisis (X) develops as the Mendelsons attempt to deal with each new recurrence of depression and the accompanying social stigma. As the family perceives an imbalance of demand and resources, it is aware that adaptation is required.

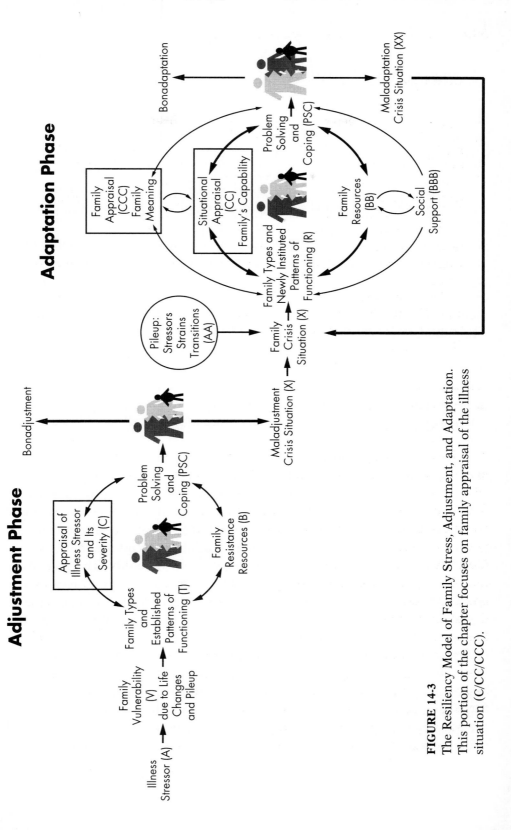

FIGURE 14-3

The Resiliency Model of Family Stress, Adjustment, and Adaptation. This portion of the chapter focuses on family appraisal of the illness situation (C/CC/CCC).

Sources of Social Stigma

For centuries people have misunderstood the nature of mental illness. This has led to the fear, embarrassment, shame, and guilt connected with mental illness. Patients and families have thought of it as a punishment that God imposes on sinners, as a spiritual torment due to possession by the devil, or as a moral defect due to weakness of will. In earlier centuries the mentally ill were burned at the stake or crushed to death because they were thought to be "possessed." Others were chained in filthy cells for much of their lives. Only a century ago people amused themselves by watching the inhabitants of Bedlam, as if the mentally ill were animals in a zoo. These accounts appear far removed from the Mendelsons' experiences.

In the 1990s the mentally ill are no longer put into chains. Yet these people and their families are still victims of subtler versions of social stigmatization, cruelty, and prejudice. This prejudice grows out of ignorance and misunderstanding about mental illness. Many people fail to realize that mental illness is partly caused by biological forces, not by moral turpitude. Sontag (1977) describes the fear surrounding any disease that is not understood in an era when medicine's central premise is that all diseases can be cured. In Jeremiah's situation, recall the "looney bin" remarks made by his staff and neighbors.

People cannot afford to remain ignorant about mental illness because it affects almost everyone's life. It is possibly the most common type of illness today. Yet the pandemic incidence of mental illness leads to ambivalent feelings. On the one hand, people are genuinely curious to learn more and to understand the facts. On the other hand, they are frightened and embarrassed. Fear and embarrassment lead them to ignore, to deny, and even to dislike anything pertaining to psychiatric health care. For many people, "You need to see a shrink" is still the ultimate insult. Consequently, families may not trust the available health-care services. As in Jeremiah's case, families may discontinue treatment or change health-care professionals.

The family and the ill member with mental illness are left to feel guilty about the episodes of mental illness and to worry about the professional and social consequences of seeking treatment. This is unfortunate, since some illness episodes respond well to treatment. Society often penalizes those people who admit they are ill and are seeking treatment again. Persons with a history of mental illness, including depression, are passed over for promotions, not hired, or not accepted into schools. These persons are considered less reliable, responsible, and stable, as well as more emotional, than others. The mentally ill are stigmatized; the general public expects them to be generally incompetent, disruptive, and incurable (Segal & Baunmohl, 1988). Because of mental illness, people distance themselves, avoid, or even disdain, the patient. As a resilient family, the Mendelsons are able to give and receive positive support from one another. Unfortunately, several of their neighborhood friends now avoid them and exclude them from the usual dinner invitations.

These perceptions not only have colored personal and professional attitudes about mental illness, but also have influenced society's investment in various treatment programs for the mentally ill. The mentally ill are treated in the hospital rather than in community-based programs. Only in recent years has the focus of care shifted to the community. Family care has not been the intent of Western culture. Yet an estimated 65% of patients return home to live with their families (Goldman, 1982). Only about a quarter of the U. S. population has access to a community mental health center despite numerous recent attempts at the federal level to legislate universal mental health programs (Mosher & Burti, 1989). Jeremiah is fortunate to have the resources to seek private treatment.

In summary, society's attitude toward mental illness (contributing to CCC of the Resiliency Model) can be a destructive force in a family's ability to cope. Many patients, family members, health professionals, and potential sources of support hold these negative viewpoints. Therefore families find it difficult to obtain needed resources to reduce the stress of caregiving, of seeking treatment and residence, and of resolving problems associated with mental illness.

◆ ◆ ◆ ◆ ◆

In appraising Jeremiah's depression, the Mendelson family was concerned about the negative impression the diagnosis of depression would create in the community. However, being a resilient family, they decide to learn how to overcome this challenge to their family's happiness. They discuss the meaning of the illness with Jeremiah's psychiatric nurse. They attend meetings of the local chapter of the National Alliance for the Mentally Ill, and seek the support of their clergyman. After a "crash course" in depression and its treatment, the Mendelsons appraised Jeremiah's illness as a serious problem that could be managed.

✦ FAMILY INTERVENTIONS

Application of the Resiliency Model to the Mendelsons' family situation with depression provides health-care professionals with important guidelines for intervention. During this recurrent illness, health-care professionals will have several opportunities to influence changes in the family situation. Key times for these opportunities are likely to be during the initial diagnosis, engagement in treatment, reentry to the community, and during recurrent episodes. The Mendelsons' primary needs will be for information and support to manage depression's demands for family reorganization and resources. The health-care professional can assist families by attending to the family *appraisals* (C/CC/CCC) and to the presence of *resources* (B/BB/BBB) at these key times. The family appraisal and the resource components of the Resiliency Model influence and contribute to the family's problem-solving capacities (PSC) and therefore govern the level of family adjustment and adaptation (Fig. 14-3; see McCubbin & McCubbin, Chapter 2). During an illness situation, the family-oriented health-care professional's primary focus is to assist the family to develop *manageable, positive appraisals* and to maximize the application and development of *individual, family,* and *community resources.* The overall goal of this focus is to increase the opportunity for family bonadjustment and bonadaptation and to decrease the potential for maladjustment and maladaptation.

Developing Manageable, Positive Appraisals

Due to the negative social stigma of mental illness, health-care professionals may observe a number of potentially maladaptive behaviors in families who are helping a family member with mental illness. Family embarrassment may be devastating, and guilt fostered by social stigmatization may arise. Family members may then feel low member satisfaction and display this overtly or covertly. Social stigma has in effect produced a negative family appraisal that impacts family and individual self-esteem.

Another common and obvious difficulty is that the family cannot maintain a balance as it passes through the usual transitional stages of family life and periods of stress. Each transitional stage seems to prompt a crisis. As the ill member reaches another developmental stage, the family finds itself in a state of chaos with little understanding or forewarning that this could occur. The crisis often follows each transition that the ill member attempts. Depending on the family dynamics, crisis may occur because the family appraisal involves the belief that the emotional problems reside in the identified patient, rather than seeing them as a function of each person in the family. In some cases family therapy may be needed to overcome these difficulties and alter the appraisal.

Sometimes the family can be overprotective of its ill member. In part, this may be a reaction to protect the family from negative social status related to the embarrassing and socially unacceptable behaviors of the ill person. If this overprotection occurs to the extent that the once ill family member is prevented from taking age-appropriate responsibility or obvious overcloseness or fusion exists between family members, then the family is maladapting. Emotions need expression when they are felt. Peace cannot be maintained at any price. The family must become adept at balancing affective expression, careful rational thought, relationship focus, care-taking, and object orientation. Thus the overinvolved and overprotective family is not the healthiest for the member with mental illness. Maladaptation also can occur when problems are approached with distance and avoidance. Health professionals facilitating an appraisal that frames the family within close to normal expectations without overprotecting or ignoring the mentally ill member can foster family bonadaptation (Saylor, 1990).

The emotional contact maintained across generations and between family members is an important component. When lines of authority and generational identity are ill defined and members are acting out because of a lack of effective limit-setting by agreed- on family figures, then role expectations can be difficult to achieve and also confusing to the patient. The family confronting mental illness needs to solve numerous problems, and that process is an important function. Maladaptive behaviors are those that occur when problems are rarely addressed, or left to a third person, or members take opposing sides. Yet differences between family members are a healthy characteristic to encourage for personal growth and creativity. A family appraisal that tolerates differences and is able to reconcile differences around problems will allow better flexibility for adaptation.

Positive family appraisals can be developed by creating a spiritually fulfilling philosophy of life. A philosophy with personal meanings that support efforts and provide understanding and forgiveness for their limitations will be especially valuable. This philosophy may contain a belief that encourages their feelings of worth and that of respect for others. Family members need to have some challenges and exciting things to do. Focusing on important tasks, directions, and people in their lives can be a great source of energy and satisfaction. It is important for family members to acknowledge that they cannot take good care of others if they do not take care of themselves. When they are not acting in their own best interest, they are modeling how not to live successfully.

Maximizing Family Resources

How well families manage mental illness can depend on the adequacy of the community supports available and how well the families use them. Families dealing with mental illness need community resources similar to those identified by Hatfield (1979) to cope with their situation. These resources are in the form of *education, formal and informal support, respite care,* and *crises services.* Giving support to families depends on the degree to which professionals understand the family experience. Grunebaum and Friedman (1988) point out that health-care professionals need to have a nonjudgmental attitude and should try to collaborate with the family. Interventions that seem most useful center around an effort to find the family community support that meets family needs. The health professional needs to help the family balance the demands of mental illness with available resources.

Health professionals need to educate the family about mental illness and encourage the family's active participation in the patient's treatment (Francell, Conn, & Gray, 1988). The professional assists relatives in assigning priorities to their concerns and teaches them basic behavioral techniques for dealing with the patient. The professional facilitates self-help and support among families with similar concerns. Support is offered by the professional, assuming the role of ombudsman for the family and avoiding assignment of blame for the patient's problems. The professional is an essential link with other parts of the health-care system, helping to identify community resources or to alert the community to the need for a new service. In sum, professionals serve as a role model of effective communicators, educators, advocates, and facilitators for the family.

Education. One important resource health-care professionals can provide is the knowledge that comes from education about mental illness. Families need to understand the patient's behavior and know how to respond helpfully to disturbed behavior. They benefit from a clear, nontechnical explanation of the illness, as well as from a prognosis that is as accurate as possible. Families need to know the available treatments, the medication regimen, and the best way to manage the problems of day-to-day living (Chesla, 1989). One particularly perplexing problem for families is to learn how to be sufficiently involved and interested without being either too intrusive or too distant. Feedback on family interactions can be provided with models of effective communication skills. In some families the interactions are disturbed enough to require family therapy.

Specific strategies can be taught by health professionals to help families deal with a mentally ill member. One such strategy involves understanding and controlling one's responses. For example, it may be difficult not to respond to behavior that is disturbing or annoying, but is not harmful to the ill person or to anyone else. It is more useful to focus on harmful or destructive behaviors. Learning what to respond to and how to respond can be accomplished by family members willing to learn from knowledgeable professionals. Families can begin to achieve this skill through open discussion of their feelings and reactions with other family members and friends. This prevents the buildup of indifference and resentment. This technique is especially useful when dealing with a family member who generates strong feelings. This strategy makes it possible to focus energy in more useful directions. The ability to establish this strategy brings a new perspective and a new resolve to engage a disabled family member in more important ways.

Families need to understand that it takes time to learn and establish strategies taught to them by health professionals. If families have not been coping successfully or have been feeling especially stressed, 2 to 3 years of effort may be necessary to turn their lives around. Change involves a decision, but it also involves learning of new behaviors, a great deal of practice, and substantial support.

Finally, families need education about patient behaviors that could indicate a recurrence so that they know when to encourage the patient to seek help before hospitalization is required. Available resources in the community should be identified early in the illness. Group education sessions for families can be worthwhile because participants can share experiences while they learn.

Support. The importance of support and support groups has been mentioned throughout this text. Families of the mentally ill rely on support from health-care practitioners, friends, and community resources. The National Alliance for the Mentally Ill (NAMI) is a group that has done most of the promoting of peer support groups for families of the person with mental illness. Family members can join a peer support group for emotional support, problem solving, and advocacy. Some families even learn to develop more skills to manage their lives adequately. Regular meetings help family members to talk about painful experiences and to look for personal and organizational solutions. The group process helps family members to deal directly with their internal and external sources of stress. Families are helped to face the fear and the pain in their lives rather than deny it or feel victimized.

In addition to emotional support, these organizations also have helped families become involved in direct advocacy or problem solving for their disabled member. Families learn new options for coping with mental illness. For example, families are no longer willing to accept the blame for the disability of their family member, but they are willing to look at how they might be contributing to stressful situations. They are also concerned about the contribution of society to mental illness. The family's ability to reach out for help and to develop relationships with helpful organizations should be encouraged.

Respite care. Another valuable resource is respite care, which provides supervision for the patient in a community setting when the family needs relief. The family may take a vacation or spend a short time away from the patient without feeling the guilt associated with rehospitalization. Respite care provides a basis for a positive association between the patient and the organization or family that provides the care (Geiser et al., 1988).

Crises services. The final important resource is crises services, including home visiting. It is sometimes difficult for a family to persuade a disturbed member to go to a treatment facility, especially if the patient has been hospitalized in the past and suspects a possible readmittance. Families should not have to wait until the situation becomes so serious that they must call the police to take the patient into custody. This also has a destructive effect on the patient. Crises intervention in the home can avert this distressing situation. Home health care is a good service for patients and families who are unwilling or unable to participate in other forms of outpatient care.

Specific Intervention — Depression

The following is an example from the Mendelsons' situation and interventions that the health-care professional might employ to facilitate the formation of a manageable family appraisal and to maximize family resources. The reader now encounters the Mendelsons during the initial onset and diagnosis of Jeremiah's depression. This time is critical for family intervention, since the Mendelsons are forming new patterns but are not yet entrenched or committed to them. Maladaptive family behaviors are more easily prevented at this time (Halm, 1990). The family is also more open to new ideas and support at this time (McCubbin & McCubbin, 1989).

✦ ✦ ✦ ✦ ✦

Margaret encourages Jeremiah to get a complete physical checkup. For the past 2 months he has had a poor appetite, has lost 10 pounds, cannot sleep in the early morning hours, and feels nervous and generally old and useless. The family physician completes Jeremiah's comprehensive physical. Examination results and laboratory tests indicate that Jeremiah is a physically healthy 59-year-old. The physician shares his findings with Jeremiah. Jeremiah is perplexed with the absence of negative findings and relays this to his physician. They discuss his concerns late one afternoon. Jeremiah cannot believe that no source for his weight loss, sleeplessness, and worries has been discovered. He worries that his physician overlooked something or that the tests are falsely positive. The family physician listens to Jeremiah's concerns and asks him more about all of his worries. They discuss his feelings that he is falling apart and feeling guilt about putting his mother in a nursing home. The physician informs Jeremiah that he appears to be suffering from depression and that it would be best if his concerns are discussed with a specialist—a psychiatrist.

Jeremiah is a bit angry and insulted by his family physician's suggestions. He storms out of the health office and drives home to discuss this with Margaret. Margaret is very sympathetic and quietly listens as Jeremiah complains about the inadequacy of health care these days. He is angry that his physician is passing off these concerns as "all in his head" and further has the audacity to pass him off to a "shrink." He remembers his mother telling him about a similar instance involving her father. Actually, his grandfather ended up in the state mental institution for awhile.

A week passes, Jeremiah's anger lessens and turns more into worry. He begins to fear that he will end up like his grandfather. He has more difficulty sleeping and tosses and turns for several nights. He feels totally exhausted. Margaret is now even more concerned about his health and talks him into returning to the family physician. She asks if she may go with him to hear what the physician thinks is wrong with Jeremiah.

When Jeremiah and Margaret make the return appointment, the physician encourages Margaret's presence and asks if all family members can attend this meeting. Jeremiah and Margaret are the only ones available at this time. During the meeting the family physician describes the details of Jeremiah's recent checkup. He encourages Jeremiah and Margaret to be forthright about their reactions and opinions. Jeremiah describes his feelings of embarrassment and disappointment in the health-care system. The physician is supportive of these reactions. He encourages more discussion, listens patiently to the couple's fears, and spends the remainder of the time teaching the Mendelsons about depression.

The family physician describes Jeremiah's symptoms and compares them with the major symptoms and common prevalence of depression. He explains to Jeremiah and Margaret that 80% of people with serious depression can be treated successfully. He describes medication and psychological therapies and combinations of both usually relieving symptoms in weeks and that often half of the people with major depression can be completely free of symptoms in 4 to 8 months. He explains that specialists such as psychiatrists are best to treat depression, since they are more informed about the latest treatment, medications, and laboratory tests that may delineate further treatment selection.

The Mendelsons listen carefully to their family physician. Margaret takes notes. They leave the health office a bit stunned and overwhelmed but hopeful that Jeremiah may be able to get help even though he will have to go to a specialist.

Jeff Mendelson comes home for a week's vacation from college. He is shocked at the change in his father. Jeremiah is embarrassed to tell his son about the depression. He avoids neighbors and stays in his den, coming out only for Margaret's meals. Margaret answers the phone for Jeremiah and turns down all social invitations. Finally, Jeff demands to know what is wrong, so Margaret updates him on the visit to their family physician. Jeff calls the physician and asks him for the name(s) of suggested psychiatrists. Jeff encourages his parents to seek help and goes with them to the first visit. The Mendelsons are pleased with their first visit to the family psychiatrist, as they are encouraged to talk further and are received warmly. The staff appears very professional, although they do not dress in uniforms or white coats. The family psychiatrist helps the family through the initial time and, after several family sessions, introduces them to another family who has experienced a similar problem.

In the Mendelsons' situation health-care professionals have concentrated on helping the Mendelsons gain a manageable perception of depression and discard their prejudice about seeking psychiatric help. This manageable family appraisal is crucial during the initial diagnosis of depression because of the stigma of mental illness can hamper treatment. The health-care professional is the major resource for educating the family at this time. It takes the family time to mobilize and seek the care of a psychiatrist. Each family member's feelings and reactions to the diagnosis of mental illness are dealt with as they surface. After open discussion with the family, the health-care professional can understand the impact on and meaning this illness has for the Mendelsons including their view of the social stigma involved. During these initial contacts, the health professional gains valuable information to guide further family interventions.

Attention to the family's appraisal begins the process of readying the family to maximize resources. Education about depression and its treatment enables them to use existing community resources. They now have a greater opportunity to find a balance between demands and resources. The Mendelsons gain an increased self-awareness and sense of control over depression and dealing with its impact. Depression will appear less threatening because of this early family intervention. Family coping patterns and community resources for future use are established.

This chapter has illustrated the application and usefulness of the theoretical components of the McCubbin & McCubbin Resiliency Model of Family Stress, Adjustment, and Adaptation. It demonstrates the powerful influence family perceptions of mental illness and family solutions can have on the family's ability to cope.

REFERENCES

American Psychiatric Association (1989). *Treatments of psychiatric disorders*. Vol. 3. Washington, D.C.: American Psychiatric Association.

Boyer, J. L., & Guthrie, L. (1985). Assessment and treatment of the suicidal patient. In E. E. Beckham & W. R. Leber (Eds.), *Handbook of depression: Treatment, assessment, and research* (pp. 606-633). Homewood, IL: Dorsey.

Cassem, E. H. (1987). When symptoms seem groundless. *Emergency Medicine, 19*(12), 62-87.

Charney, E. A., & Weisman, M. M. (1988). Epidemiology of depressive and manic syndromes. In A. Georgotas & R. Cancro (Eds.), *Depression and mania* (pp. 26-52). New York: Elsevier.

Chesla, C. A. (1989). Mental illness and the family. In C. L. Gilliss, B. L. Highley, B. M. Roberts, & I. M. Martinson (Eds.), *Toward a science of family nursing* (pp. 374-393). Menlo Park, CA: Addison-Wesley.

Derogatis, L. R., & Wise, T. N. (1989).

Anxiety and depressive disorders in the medical patient. Washington, D.C.: American Psychiatric Press.

Fish, M., & Snyder, M. D. (1985). Symbolic interactionism: A framework for interventions with the hospitalized suicidal patient. In C. A. Rogers & J. Ulsafer-Van Lanen (Eds.), *Nursing interventions in depression* (pp. 111-123). Orlando, FL: Grune & Stratton.

Francell, C. G., Conn, V. S., & Gray, D. P. (1988). Families' perceptions of burden of care for chronic mentally ill relatives. *Hospital and Community Psychiatry, 39*(12), 296-300.

Geiser, R. G., Hich, L., & King, J. (1988). Respite care for mentally ill patients and their families. *Hospital and Community Psychiatry, 39*(3), 291-295.

Goldman, H. H. (1982). Mental illness and family burden: A public health perspective. *Hospital and Community Psychiatry, 33*(7), 557-560.

Group for the Advancement of Psychiatry (1986). *A family affair—helping families cope with mental illness: A guide for the professions.* New York: Brunner/Mazel.

Grunebaum, H., & Friedman, H. (1988). Building collaborative relationships with families of the mentally ill. *Hospital and Community Psychiatry, 39*(11), 1183-1187.

Halm, M. A. (1990). Effects of support groups in anxiety of family members during critical illness. *Heart and Lung, 19*(1), 62-71.

Hatfield, A. B. (1979). The family as partner in the treatment of mental illness. *Hospital Community Psychiatry, 30*, 338-340.

Kaplan, H. I., & Sadock, B. J. (1981). *Modern synopsis of comprehensive textbook of psychiatry* (3rd ed.). Baltimore: Williams & Wilkins.

Lindenthal, J. J. (1988). The empirics of suicide. In C. S. Thomas & J. J. Lindenthal (Eds.), *Psychiatry and mental illness science handbook* (pp. 165-180). St. Louis: Warren H. Green.

McCubbin, M. A., & McCubbin, H. I. (1989). Theoretical orientation to family stress and coping. In C. R. Figley (Ed.), *Treating stress in families* (pp. 3-43). New York: Brunner/Mazel.

Montgomery, S. A. (1990). Anxiety and depression. Peterfield, Hampshire, Great Britain: Wrightson Biomedical.

Morgan, S. L. (1989). Families' experiences in psychiatric emergencies. *Hospital and Community Psychiatry, 40*(12), 1265-1269.

Mosher, L. R., & Burti, L. (1989). *Community mental health: Principles and practice.* New York: W. W. Norton.

Munoz, R. F. (1987). *Depression prevention research directions.* New York: Hemisphere.

Saylor, C. (1990). Stigma. In I. M. Lubkin (Ed.), *Chronic illness: Impact and interventions* (2nd ed., pp. 65-85). Boston: Jones & Bartlett.

Segal, S. P., & Baunmohl, J. (1988). No place like home: Reflections on sheltering a diverse population. In C. J. Smith & J. A. Giggs (Eds.), *Contemporary perspectives on mental health care* (pp. 249-263). Boston: Unwin Hyman.

Sontag, S. (1977). *Illness as metaphor.* New York: Vintage.

Taylor, C. M. (1990). *Mereness' essentials of psychiatric nursing* (13th ed.). St. Louis: Mosby—Year Book.

Tessler, R. C., Bernstein, A. G., Rosen, B. M., & Goldman, H. H. (1982). The chronically mentally ill in community support systems. *Hospital and Community Psychiatry, 33*(3), 208-211.

United States Department of Health and Human Services, Public Health Service, Alcohol, Drug Abuse, and Mental Health Administration (1986). *Psychiatric–mental health nursing:* Proceedings of two conferences on future directions. DHHS Publication No. (ADM~) 86-1449: 4-6.

Appendix

Family
Profile
Resiliency Model©

	Family Raw Scores	Low	Medium	High	Family Classification
Family Changes		0 - 3	4 - 5	6 - 15	L M H
Family Coherence		0 - 11	12 - 14	15 - 16	L M H
Family Flexibility		0 - 21	22 - 26	27 - 35	L M H
Family Bonding		0 - 28	29 - 33	34 - 35	L M H
Family Social Support		0 - 53	54 - 63	64 - 88	L M H

Directions:

Have the family member complete the five questionnaires, the Family Changes, Family Coherence, Family Flexibility, Family Bonding, and Family Social Support scales. Make sure every question has been answered. Add up the numbers circled on each scale and put the total for that scale in the Total Score box at the bottom of the page. Transfer the total score from each scale into the Family Raw Scores boxes above. Now compare the number in the Family Raw Scores box to the scores in the Low, Medium and High boxes. This will determine your family's classification; circle the L for Low, the M for Medium, or the H for High which fits your family's classification. This will provide your family with a profile of changes, coherence, flexibility, bonding and support. A profile of Resiliency.

Family Changes ©

Directions: Decide whether or not each of the changes listed below happened in your family, including yourself, during the past year. After you have decided and selected a number (0 or 1), put that number in the box to the right marked Family Score.

During the past year has this happened in your family?	No	Yes	Family Score
1. A family member gave birth to or adopted a child	0	1	
2. A family member stopped working, lost or quit a job (e.g. retired, laid-off, etc.)	0	1	
3. A family member started or returned to work	0	1	
4. A family member changed to a new job/career, or was given more responsibilities at work	0	1	
5. Family moved to new home/apartment	0	1	
6. A family member, relative or close friend became seriously ill or injured	0	1	
7. A family member or close relative became physically disabled, chronically ill, or was committed to an institution or nursing home	0	1	
8. A family member, close relative or close friend died	0	1	
9. Married son or daughter was separated or divorced	0	1	
10. A family member left home or moved back home	0	1	
11. A family member appeared to have emotional problems	0	1	
12. A family member appeared to depend on alcohol and/or drugs	0	1	
13. Physical and/or psychological violence in the home	0	1	
14. Increased difficulty in finding and/or keeping quality child care	0	1	
15. Husband and wife separated or divorced	0	1	
		Total Score	

Family Coherence©

Directions
Decide to what degree you either agree or disagree with each statement about your family. 0 = Strongly Disagree, 4 = Strongly Agree.

We cope with family problems by:

	Strongly Disagree	Disagree	Neutral	Agree	Strongly Agree
1. Accepting stressful events as a fact of life	0	1	2	3	4
2. Accepting that difficulties occur unexpectedly	0	1	2	3	4
3. Defining the family problem in a more positive way so that we do not become too discouraged	0	1	2	3	4
4. Having faith in God	0	1	2	3	4

Total Score

Family Flexibility©

Directions: Decide for each statement listed below how often the situation described occurs in your family: **(5) Almost Never, (4) Once in a While, (3) Sometimes, (2) Frequently,** or **(1) Almost Always.** Please respond to each and every statement.

To what degree do these statements describe your family:	Almost Never	Once In a While	Some-Times	Fre-quently	Almost Always
1. Family members say what they want.	5	4	3	2	1
2. Each family member has input into major family decisions.	5	4	3	2	1
3. In solving problems, the children's suggestions are followed.	5	4	3*	2	1
4. Children have a say in their discipline.	5	4	3*	2	1
5. Our family tries new ways of dealing with problems.	5	4	3	2	1
6. When problems arise, we compromise.	5	4	3	2	1
7. We shift household responsibilities from person to person.	5	4	3	2	1

Total Score

* If you do not have children, circle the number 3.
© 1985 H. McCubbin, D. Olson, Y. Lavee, & J. Patterson. The Family Paradigm Album, Family Invulnerability Test, Stress, Strengths and Adaptation. The Family Stress, Coping, and Health Project, University of Minnesota, St. Paul

Family Bonding[©]

Directions: Decide for each statement listed below how often the situation described occurs in your family: **(5) Almost Never, (4) Once in a While, (3) Sometimes, (2) Frequently,** or **(1) Almost Always.** Please respond to each and every statement.

To what degree do these statements describe your family:	Almost Never	Once In a While	Some-Times	Fre-quently	Almost Always
1. It is easier to discuss problems with people outside the family than with other family members.	5	4	3	2	1
2. Family members feel closer to people outside the family than to other family members.	5	4	3	2	1
3. In our family, everyone goes his or her own way.	5	4	3	2	1
4. Family members pair up rather than do things as a total family.	5	4	3	2	1
5. Family members avoid each other at home.	5	4	3	2	1
6. We have difficulty thinking of this to do as a family.	5	4	3	2	1
7. Family members go along with what the family decides to do.	5	4	3	2	1

Total Score

Family Social Support ©

Directions:
Please indicate how much you agree or disagreee with each of the following statements about your community and family.

	Strongly Disagree	Strongly Agree	Not Sure	Disagree	Agree	
1. If I had an emergency, even people I do not know in this community would be willing to help.	0	1	2	3	4	
2. I feel good about myself when I sacrifice and give time and energy to members of my family.	0	1	2	3	4	
3. The things I do for members of my family and they do for me make me feel part of this very important group.	0	1	2	3	4	
4. People here know they can get help from the community if they are in trouble.	0	1	2	3	4	
5. I have friends who let me know they value who I am and what I can do.	0	1	2	3	4	
6. People can depend on each other in this community.	0	1	2	3	4	
7. Members of my family seldom listen to my problems or concerns; I usually feel criticized.	0	1	2	3	4	®
8. My friends in this community are a part of my everyday activities.	0	1	2	3	4	
9. There are times when family members do things that make other members unhappy.	0	1	2	3	4	®
10. I need to be very careful how much I do for my friends because they take advantage of me.	0	1	2	3	4	®
11. Living in this community gives me a secure feeling.	0	1	2	3	4	
12. The members of my family make an effort to show their love and affection for me.	0	1	2	3	4	
13. There is a feeling in this community that people should not get too friendly with each other.	0	1	2	3	4	®
14. This is not a very good community to bring children up in.	0	1	2	3	4	®
15. I feel secure that I am as important to my friends as they are to me.	0	1	2	3	4	
16. I have some very close friends outside the family who I know really care for me and love me.	0	1	2	3	4	
17. Member(s) of my family do not seem to understand me; I feel taken for granted.	0	1	2	3	4	®

© 1982 H. McCubbin J. Patterson and Thomas Glynn
® Computer use only.
in H. McCubbin & A. Thompson (Eds.) (1987, 1991) Family Assessment Inventories for Research and Practice, University of Wisconsin, Madison

Total Score [＿＿＿]

Glossary

✦

assimilation　a family *adjustment* coping strategy characterized by an attempt to absorb the demands of the stressor with minimal change in family structure and interactions

avoidance　a family *adjustment* coping strategy characterized by an attempt to ignore or deny a stressor in the hope it will resolve itself

balanced family　a family unit characterized as having established patterns of moderate cohesiveness and moderate adaptability

bonadaptation　the ability of the family to stabilize with instituted patterns in place, promote the individual development of its members, and achieve a sense of coherence and congruency even when stressors and substantive changes threaten established patterns of family functioning

boundary ambiguity　an uncertainty as to which members are present in a family system; a condition created out of the family system's need to be sure of its components, that is, who is inside and outside of the family boundaries, physically and psychologically

capability　the potential the family has to meet demands

coherence　a shared or agreed-on worldview underscored by a sense of manageability, comprehensibility, meaningfulness, and trust

compromise　a family *adaptation* coping strategy in which family members agree to and support a less than perfect resolution to their problems

congruency　a condition of the family unit that describes the relationship between the family's schema (that is, values, priorities, goals, rules, and expectations) and the family's instituted patterns of functioning

differentiation of families　the balance between the intellectual and emotional systems of a family group. Family members may behave in various ways, but the underlying level of differentiation remains constant

differentiation of self　the balance between the intellectual and emotional systems in an individual. This is generally conceptualized as a scale ranging from 0 to 100

distance　one manifestation of undifferentiation in which a person is totally

413

separate from the family emotional system; accomplished by means of the emotional cutoff

elimination a family *adjustment* coping strategy characterized by the family's attempt to rid itself of the stressor by changing, removing the stressor, or redefining the stressor

emotional system the portion of the brain that deals with instincts and governs automatic functions and behaviors, the most important of which are those governing emotional and relationship systems

established patterns the behaviors and routines in the family unit that evolve over time and are designed to reinforce a family's schema of values, expectations, goals, priorities, and rules

family adaptation the outcome of family efforts to bring a new level of balance, harmony, and coherence, as well as a satisfactory level of functioning, to a family crisis situation; involves coping strategies such as synergizing, interfacing, and compromising

family adjustment the ability to make short-term changes in the family patterns of functioning to manage a stressor; involves coping strategies such as assimilation, avoidance, and elimination

family appraisal the assessment the family unit makes of (1) the stressor, (2) the family's capability of managing a crisis, and (3) the family schema's ability to attach meaning that legitimizes and affirms changes in family functioning

family coping the family's strategies, patterns, and behaviors designed to maintain or strengthen the family as a whole, maintain the emotional stability and well-being of its members, obtain and use family and community resources to manage crisis situations, and initiate efforts to resolve the family hardships

family crisis a continuous variable denoting the amount of disruptiveness, disorganization, or incapacitation in the family social system; it is a state of family system disorganization and denotes a demand for basic changes in the family patterns of functioning so that stability, order, and coherence can be restored

family distress a negative state in which the family defines the demand-resource imbalance as unpleasant, destabilizing, and threatening to the current stability of the family and possibly to the future integrity of the family system

family eustress a positive state in which the family defines the demand-resource imbalance as desirable, without stress, and as a challenge that family members accept, acknowledge, and, in some cases, appreciate; the term *eustress* was originally coined by Selye (1956) in describing the general adaptation syndrome (GAS)

family hardiness the internal strengths and durability of the family unit; characterized by a sense of control over the outcome of life events and hardships, a view of change as beneficial and growth producing, and an active rather than passive orientation in responding to stressful situations

family meanings   the explanations families create and share to justify, legitimate, and affirm changes in family functioning brought about by a crisis situation in an effort to achieve a satisfactory level of adaptation

family resiliency   the family's potential to recover from crisis, change, or other stressors facing the family unit

family strain   a manageable level of family tension produced in response to a stressor

family stress   a state of tension that arises when an actual or perceived imbalance exists between the demands placed on the family and the family's resistance resources and capabilities; a nonspecific demand for adjustment or adaptation

family system   the perspective that the family is a holistic entity and that all members are attached to previous generations and to one another through the emotional system

family typology   a set of basic family patterns of behavior that characterizes and explains how the family system typically operates and behaves

fusion   one manifestation of undifferentiation in which a person is enmeshed within the family emotional system

instituted patterns   newly created, developed, or adopted behaviors and routines designed to facilitate family adaptation in a crisis situation

intellectual system   the portion of the cerebral cortex that allows people to think, reason, and reflect on their behaviors and plan their lives

interfacing   a family *adaptation* coping strategy that families undertake to fit and integrate with their communities

maladjustment/maladaptation   a negative family adjustment/adaptation that produces a family crisis requiring changes in the family's established patterns of functioning

multigenerational transmission process   the mechanism whereby the family relationship system is transmitted from generation to generation

normative transitions   a predictable and expected series of changes in the family as the result of the growth and development of its members, of changes in the extended family system (birth of children and death of grandparents), and of predictable family life cycle changes (children entering school, adolescence, the empty-nest state, retirement, and so forth)

pileup   the accumulation within the family of demands, transitions, strains, hardships, and ambiguities overlapping with the impact of an illness or another stressor straining the family's efforts to adjust or adapt to a stressor

prior strains   a residual of tension that may result from unresolved hardships from earlier stressors, transitions, and crises, or may be inherent in ongoing roles such as parenthood and employment

problem solving   the family's ability to organize a stressor into manageable components, to identify alternative courses of action to deal with each component, to initiate steps to resolve the issues, and to develop and cultivate patterns of problem-solving communication needed to bring about family problem-solving efforts

regenerative family typology   a pattern of family functioning characterized by family coherence and hardiness

relationship system   the specific emotional relationships within a family that express the level of differentiation; it governs who is close, who is distant, and what behaviors are allowed within a family

Resiliency Model   a theoretical model to guide educators, practitioners, and researchers in understanding the family's response to a stressor and recovery from crisis

resilient family typology   a pattern of family functioning characterized by family bonding and flexibility

resistance resources   the family's capabilities and strengths to manage a stressor while maintaining established patterns of functioning

rhythmic family typology   a pattern of family functioning characterized by an emphasis on family time and routines and the valuing of these patterns

schema   a family's blueprint for functioning that encompasses shared or agreed-on values, expectations, goals, priorities, and rules

sibling position   the place a person occupies with regard to siblings

social support   the information exchanged among persons or between groups of persons outside the family system intended to enhance emotional well-being and esteem and promote an overall sense of belonging and affirming appraisal

stressor   a demand placed on the family unit that produces or has the potential of producing changes in the family system

synergizing   a family *adaptation* coping strategy wherein the family works together to accomplish a shared orientation and life-style that could not be brought about by one member alone

triangle   a three-person emotional system in which two people are comfortable and the third person is distant

vulnerability   the interpersonal and organizational weakness of the family system at the onset of an illness or other stressor or concurrent with the course of the illness or other stressor; it is shaped by pileup of demands within the family and the family life-cycle stage with its normative demands

Credits for Chapter Opening Photos

✦

Chapter 1: Courtesy of Pat Watson. From Stanhope M and Lancaster J: *Community health nursing: process and practice for promoting health*, ed 2, St Louis, 1988 Mosby–Year Book.

Chapter 2: From Whaley L and Wong D: *Nursing care of infants and children*, ed 3, 1987, St Louis, Mosby–Year Book.

Chapter 3: From Whaley L and Wong D: *Essentials of pediatric nursing*, ed 2, St Louis, 1985, Mosby–Year Book.

Chapter 4: Courtesy of Dottie Kauffmann. From Giger J and Davidhizar R: *Transcultural nursing: assessment and intervention*, St Louis, 1990, Mosby–Year Book.

Chapter 5: Source unknown.

Chapter 6: From Potter PA and Perry AG: *Fundamentals of nursing: concepts, process, and practice*, St Louis, 1989, Mosby–Year Book.

Chapter 7: From Whaley L and Wong D: *Nursing care of infants and children*, ed 3, St Louis, 1987, Mosby–Year Book.

Chapter 8: Courtesy of Dottie Kauffmann. From Giger J and Davidhizar R: *Transcultural nursing: assessment and intervention*, St Louis, 1990, Mosby–Year Book.

Chapter 9: From Whaley L and Wong D: *Essentials of pediatric nursing*, ed 2, St Louis, 1985, Mosby–Year Book.

Chapter 10: Courtesy of Pat Watson. From Whaley L and Wong D: *Nursing care of infants and children*, ed 3 St Louis, 1987, Mosby–Year Book.

Chapter 11: Courtesy of Carol Danielson.

Chapter 12:   Courtesy of Dottie Kauffmann. From Giger J and Davidhizar R: *Transcultural nursing: assessment and intervention,* St Louis, 1987, Mosby–Year Book.

Chapter 13:   From Potter PA and Perry AG: *Fundamentals of nursing: concepts, process, and practice,* ed 2, St Louis, 1989, Mosby–Year Book.

Chapter 14:   From Whaley L and Wong D: *Essentials of pediatric nursing,* ed 3, St Louis, 1989, Mosby–Year Book.

Index

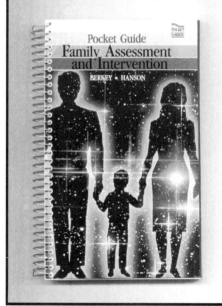
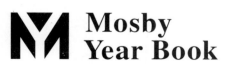

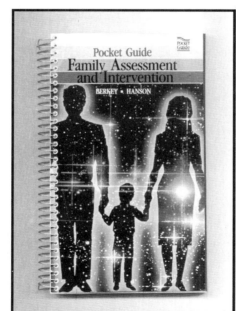
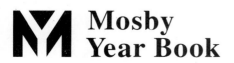